PRAISE FOR GOING MENOPOSTAL

"I met Amy Alkon at a behavioral science conference over 20 years ago, the only nonacademic there, voraciously consuming knowledge and asking all the right questions in the pursuit of applying behavioral science to real-world problems. In this book, she will empower you to use science to advocate for yourself and get relief from hot flashes, insomnia, brain fog, and other life-altering symptoms.

In *Going Menopostal*, she exposes the truth about the medical neglect and mistreatment of women in perimenopause and menopause. But more than that, she gives you the language and strategies to advocate for yourself with your doctors without antagonizing them, making them partners in your healthcare, so that you get the evidence-based care you deserve."

—Catherine Salmon, PhD, Professor of Psychology at the University of Redlands and coauthor of *The Secret Power of Middle Children*

"Amy Alkon's *Going Menopostal* is a groundbreaking book that sheds light on the inequities in medical research and care, particularly for women from underrepresented communities. As a family doctor serving the South Side of Chicago, I see firsthand the metabolic health challenges faced by women in predominantly African American communities, where social determinants of health often amplify disparities.

Alkon courageously addresses how much of the existing research is centered on white, middle-class women, leaving the unique needs of women from diverse backgrounds inadequately explored and understood. This book empowers readers with vital information to advocate for better care, challenges systemic inequities, and gives voice to women who have long been overlooked. By doing so, it fosters greater empathy and paves the way for a more inclusive approach to women's health."

—Dr. Tony Hampton, Family and Obesity Medicine Specialist at Advocate Health, author of *Fix Your Diet, Fix Your Diabetes*, and host of the *Protecting Your NEST* podcast

"A fiercely edgy and heartfelt storyteller, Amy Alkon exposes the inadequacies of traditional menopause care in the United States through her raw, personal journey. Her perspective as a high-functioning professional woman is both poignant and deeply relatable, shining a light on the frustration many women face when they feel disconnected from themselves during this pivotal time.

Amy Alkon skillfully unpacks the long-standing impact of the Women's Health Initiative (WHI), revealing how it has perpetuated fear and confusion around hormone therapy. The book also critiques the overreliance on clinical practice guidelines, which, while ensuring uniformity and legal protection, often stifle innovation and leave little room for individualized care. A compelling call to action, this work challenges clinicians to move beyond the status quo and empower women with solutions grounded in both evidence and empathy."

—Dr. Andréa Salcedo, ob-gyn, Assistant Professor of Gynecology and Obstetrics at Loma Linda University School of Medicine, and host of YouTube: Conscious Gynecology—Low Carb Nutrition and Metabolic Health

"*Going Menopostal* is essential reading for women navigating perimenopause and menopause—critical life stages overlooked by the medical community. Veteran science writer Amy Alkon brings an outsider's objectivity and cuts through outdated advice with a rigorous, evidence-based approach. Infused with warmth, wit, and compassion, she tackles everything from hot flashes and weight gain to mood changes and insomnia, offering clear, science-backed solutions. This book is a vital resource for women seeking real answers in a field that has long been underserved."

—Nina Teicholz, PhD, internationally bestselling author of *The Big Fat Surprise* and science journalist

"Amy Alkon's *Going Menopostal* is a masterpiece of scientific inquiry and clarity, cutting through decades of misinformation and fear around menopause. Clinical studies have been misinterpreted and menopausal symptoms have not been given enough attention. With her keen scientific mind and her ability to examine clinical and epidemiological evidence honestly, critically, and objectively, she has created a work of great importance for women struggling with menopause and perimenopause.

With writing that is sharp, biting, and on point, Alkon empowers women to understand the research and advocate effectively to be given evidence-based care. This book is a much-needed resource for addressing the medical neglect women have endured for far too long."

—Dr. Kevin B. Knopf, MPH, Clinical Assistant Professor of Medicine, University of California San Francisco School of Medicine

GOING MENOPOSTAL

ALSO BY AMY ALKON

Unf*ckology: A Field Guide to Living with Guts and Confidence

Good Manners for Nice People Who Sometimes Say F*ck

*I See Rude People: One woman's battle to beat
some manners into impolite society*

GOING MENOPOSTAL

WHAT YOU (AND YOUR DOCTOR) NEED TO KNOW ABOUT
THE REAL SCIENCE
OF MENOPAUSE AND PERIMENOPAUSE

AMY ALKON

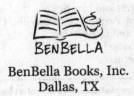

BenBella Books, Inc.
Dallas, TX

This book is for informational purposes only. It is not intended to serve as a substitute for professional medical advice. The author and publisher specifically disclaim any and all liability arising directly or indirectly from the use of any information contained in this book. A healthcare professional should be consulted regarding your specific medical situation. Any product mentioned in this book does not imply endorsement of that product by the author or publisher.

Going Menopostal copyright © 2025 by Amy Alkon

All rights reserved. Except in the case of brief quotations embodied in critical articles or reviews, no part of this book may be used or reproduced, stored, transmitted, or used in any manner whatsoever, including for training artificial intelligence (AI) technologies or for automated text and data mining, without prior written permission from the publisher.

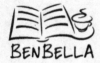

BenBella Books, Inc.
8080 N. Central Expressway
Suite 1700
Dallas, TX 75206
benbellabooks.com
Send feedback to feedback@benbellabooks.com

BenBella is a federally registered trademark.

Printed in the United States of America
10 9 8 7 6 5 4 3 2 1

Library of Congress Control Number: 2024054640
ISBN 9781637742457 (trade paperback)
ISBN 9781637742464 (electronic)

Copyediting by Scott Calamar
Proofreading by Rebecca Maines and Lisa Story
Text design and composition by PerfecType, Nashville, TN
Cover design by Emily Weigel and Little Shiva
Cover photography by Emily Weigel
Printed by Lake Book Manufacturing

Special discounts for bulk sales are available. Please contact bulkorders@benbellabooks.com.

In memory of Julia Reyes Taubman
who lived with gorgeous ferocity
until breast cancer stole her from us

Julie was an insurrectionist against untapped potential—a creative visionary
who saw and refused to accept where the world was beige
and lacking and filled it with lights and fireworks and art museums.

She'd hound you into greatness
(and you'd secretly love it while complaining to her
that whatever she was asking for
couldn't be done—until you eventually just did it).
Because there was no turning down a motivated Julie Taubman.

Julie was the most fully alive person I've ever known,
fiercely loving and loyal, principled, brave—and fiercely fun.

In the spirit of her relentless drive for *what could be*,
this book dedication is about 197 words longer than it "should" be.

I do this in hopes her extraordinary Julieness will live on
as a template for what's possible for each of us:

> Refusing to accept the "acceptable"
> and seizing life with everything we have.

> Living transformatively—audaciously alive, jam-packing in
> all the joy, love, beauty, fun, and adventure we can.

> Being bold and brave enough to try our guts out and fail,
> and then (that's Julie hounding us from the beyond!)
> getting up and trying our guts out again.

Julie would have respected the hell out of all of that.

Julia Reyes Taubman: 1967–2018…and beyond.

CONTENTS

FOREWORD xv

— PART 1 —
THE MEDICAL NEGLECT AND MIS-TREATMENT OF WOMEN IN MENOPAUSE AND PERIMENOPAUSE

1. **THE AWAKENING** 3
   (All night, every night)

2. **WHY YOU WON'T WANT TO BELIEVE ME AND WHY YOU SHOULD** 11

3. **THE MAJOR ERROR DOCTORS AND RESEARCHERS MAKE BY VIEWING PERIMENOPAUSE AS MENOPAUSE LITE** 27

4. **PERIMENOPAUSE AND MENOPAUSE** 39
   Two distinct symptomatic stages, not one big meno-blob

5. **PERIOD DRAMA** 49
   The vital prequel to understanding perimenopause and menopause

6. **JOAN OF ENDOCRINOLOGY** 59
   Dr. Jerilynn Prior's crusade to have perimenopause recognized, studied, and treated appropriately

7. **IT'S NOT THE MONEY, IT'S THE MONEY** 73
   Women are prescribed a cheap progesterone imitator with multiple awful side effects—including increased cancer risk

8. **A BRIEF HISTORY OF A SCIENTIFIC MESS**   **85**
   *Why progesterone got misclassified as a progestin
   and how that still misinforms our medical care today*

— PART 2 —

SYMPTOMS, SYMPTOMS GO AWAY

Introduction   **105**
SYMPTOMS ARE JUST THE STARTING GATE
Alleviate—and then protect

Hot, Sleepless, and Hurling

9. **NOW I LAY ME DOWN TO THRASH**   **109**
   Insomnia all night, brain fog all day

10. **HOT FLASHES AND NIGHT SWEATS**   **123**
    There's a dumpster fire burning and it's inside us

11. **BLOW UP AND THROW UP**   **141**
    Nausea, migraines, bloating, and inflammation run wild

The "Down Under"
Fibroidzillas, Desert Vagina, and Clitty-Clitty Dead Zone

12. **NEEDLESS GUTTING**   **155**
    *Countless unnecessary hysterectomies
    for fibroids and heavy menstrual bleeding*

13.	**MENOPAUSE BY SCALPEL**	173
	Side-effect-laden gyno cancer protection	
	for high-risk women promiscuously applied to all	

| 14. | **SEX, LIBIDO, AND DESERT VAGINA** | 181 |

It's All In Your Head
Menopause and Perimenopause: Not as Bad as Brain-Eating Zombies

| 15. | **CRAZY IS SOMETIMES A STATE OF OVARIES** | 201 |
| | *Mental and cognitive health* | |

| 16. | **MENOPAUSE BRAIN** | 217 |
| | *Untangling what estrogen does and doesn't do* | |

— PART 3 —

LONG-TERM HEALTH PROTECTION
Estrogen, Progesterone, and Hearts, Breasts, and Bones

| 17. | **RETHINKING ESTROGEN** | 233 |

| 18. | **DROP DEAD, GORGEOUS** | 249 |
| | *There's a heart-eating serial killer on the loose* | |

19.	**SISTER SLUDGE**	257
	Estrogen and progesterone prevent	
	blocked arteries and an early exit	

20. THE ESTROGEN, DIET, AND EXERCISE TRIFECTA — 277
Kill inflammation overload and insulin resistance so they can't kill you

21. THE TROPIC OF BREAST CANCER — 299

22. DEM BONES — 315
How to avoid smoking a hip joint

— PART 4 —

HOW TO HELP YOUR DOCTOR GIVE YOU EVIDENCE-BASED CARE

23. CLUELESS-CARE FOR MENOPAUSE AND PERIMENOPAUSE — 335
Is your gynecologist qualified to treat you—or required to act the part?

24. THE KEY TO THE GATEKEEPER — 343
Shifting the doctor-patient power imbalance

25. HOW TO TALK TO YOUR DOCTOR — 353
How to partner with your doctor to get evidence-based care (despite their institution's myth-based practice standards)

26. DIY MEDUCATION — 361
What your doctor doesn't know can hurt you

27. GENERIC DRUGS ARE THE SAME AS BRAND DRUGS (EXCEPT WHEN THEY'RE NOT) — 371
How to know when you've gotten a bum generic and get it replaced

— PART 5 —
MENOPOWER!

28. THE AMAZING ERASE — 379
Rebelling against the mass cancellation of women in menopause

29. OLD IS THE NEW BLACK — 385

ACKNOWLEDGMENTS — 393
SELECTED BIBLIOGRAPHY — 397
INDEX — 409

FOREWORD

As a medical school professor and physician for over two decades, I've come to a sobering realization: Much of what we teach in medical school is wrong. This isn't to say that my colleagues and I are intentionally misleading our students. The problem is more insidious. We're trapped in a system that prioritizes tradition over evidence, profits over patients, and dogma over critical thinking.

Nowhere is this more apparent than in the field of women's health.

Amy Alkon's *Going Menopostal* is a much-needed antidote to this prevailing dysfunction. It's a book that every woman—and every doctor who treats women—needs to read. Alkon isn't a doctor, and that's important. This allows her to turn a critical eye on the medical status quo in treating menopause and perimenopause in a way that's near impossible if you're part of the system.

Vitally, Alkon is a rigorous evaluator and translator of science—with a razor-sharp intellect, a relentless curiosity, and a deep empathy for those who've been failed by the very system that's supposed to heal them. These qualities make her the ideal person to write this book.

Unconstrained by the blinders of medical orthodoxy, she brings a fresh perspective and an uncompromising commitment to following the evidence wherever it leads, no matter how inconvenient or controversial those findings might be. Her writing is crystal clear, highly engaging, and often very funny—making even the most complex scientific concepts accessible to everybody.

Like Alkon, I've come to recognize the limitations of conventional medical wisdom. In my book, *Lies I Taught in Medical School*, I explore the many ways in which our current medical model is failing to address the root causes of chronic disease. One of the key arguments I make is that the human body is a complex system, and we can't hope to understand it—or treat it effectively—if we only view it through the narrow lens of a single discipline. We need to be willing to consider insights from a variety of fields, including evolutionary biology, anthropology, psychology, and sociology.

Alkon embraces this transdisciplinary approach in *Going Menopostal*. She recognizes that menopause is not merely a medical issue. It's a multifaceted phenomenon with biological, psychological, social, and cultural dimensions. This nuanced understanding is reflected in her discussion of some of the meaningful physiological differences in women of color—all too neglected by the medical establishment, but not Alkon.

Alkon doesn't shy away from exposing the ways in which women have been misled and mistreated by the medical establishment when it comes to menopause and perimenopause. Meticulously dissecting the flawed science behind many common medical recommendations, she reveals how they have led to unnecessary suffering and increased health risks for millions of women.

But she doesn't just point out the problems. Using her background in behavioral science, she details a clear and actionable plan for women to get the evidence-based care they deserve. She provides women with practical strategies for navigating the medical system, asking the right questions, and advocating for their needs.

Alkon's book is particularly valuable for its focus on patient empowerment. She knows firsthand how difficult it can be to get appropriate care from the medical system, and she gives women the language and tools to demand transparency and accountability from their doctors.

Alkon understands that knowledge is power. *Going Menopostal* is more than just a book about menopause. It's a call to arms. It's a manifesto for women to reclaim their health, challenge the medical status quo, and demand better care for themselves.

Amy Alkon's work is not only necessary but groundbreaking. This is a book that has the potential to change the lives of millions of women. It's a book that I'm recommending to all of my female patients—and to all of my colleagues as well.

—Robert Lufkin, MD
New York Times bestselling author of *Lies I Taught in Medical School*
www.robertlufkinmd.com

PART 1

THE MEDICAL NEGLECT AND MIS-TREATMENT OF WOMEN IN MENOPAUSE AND PERIMENOPAUSE

— 1 —

THE AWAKENING

(all night, every night)

IT MADE SENSE that I was having sleep problems.

My best friend dumped me. She's a professor in the Midwest who called me her "BFF," Best Friend Forever. I find "BFF" embarrassing when used unironically by anyone over 12, but it was a way of saying I meant a lot to her, so I went with it and even BFF-ed her back.

We'd met 10 years before, in 2008, when she was giving a talk in LA. We sat down for drinks, and 20 minutes in we felt like we'd been friends all our lives. I sometimes pictured us as old bags together in The Home, talking science in scratchy grandma voices and racing each other down the corridors in groovy matching wheelchairs painted with hot rod flames.

And then, one Sunday, an email. Some stuff about her beloved cat that had just died, then eight words: "I think we should go our separate ways." There was no explanation. There was just the axe, like I was some stranger she'd once exchanged sharp words with in the grocery store.

I never heard from her again.

Getting dumped by a friend is worse than getting dumped by a man, because you kind of expect that could happen. There's also a predictable set of reasons a man ends it with you: Sex got boring. You got boring. He's in love with your sister. He's in love with your sister's husband. I just couldn't figure out what might've gone so wrong for my ex-BFF, and it left me obsessed. I would be washing a dish or getting the mail, and my mind would leap to "Why?! What happened?!" I regularly woke up at 2 or 3 a.m. asking myself these questions.

When I wasn't waking up wondering about her, I woke up worrying about bills. Money had begun steering clear of me. I used to earn a nice middle-class living, but I had a recently-failing business model: writing a science-based syndicated column for newspapers, publications going out of business right and left—or cutting content in a "Try anything!" push to avoid it. I knew I had to find new ways to earn, but everything I tried turned out to be a way to work for free or close to it. I was afraid I'd end up in a tent under an overpass, eating old rolls out of dumpsters.

Piling onto my stress about money and the mysterious amputation by my supposed BFF was the looming deadline for my science-based book on confidence. The research behind it was way more complex and required more synthesis across disciplines than I'd initially thought. I joked to friends that the book kept trying to kill me, but as I careened toward my deadline with too many pages still blank, that seemed less and less like a joke.

WAKE AND BAKE

With all I had gnawing on me, I wasn't surprised when I began waking up once or twice a night. Stress'll do that to you, right? But by January of 2016, it was five or six times a night. I'd lie angrily awake, thrashing into different sleeping positions, as if I just had to arrange my body in the correct magical way and a wizard would let me sleep.

This fitful, all-night insomnia was emotional and physical torture, and it should have been worrisome, but I clung to my assumption that I was just really stressed. And then, one afternoon in May, I was sitting at my desk in breezy Venice, California, on a perfectly cool day, when—whoa, Mamacita! A blast of heat shot through me and my body temp spiked to "locked in a car trunk in the Everglades."

Could that be...a hot flash?

And then it hit me—at 52, menopause was finally creeping up.

Hot flashes began blasting me seven to 10 times daily. After I'd hit the pillow, their co-workers—drenching night sweats—made it feel like I'd wet the bed, but through every pore of my body.

I wondered how long this hormone-run circus might go on. I called my mother, who was about to turn 81, and asked when she stopped having periods. "I'm not sure," she said. "Maybe at 70."

"Mom, you were not having periods at 70!" (But thanks so much for your help.)

I knew almost nothing about menopause. Ugh. I suddenly had a lot of reading to do. I mostly read behavioral science and some dietary science for my books and column. However, for about 15 years, I'd become increasingly informed about serious failings in much of our medical care. For instance, treatments and procedures that are useless or harmful—including common types of knee, spine, and heart surgery!—are given to patients for years or even decades after research finds them to be ineffective, injurious, or deadly. Knowing this, when I have a medical issue, I protect myself by reading the research in the area *before* I go to the doctor.

My cute little one-bedroom house turned into a walk-in file cabinet as I printed and piled up hundreds of journal articles on my living room floor. I ran out of floor space, and these paper Towers of Pisa soon took over any flat surface that didn't have kitchen appliances or shake when flushed.

The more I read, the angrier I got. There was a huge gap between the evidence I saw in the research findings and the medical advice and treatment being given to women in and around menopause.

"EVIDENCE"-BASED MEDICINE

Many women in their 40s start feeling mysteriously unwell. "Mysteriously" because their symptoms sneak up on them, little by little, and seem unrelated since they don't trace to a single identifiable cause.

At first, a woman might mistake some symptoms for mean ole PMS—until it occurs to her that *premenstrual* syndrome isn't supposed to be endless. She's bloated and achy—not just at tampon time, but throughout the month. Every day, her boobs feel like overfilled water balloons, and they hurt every time she takes a step. And whoa! Is that her period or a test run for bleeding to death?

Eventually, sleeping through the night becomes a battle—one she usually loses. Then there's the bottomless hunger. No matter how much she eats, she remains monstrously hungry—like a starving wild animal—and she's got the depressing rapid weight gain to show for it. And while we all have the occasional "I HATE EVERYONE AND EVERYTHING!" bad day, hers start coming daily. She's wired and angry—for no apparent reason—and spends much of her time wishing a gory death on people who commit horrific crimes, such as humming while in line at the hardware store.

Notice something? *No one symptom* stands out as frighteningly worrisome. (Nobody dies of sore boobs.) It is important to note that some lucky women experience few symptoms or none at all—or fewer and less intense symptoms. However, for those of us who *do* get slammed, the collective mystery is the problem: the sudden "new normal" of feeling like something the dog threw up on the rug—without a clue as to why.

We can come to terms with facts we know—even devastating facts like "It's cancer." The medical unknown, on the other hand, dumps us and our imagination into a bottomless pit of worry about all the terrifying things that could be wrong with us.

Take me, for example. Until the summer of 2016, when I got that first hot flash (at age 52), I'd spent six to eight years not noticing I was slowly but increasingly feeling pretty terrible. Eventually, it hit me, and I got really scared. After a lifetime of barely going to the doctor, I seemed to be falling apart in a disturbing variety of ways—but why? Do you get, like, 40-some years of good health, and then some dark figure checks their watch and says: "Happy birthday! Welcome to 'Feel Like Total Crap Till You Die!'"?

If only I'd known that my menstrual cycle hormones—estrogen and progesterone—were the perps behind my mental and physical symphony of suck. Many women suffer hormone-driven symptoms not just after their periods stop—the phase called "menopause"—but in the three to 10 years leading up to it: the phase I'd been in, called "perimenopause." These symptoms can show up as early as age 35, but they usually rear their nasty little heads in a woman's 40s.

Some women do bring their symptoms to their doctor. Unfortunately, their reward is seldom relief. Perimenopausal symptoms are consistently dismissed, misdiagnosed, and mis-treated—by well-meaning doctors who have every intention of helping their patients.

The problem is this: Treatment guidelines for women in perimenopause are based on a major error—the long-held, unquestioned assumption that estrogen levels in perimenopause are *low*, as they are in menopause.

They aren't.

In perimenopause, estrogen levels can actually soar, making many women sick and putting them at increased risk for breast and endometrial cancer. Yet, women in perimenopause are prescribed estrogen—potentially overdosing them on the hormone causing their suffering—when the actual problem is not that they are low on estrogen, but that their bodies have stopped producing enough of its vital counterbalancing partner hormone, progesterone.

Doctors will pair the estrogen prescription with what many—wrongly—believe to be progesterone. However, instead of prescribing safe, FDA-approved progesterone—chemically identical to the progesterone produced by our bodies—they often prescribe an el cheapo synthetic knockoff, medroxyprogesterone acetate. This drug not only fails to do the job progesterone does to dial down perimenopausal insomnia and other life-trashing symptoms, but it increases a woman's risk of breast cancer, heart attacks, and strokes.

In menopause, estrogen levels bottom out, and with the loss of estrogen, many of us get socked with daily misery from hot flashes, vaginal dryness, and other symptoms. Prescription estrogen alleviates these symptoms. In fact, once we hit menopause, it's the most powerful hot flash relief we've got, and it's near miraculous at rehydrating the parched desert territory formerly known as our naturally lubricated vagina. In addition, research increasingly suggests estrogen protects and preserves the long-term health of our bones and our cardiovascular system.

However, for over 20 years, women were denied these benefits—and continue to be because estrogen continues to be baselessly demonized. This is a lingering effect of the methodologically terrible Women's Health Initiative study (WHI) and the inexcusably distorted way it was announced to the public in 2002—basically amounting to "Hey, Ladies! ESTROGEN WILL DESTROY YOUR BREASTS AND EAT YOUR BRAIN AND THEN TAKE YOU OUT IN A MASSIVE HEART ATTACK!"

As I'll detail in Chapter Sixteen, the WHI researchers' claim was a gross misrepresentation—a finding of harm made out to apply to *all* menopausal women when it was drawn from a highly atypical and unrepresentative subset: a substantial number of elderly women (up to age 79). These women had no menopausal symptoms and were so old and in such poor health that the estrogen the researchers gave them had no possibility of helping them and likely harmed them, like by increasing the plaque buildup in already-narrowed arteries (the Heart Attack Highway).

Elderly, unhealthy women should never have been treated with hormone therapy appropriate for healthy, just-menopausal, symptomatic women, and would never have been—by any doctor with a medical license generated by the state rather than Photoshop.

These women were falsely described to the public as "healthy" by the WHI researchers—most sickeningly, right in the title of the study: "Risks and benefits of estrogen plus progesterone in healthy postmenopausal women."

This was criminally misleading. The cardiovascular and other risks to elderly, chronically ill women do not apply to healthy just-menopausal women who are prescribed estrogen. In fact, taking estrogen immediately upon going into menopause is the single best protection we have against the biggest killer of women: heart disease. Unbeknownst to most of us, heart attacks, strokes, and ride-along diseases like diabetes now kill one in five women and will soon kill a whopping one in three.

We also are not told there's a clock on protecting ourselves; for example, a short window of time after we hit menopause when estrogen is helpful and protective for our cardiovascular system. If we start taking it within that window, we set ourselves up to be helped and protected by it throughout our lives. If, like the older women in the WHI, we miss that window, estrogen can be unhelpful or destructive.

Sadly, while the initial 2002 WHI results leapt onto front pages across the globe with the simple horror story, "ESTROGEN WILL KILL YOU: HERE'S HOW!", the later corrective studies were complicated to explain: "Estrogen might kill you if you take it as an unhealthy elderly lady, but it'll probably help you if you take it just after hitting menopause when your arteries aren't sludged up like a drainage ditch after a mudslide."

The corrective story's lack of media "legs" has left women and their doctors trapped in scientific 2002 *for two-plus decades*—and continues to do so. Back in 2002, in the wake of the deceptive WHI announcement, a sucking riptide of mass panic over hormone therapy blew around the globe—and not just among women. Doctors, understandably, were petrified at the prospect of harming their patients with hormone therapy and being hit with huge malpractice suits.

Newly-menopausal healthy women *whom the announced risks did not apply to* were frightened into believing they couldn't do anything *stupider* than start hormone therapy. Women who had previously been helped by hormone therapy abruptly stopped using it—of their own volition or because their doctors flat-out refused to continue prescribing it.

HOW FAR WE HAVEN'T COME

Even now, if you mosey around the posts on the Menopause Reddit, you'll see that many doctors *still* refuse to prescribe hormones. Perimenopausal and menopausal women suffering debilitating emotional and physical symptoms are shut out of the daily rescue that hormone therapy could provide—leaving some to practically melt from severe hot flashes. These women are likewise robbed of the crucial cardiovascular protections afforded by hormone therapy and the ensuing benefits for overall health, well-being, and longevity.

Again, not every woman is symptomatic or disturbingly symptomatic (to the point of longing for pharmaceutical rescue). However, due to the vast gap between current science and medical practice standards, asymptomatic women are led to believe there's no benefit for them from hormone therapy in perimenopause and menopause. While these biologically blessed ladies may be strangers to hot flashes, they still have hearts, bones, brains, and other organs and tissues that are worthy of the benefits and protections provided by progesterone in perimenopause, and, in menopause, estrogen plus progesterone.

There *are* many women who bristle at the idea they'd take a drug. Confession: I was one of them! It was irrational, fear-driven nonthink on my part—a handed-down prejudice from my parents that I realized was unfounded and counterproductive to being at my functional best. My blanket anti-drug stance led me to have a prejudice against taking estrogen in particular. I now see it as a sort of mental infectious disease I'd caught from the mass panic about estrogen in the wake of the WHI, back when I was too far from menopause and too immersed in behavioral science to pay attention to research in this area.

Once I started writing this book, it was time to dive into the research on estrogen. After I got reading, you could say *I* changed my mind. But, really, the science changed it for me.

YOUR EMPOWER TRIP STARTS HERE

My goal in writing this book is to help *all* women have access to the evidence-based care I fought for and eventually got: the safe, symptom-quashing, health-protecting treatment that every woman deserves.

But access alone isn't enough. We patients are too often treated like children, given a prescription or told we need surgery with little more than: "Here's what you should do—take my word for it." We deserve so much better.

We deserve to *understand* the reasons behind a diagnosis and course of treatment so we aren't just taking a blind leap—so we can make informed choices about our health. And we *can* do this—all of us—even if our "medical background" amounts to taking a shortcut past a med school when we're late to work. I've done my best to explain even the most complex research findings and facts about the body in clear, everyday language that you don't need a science background to understand.

Ultimately, I wrote this book to empower you with knowledge—real understanding—so instead of simply crossing your fingers and *hoping* for evidence-based care, you're armed with the information to ask for it.

— 2 —
WHY YOU WON'T WANT TO BELIEVE ME AND WHY YOU SHOULD

*I don't want to believe you. Because if I do,
it's terrifying. It means I can't trust my doctor.*
—KL

KATIEDID LANGROCK SAID that to me. She's one of a few non-scientists I asked to read an early version of this book. Though Katie's a TV writer and show developer, she has an insider's view of the obsessive work I put in to get the science right because her husband copyedited my weekly science-based advice column from 2011 to 2019.

"I *know* I can trust both you and your work," she said. "But, holy hell. I deeply want not to—because I want to believe that my doctor is giving me care that is scientifically founded and not myth-based and ultimately harmful to my body."

I completely get it. When that hot flash hit me, I wanted to go to my gynecologist and say, "Hi, here's my problem; what should I do?"—not go, "Oh, great. Now, I'll embark on an eight-year excavation of the research on menopause and perimenopause to figure out what treatment my gynecologist *should* be giving me."

The truth is, I only understood the need for this because I happened to be free one night in 2007 when a science writer friend called me. He had dinner plans with UCLA professor Sander Greenland and invited me to join them.

Greenland is one of the world's top epidemiologists and statisticians and the co-author of the seminal textbook in his field. He has spent his career going after errors, distortions, and fraud in medical research and pushing for reforms. While many researchers—understandably!—reserve their time for work that amps up their stature in their field, Sander is incredibly generous to *anyone* who expresses a sincere interest in assessing scientific studies and developing appropriate skepticism.

I started sending him my science-based syndicated column every week, and he began educating me in how to vet scientific research. Over the years, he's opened my eyes to how *unscientific* much of our medical care is; that is, not driven by some sort of proof it actually works.

"Much of our medical care" sounds like a sloppy exaggeration on my part. I wish it were. A 2011 US National Academy of Medicine report suggests that more than half of the care we get may not be based on or supported by "adequate evidence."

Surgeon and professor of public health Atul Gawande, MD, writing in *The New Yorker*, concurs. Millions of Americans are given "pointless medical care"—"drugs that aren't helping them, operations that aren't going to make them better, and scans and tests that do nothing beneficial for them, and often cause harm."

Patients "have little ability to determine the quality of the advice they are getting," he explains. "We [doctors] can recommend care of little or no value because it enhances our incomes, because it's our habit, or because we genuinely but incorrectly believe in it, and patients will tend to follow our recommendations."

This isn't to say you should bring your medical concerns to the shaman with the card table outside the health food store. But at least that dude'll tell you he got his information from the clouds or the elders; he won't lead you to believe there's any scientific anything to back it up.

MEDICAL FANTASY VS. MEDICAL REALITY

There are three big myths we believe about our medical care:

Myth #1: Doctors make decisions about drugs and treatments to give us based on scientific evidence.

Myth #2: Doctors are highly trained in and skilled at diagnosis, the reasoning process to determine the underlying cause of a patient's symptoms.

Myth #3: Doctors do a careful risk-benefit analysis when considering a treatment for a patient.

Admittedly, it isn't easy for a doc to stay current with the evidence base. "Medical knowledge grows every day" and "previously accepted facts rapidly become old," explains medical informatics professor Izet Masic, MD.

Epidemiologist David Sackett, MD, called the "father of evidence-based medicine," told doctors: "Half of what you'll learn in medical school will be shown to be either dead wrong or out of date within five years of your graduation; the trouble is that nobody can tell you which half, so the most important thing to learn is how to learn on your own."

Most important—and *largely neglected.*

There's a good chance your doctor hasn't read many (or any) scientific studies since they got out of medical school—perhaps 20 or more years ago. Like Katiedid Langrock, we don't want to believe we're putting our health in the hands of doctors who last rubbed noses with the science decades ago.

Newly-minted doctors offer no more hope. Cardiologist Milton Packer, MD, writes at MedPage Today about polling a group of nearly 200 young doctors at a medical conference he spoke at in 2018:

> "I asked how many actually read an issue of any [medical] journal that was delivered to them, electronically or physically."
>
> *Answer: Zero.*
>
> "Did they at least read the titles of the lead papers in the *New England Journal of Medicine* every week?"
>
> *Not one did.*

"Did they pick one journal in their field of interest and try to keep up?"

Nope.

"Then I asked the most revealing question of all. When is the last time that you read any single paper on any topic from start to finish?"

The response? Silence.

Packer was shaken. "I asked why no one was reading any papers. The answer was: We don't know how to read them. And most papers will subsequently get contradicted by another paper published somewhere else. So it makes no sense to read any single paper."

The young doctor who told Packer they don't know *how* to read medical science probably meant that they have no idea how to understand and evaluate it.

"Doctors are trained to treat patients. They're not trained to evaluate research claims," explains statistician Andrew Gelman in a blog post. "Sure, in medical school I guess they get some lectures on statistics or whatever." Ultimately, Gelman writes, "It's kind of silly for people to think that going to medical school for a few years will give you the skills necessary to be able to evaluate research claims in medicine or anything else."

The thing is, going to medical school *should* give you those skills. In fact, med schools have a "moral responsibility" to patients to stop churning out entire classes of doctors who are both *scientifically* illiterate and *statistically* illiterate, asserts behavioral scientist and statistician Gerd Gigerenzer, director of the Harding Center for Risk Literacy in Berlin.

Scientifically illiterate doctors lack "research literacy"—meaning they lack the ability to understand, critically evaluate, and interpret scientific research. In other words, they are unable to diagnose and treat us based on the best current evidence—the defining principle of the "evidence-based medicine" we believe we're getting!

It is not just newbie doctors who are lost dogs in the scientific woods. Experienced clinicians are right there with them. Research from 2002 to 2017 by epidemiologist John Ioannidis suggests "*Most* healthcare professionals lack the skills necessary to evaluate the reliability and usefulness of medical evidence." (Italics mine.)

Statistically illiterate doctors, on the other hand, lack the basic statistical skills and understanding needed to correctly calculate an individual patient's risk—the chances that something bad will happen to them from a drug, test, or treatment. (This "basic statistical competency," as Gigerenzer describes it, is also essential for assessing potential benefits from tests or treatments.)

Research across medical disciplines suggests *most* doctors are statistically illiterate—including those who have been practicing for decades! For example, in a 2012 study testing the statistical acumen of 4,713 US ob-gyn residents—most of whom are the practicing ob-gyns of today—public health researcher Britta L. Anderson found only 12 percent were able to give correct answers to a pair of very easy questions. (Stats 101-level! One true-or-false and the other multiple-choice!)

If your doctor is one of the statistically illiterate, you're in trouble. "Minimum statistical literacy" is required for "every medical decision, from whether a child's tonsils should be removed to whether an adult should take cholesterol-lowering medication," writes Gigerenzer.

The many doctors who cannot understand health statistics and calculate a patient's actual level of risk are predisposed to practice "defensive medicine," Gigerenzer explains. This involves (consciously or subconsciously) recommending excessive drug treatment or surgical intervention because their obligation to protect patients is tainted by their desperation to protect themselves from being sued.

Statistically illiterate doctors are also easily induced to overtreat patients by the sneaky, misleading ways study results are often announced in the press and in pharma leaflets—for example, with big honking percentages that make relatively minor risks seem vastly bigger and scarier than they actually are. Doctors who lack statistical competency are prone to prescribe drugs with serious and even terrible side effects that either have no benefit for their patient or a potential benefit so ridiculously minuscule as to be meaningless.

For an example of the harm those "big honking percentages" can do, Gigerenzer tells the story of the 1995 birth control pill scare in the UK—caused by top experts, doctors, and pharmacists on the UK government's Committee on

Safety of Medicines. This committee sent a terrifying "Dear Doctor" letter to 190,000 UK physicians and other health professionals and alerted the media, warning that third-generation birth control pills led to a whopping 100 percent increase in life-threatening blood clots in the legs or lungs.

Technically, the announced 100 percent increase wasn't wrong. But it's a result from a statistical measure called "relative risk" that's used for comparing one group to another: *relative*, because it's the risk of one group *relative* to that of another. It's useful for population health researchers, but *meaningless* for determining the actual risk to an individual, called *absolute risk*, and what their best course of action might be. *(See absolute versus relative risk, Chapter Sixteen.)*

Women across the UK panicked, and garbage bins and toilet bowls far and wide suddenly found themselves protected against unwanted pregnancy. It didn't have to be this way—and wouldn't have been, if only the committee had stated the numbers that matter for meaningfully assessing risk. Those numbers were right there in the studies behind their recommendation: 1 in 7,000 women on the second-generation pill developed a blood clot—compared with a whopping 2 in 7,000 on the third-generation pill! So, sure, there *was* a 100 percent increase in going from 1 woman up to 2—but nothing for anyone to pitch their pills over.

However, stating the risk with this 100 percent figure rather than announcing the actual numbers—a rise from 1 woman to 2—caused massive harm. "The pill scare" and pill dumping that ensued "led to an estimated 13,000 additional abortions [!] in the following year in England and Wales," writes Gigerenzer. Abortion rates, which had been declining, increased for years afterward. "For every additional abortion, there was also one extra birth, and the increase in both was particularly pronounced in teenagers, with some 800 additional conceptions among girls under 16."

He ends with the sickening irony: Pregnancies and abortions are associated with a stroke risk exceeding that of the third-generation pill!

There's another vital skill that isn't taught in med school: the critical thinking needed to correctly diagnose patients. "At most [med] schools, believe it or not, there is no course on diagnosis or how to avoid diagnostic error," explained SUNY Stony Brook professor emeritus of medicine, Mark L. Graber, MD, in 2016.

Med students supposedly pick up diagnostic reasoning skills by observing the faculty in their medical rotations in their last two years of med school.

Supposedly. In fact, it's outrageous to expect med students to pick up this ability in passing—like dog hair sticking to a cashmere sweater. Diagnostic reasoning is medical detective work: a thinking and skill set that requires formal education and practice.

"There are way too many patients being harmed" because doctors lack this formal training, Graber observes. "The best estimate from autopsy studies is that there are 40,000 to 80,000 deaths a year from diagnostic error" (though he suspects vastly more patients are injured). He explains that many of these errors involve doctors impulsively settling on a diagnosis because the symptoms "in front of them" happen to fit with a particular condition. Classes in diagnostic decision-making would help doctors avoid this common reasoning error, called the "availability bias": diagnosing based on the facts most "available" to the mind without looking for other symptoms or considering other possible conditions the same symptoms could point to.

Considering various possibilities is called "differential diagnosis." If, like me, you've never missed an episode of *House*, you've seen this in action, with lots of scribbling of disease names on a big whiteboard. The doctors then "differentiate" between the various conditions that the symptoms could show up in, exploring the likelihood of each for the particular patient. They eventually drill down to which condition it's most likely to be—which tells them how to treat it.

There *are* some doctors who study and become skilled at diagnostic reasoning on their own. Additionally, artificial intelligence is beginning to improve diagnostic accuracy in some specialties. But Graber, who founded the Society to Improve Diagnosis in Medicine in 2011, is determined to formalize diagnostic training in med schools with a comprehensive curriculum.

Med schools are increasingly developing diagnostic training programs. (Super-duper news for patients who get sick five or 10 years from now!) However, in a 2015 survey of med school faculty members, "only a minority reported having teaching sessions devoted to clinical reasoning."

MEDICAL PAINT BY NUMBERS
The often-outdated treatment guidelines doctors are required to follow

If most doctors don't keep up with the research and can't assess risk, and House-like diagnostic wizardry requires skills they haven't been taught, how *are* doctors determining what's wrong with us and how to treat it?

The answer is "practice standards"—a set of diagnostic criteria and treatment standards developed by medical practice organizations (and often, government healthcare institutions) that medical providers require their doctors to follow. For example, the American College of Obstetricians and Gynecologists (ACOG) publishes guidelines for diagnosing and treating menopause and perimenopause, and some version of those guidelines will be adopted by the institution employing your doctor.

You'd think a provider's practice standards would be updated pronto in the wake of scientific discoveries, so even doctors who *aren't* up on the research can provide evidence-based care. In fact, practice standards often remain almost mummified: untouched for years or even decades by scientific advancement—including research exposing long-recommended treatments as ineffective or even harmful!

Take the surgical procedure a Kaiser Permanente orthopedist proposed for me. In my late 40s, my right knee decided I'd gone way too long without constant searing pain when I walked more than a few blocks.

The orthopedist told me I had osteoarthritis in my knee, probably from my years of running. He said if the pain got worse, he could do arthroscopic surgery—surgery with a tiny incision, guided by a tiny camera—to shave down the nasty bits inside the knee.

Actually, no, he could *not*—not on me, anyway—thanks to the daily swim I'd been taking in the knee research sea. Starting in 2002—12 years prior to my appointment!—rigorous scientific trials found arthroscopic knee surgery *worthless for most patients* (those with knee pain from osteoarthritis or wear and tear over time).

Though many patients who've had this surgery "report relief from pain," there's no physiological basis for this—no evidence that arthroscopy cures or slows osteoarthritis, explains Nelda P. Wray, MD, who led the 2002 study. Chances are those patients were experiencing the "placebo effect": the *perception* of benefit from a treatment due to the mere *belief* it is effective.

The Wray team gave one randomly chosen group of research participants the actual surgery and the other group, the placebo: sham knee surgery. (A "placebo" itself is a fake drug or treatment that appears to be the real deal, used to determine how much of a study result is from the intervention and how much is just psychological.)

In the placebo group, the surgeon made the usual arthroscopic incision in the patient's knee, but merely simulated the surgery by asking for instruments and manipulating their knee as if the real procedure were being performed. All the patients were monitored over a two-year period. The result? At no point during that time did the patients who got the real-deal surgery report having less pain or better knee function than patients who got the pretend surgery!

Yes, you're reading that right: The actual surgery was no better than the fake surgery! And the real kind costs $10K or more and involves weeks or months of recovery time, plus there are risks like a potentially deadly blood clot (thankfully rare) or long-term damage to your knee.

Depressingly, the rate of these useless knee surgeries continued to increase for almost a decade after the 2002 study—and even longer, according to some studies. And yes, as of 2024, there are doctors who continue to recommend it and perform it on their patients!

KEEPING THE BLIND FAITH
Sometimes it's the science itself that's in need of updating

People will tell you—with a completely straight face—that science is "self-correcting," meaning that new evidence that reveals errors in previous conclusions will lead researchers and institutions to update their understanding and practices accordingly. ASAP!

Scientist and biologist Douglas Allchin practically rolls his eyes at the absurdity: "Researchers supposedly examine each other's results critically. Any mistake is soon exposed. It cannot persist for long. Progress toward truth is restored. So they say."

In fact, over here in Realityville, "Science has no inherent mechanism for self-correction," Allchin writes. "Errors can persist, sometimes famously for decades." Contributing to this, daring to challenge the scientific status quo—even when armed with strong evidence—can be toxic to a researcher's career.

Allchin points to the belief by doctors "for much of the 20th century" that gastric ulcers—searingly painful open sores in the stomach lining or small intestine—were caused by stress, spicy foods, and too much stomach acid.

Their patients with ulcers suffered unrelenting digestive torture: burning stomach pain, indigestion, bloating, burping, and nausea and sometimes vomiting. There was no cure; just temporary relief from constantly popping antacids: chalky acid-neutralizing tablets doctors prescribed that coated and soothed the stomach for a few hours.

In the early 1980s, Australian scientists Barry Marshall and Robin Warren, both doctors, discovered that 80 to 90 percent of stomach ulcers (as well as some stomach cancers) are caused by the bacterium Helicobacter pylori (H. pylori) and could be cured with a course of antibiotics. *Cured!*

There was a problem. "To gastroenterologists"—stomach doctors—"the concept of a germ causing ulcers was like saying that the Earth is flat," Marshall told *Discover* magazine's Pamela Weintraub. Marshall and Warren's finding was widely dismissed and even ridiculed by the medical community until the early 1990s—causing nearly a decade of unnecessary suffering by patients whose doctors kept prescribing antacids that the bacteria simply ignored.

In 2005, Marshall and Warren were awarded the Nobel Prize in Medicine. The Nobel committee wrote: "Thanks to the pioneering discovery by Marshall and Warren, peptic ulcer disease is no longer a chronic, frequently disabling condition, but a disease that can be cured by a short regimen of antibiotics and acid secretion inhibitors."

In fact, it was *not* thanks to their "pioneering discovery" that the science eventually prevailed, but their unrelenting refusal to let their discovery be dismissed and kept from patients by the medical fraternity deriding them. For a long time, there was *only one doctor* who believed in what they were doing—Warren's psychiatrist wife, Win—but they maintained their near-fanatical commitment to having their finding accepted by the field. Marshall, especially, fought fiercely for years to have their research published and given fair hearing, even infecting himself with H. pylori to prove once and for all the nasty little buggers were the cause of ulcers.

Had Marshall and Warren been *just a little less driven*, millions of people might still be suffering searing gut pain and digestive distress every day—with not a clue they could put an end to it with a short course of pest control.

MEDICAL OUTSIDERS
The light at the end of the tunnel vision

Science can't do its job—be a search for truth with a vigorous openness to being proven wrong—when scientists' minds are made up like beds with the sheets glued down.

Because *believing* is a major obstacle to *seeing*—to being open to the possibility of errors in long-accepted thinking and practices—voices from outside a field are vital for spotlighting its scientific shortcomings.

This sort of spotlight from medical outsiders—investigative science journalists Gary Taubes and Nina Teicholz, among others—has revolutionized the way many Americans eat. For decades, we were advised to avoid saturated fat and stick to a low-fat, high-carbohydrate diet, which would supposedly keep us lean and healthy and prevent heart disease. It instead led to an epidemic of obesity, diabetes, and heart disease.

In 2002, Taubes published *The New York Times Magazine* cover story, "What If It's All Been a Big Fat Lie?" It was a meticulous 8,000-word exposé, pulling the rug out from the unproven claims behind the low-fat/high-carb dietary advice for Americans.

Taubes presented compelling evidence that it is not saturated fat but sweet and starchy carbs that cause us to become obese and lead to increased risk of heart disease. Contrary to what the American Heart Association, the government, and our doctors kept telling us, cheeseburgers weren't the enemy; it was the bun, Coke, and fries that were doing us in. The evidence supporting this was right there in the research for any doctor who looked. But again, few doctors look.

Doctors' patients, however, dove into books and articles by Taubes, Teicholz, and others. They saw the evidence that saturated fat—the kind in eggs, butter, cheese, and steak—had been falsely accused as the greasy, artery-clogging means to munch our way to a heart attack. Numerous Americans cut carbs and threw the steaks back on the grill, losing sometimes massive amounts of weight, eliminating type 2 diabetes symptoms without drugs, and improving their overall health.

Doctors, bowled over by their patients' remarkable transformations, began getting on board: eating low-carb and recommending a low-carb diet to other patients—tacit acknowledgment of the lack of evidence behind the low-fat/high-carb standard. Some doctors, to their credit, are openly remorseful. Neuroradiologist and USC Keck School of Medicine Professor of Radiology Robert Lufkin, MD, is one of them, tweeting:

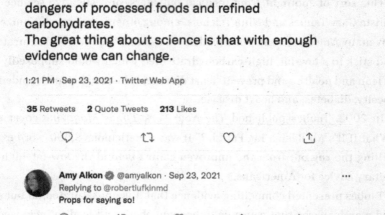

Almost 20 years after Taubes published his 2002 *New York Times Magazine* exposé, the American College of Cardiology (ACC) *finally* came around. In August of 2020, the ACC announced that their previous guidelines radically limiting saturated fat intake were "not aligned with the current evidence base."

"Saturated fatty acid-rich foods" like "whole-fat dairy, unprocessed meat, and dark chocolate" are not associated with increased risk of heart disease, diabetes, or death, they reported. "The totality of available evidence does not support further limiting the intake of such foods."

MALPRACTICE STANDARDS
Why bad science has staying power

Despite the ACC's 2020 admission that they'd wrongly demonized saturated fat, current medical practice standards remain, shall we say, *a bit retro*. As of February 28, 2023, my healthcare provider, Kaiser Permanente, was still advising patients to go stingy on saturated fat, giving the scientifically unsupported advice on their website that "No more than 10% of your daily calories should come from saturated fat."

It actually pays for a healthcare provider to look the other way when new findings conflict with the advice their doctors have been dispensing for years or decades. Telling a new evidence-based truth could require them to admit their longstanding practice standards were wrong and even harmful, potentially opening them up to lawsuits.

Of course, such admissions wouldn't be necessary if medical institutions professing to provide evidence-based care actually, you know, *provided it. Reliably*—by having panels of Sander Greenland and Gerd Gigerenzer-level experts on staff assessing the evidence, generating *actually evidence-based* practice standards, and updating them as called for by new evidence.

I'm not alone in seeing a need for this. In a 2024 Substack post, Gary Taubes calls for public health problems like the "out-of-control epidemic" of diabetes to be addressed by "committees of the brightest clinical investigators" in the country "sifting through and critically reviewing the evidence."

"Because that has not happened," writes Taubes, "the job was left to an investigative journalist and *Rethinking Diabetes* [Taubes's 2024 book] is the result." He adds that "one ambitious goal" of his book "is to see if it could generate the kind of investigative committees this public health situation seems to demand."

Kaiser (and other institutions) will protest that they *have* committees doing this—and they do. They just aren't doing the job—nor are the medical associations and government healthcare institutions that generate practice guidelines Kaiser uses—which is why Kaiser's website and Kaiser doctors make so many recommendations contrary to current evidence.

These guideline-generating committees are typically made up of medical insiders. "They have mechanisms to incorporate the latest findings, but always on the assumption that what they've done before is correct and just needs minor variations," Taubes explained to me. They "have no mechanism to rethink bad practices in their fields and why they are ineffective" and what needs to change.

In contrast, Sander Greenland and Gerd Gigerenzer operate on the principle of what I call "educated doubt," with skepticism being the prevailing culture driving their work. Ideally, they'd be paired not with myopic medical insiders—doctors and pharmacists steeped in status quo beliefs and practices—but unbiased yet deeply informed outsiders.

Importantly, outsiders are free to let the scientific chips fall where they may—in a way medical and scientific insiders are not. Outsiders, by nature, are not "trapped in the groupthink of any particular medical discipline," notes Taubes. Not being part of the system, their careers don't suffer if they "conclude that the authorities may have got it wrong—that the groupthink is incorrect." This gives outsiders the ability—and, in fact, the incentive—to be that much-needed grating voice of dissent rising out of the crowd of medical head-nodders.

What's stopping us from having panels like this right now? Gigerenzer points to a massive lack of interest in scientific reform among medical school deans, CEOs of healthcare institutions, and health insurance honchos. He predicts that "At some point in the future, patients will notice how often they are being misled...just as bank customers eventually did" during the subprime crisis. "When this happens, the health industry may lose the trust of the public, as happened to the banking industry."

As it should! And that "point in the future" should be right now.

Though some individual doctors absolutely do deserve our trust, you've seen throughout these two chapters that the medical system and our medical institutions absolutely do not. So, borrowing from Gary, "one ambitious goal" of this book is generating public conversation that lets medical institution bigwigs know we patients are no longer in the dark about the yawning gap between the evidence and medical practice, and the same goes for all the medical betrayal we see being passed off as medical care.

THE EMPEROR'S NEW LAB COAT
Calling out the bad science behind medical practice standards for menopause and perimenopause

In 2016, when I had that first hot flash and began my dive into research on menopause and perimenopause, I noted a disturbing parallel with the saturated fat debacle: researchers clinging to scientifically unwarranted beliefs about menopause and perimenopause—dismissing any pesky evidence that called their beliefs into question.

Doctors, reasonably, don't think to question the scientific basis of the research behind the menopausal and perimenopausal practice standards their department requires them to go by. (Who would imagine a respected medical institution's treatment requirements would have anything but a solid scientific foundation?)

I, however, was able to see the often-unscientific underpinnings of menopausal and perimenopausal research and medical care—not because I'm some sort of genius, but because I'm a medical outsider, coming in largely cold to the subject matter.

I approach medical science taking nothing for granted—including the foundational beliefs in a field: those "facts" everybody in the field "just knows" (like all those gastroenterologists "just knowing" ulcers were the fault of the patient for having that stressfest of a job and marital problems, too). I look not just at current studies but dig into medical history, starting with the first findings in the field and working my way up to the latest research and thinking.

Still, I was cowed by what a huge and truly terrible responsibility writing and publishing this book would be. If I'm in my usual neighborhood, behavioral science, and I do a bad job assessing the research, somebody might say the wrong thing to their boyfriend and kill their relationship. If I get medical science wrong, somebody could be harmed or maybe even *die*.

I struggled with what to do, and then it occurred to me: In writing this book, I wouldn't be without a scientific net. I would do what I do with every science-based book I write: send chapters and sections out for fact-checking by experts in each area—researchers whose scientific rigor I respect—and beg them to "hand me my ass" in any places I might've erred or fallen short.

Ultimately, I wrote this book because I couldn't live with *not* writing it.

No, I don't wear a white coat, and the last time I held a stethoscope, it was plastic and I was six. What I do have to offer you are the benefits of my drilling down in the research to find the most powerful, efficient ways for us to stay strong and healthy throughout our lives. You deserve what I was able to get for myself—evidence-based care to ease the life-chomping symptoms of menopause and perimenopause. You deserve to join me in flipping the bird to the inevitability of ill health in old age.

— 3 —

THE MAJOR ERROR DOCTORS AND RESEARCHERS MAKE BY VIEWING PERIMENOPAUSE AS MENOPAUSE LITE

THERE'S THIS FAMILY, the Laskos, who've done a lot to ease my suffering during my hormonal hellride years. Lasko is a Hungarian name, and if you know anything about Hungarian hospitality, you're picturing nice neighbors who invite me over for big soothing bowls of goulash. In fact, we've never met.

The Laskos make "tower fans": the plug-in saviors for we women whose ladyhormones have turned on us, constantly making us overheat like an old Buick.

You can't fully appreciate the intense beauty of a four-foot wind phallus until you start having hot flashes. "Flash," by the way, is false advertising, suggesting a brief blast of heat, causing an equally brief blast of discomfort. (If only!) For maybe two to five minutes, a hot flash boils your face and upper body from the inside out, making you feel like a giant pork chop being microwaved.

But my hot flashes didn't just overheat me; they confused me.

I *thought* hot flashes happened in menopause, after you stopped having periods. I was still having periods. What the hell was going on?

In reading the research, I discovered I was in *perimenopause*.

You might've seen the word "perimenopause" hanging around here and there over the years, like some weirdo skulking in the back corner of the local bar—but maybe, like me, you just blew past it. As I explained in Chapter One, perimenopause is the term for the transition years to menopause—the phase when a series of hormonal changes can lead to unpleasant, annoying, and even health-tanking symptoms.

Articles about perimenopause started popping up around 2021. But I'd been asking women, "Have you heard of perimenopause?" since around 2016. And very often, they hadn't. In a 2022 survey of UK women 40 and older by pharmacologist Joyce Harper, a whopping 61 percent said they were not informed *at all* about perimenopause. "A number of them stated they had never even heard the word perimenopause before," she writes.

Our cluelessness about perimenopause comes in large part from that major error by researchers that's been baked into medical practice standards: the sloppy, scientifically incorrect assumption that perimenopause is simply *menopause lite*, when it's actually a hormonally different stage that needs to be treated accordingly.

That's why, until that summer afternoon I got blasted with my first hot flash and then got reading, I believed what pretty much everybody believes about women's menopausal (and menopause-adjacent) years: they're a time of lowered estrogen levels.

My understanding was *partly right:* Estrogen levels *are* lower in menopause, when menstrual cycles are no more. However, as I went deeper into the research, I learned of a serious and, in fact, terrible error in much of the scientific literature, spotlighted by endocrinologist (aka hormone doctor) and University of British Columbia med school professor Jerilynn C. Prior, MD. There's been an unscientific lumping together of perimenopause, the years of *transition* to menopause, with menopause itself, *by researchers in the field*! This has led to that harmfully incorrect but widely believed assumption by both researchers and gynecologists that perimenopause and menopause have *the same hormonal makeup*: supposedly a single, uniform hormonal profile involving estrogen levels *substantially lower* than in a woman's most fertile years.

Research by gynecologist Nanette Santoro, MD, among others, shows that this view is wrong. Perimenopause is actually a time of *soaring* estrogen—estrogen rising to levels that are, on average, about 30 percent higher than those in women in their fertile 20s and 30s, explains Prior. *Thirty percent higher!*

In addition, perimenopausal estrogen levels rise and fall erratically, so, at times—in some women—they may climb to a physiologically hellish 200 percent higher and then take a dive. Adding to this hormonal turmoil, just as estrogen is soaring, a perimenopausal woman's progesterone levels tend to go the other direction—on average, ending up 50 percent lower than normal (or missing or barely there). This is significant, Dr. Prior explains, because "The most symptomatic women have higher estrogen and lower progesterone levels."

Take women who have extremely heavy perimenopausal bleeding, as I did (à la "Am I mortally wounded, or do I need to borrow a tampon from an elephant?!"). Research by endometriosis specialist Mette Hass Moen, MD, suggests that we big-time bleeders have generally higher estrogen levels: more than double the levels of women with more normal flow.

Women who experience this heavy menstrual bleeding in midlife (around age 35 and up) also have the lowest levels of progesterone, notes Dr. Prior—and the worst perimenopausal symptoms. (If only doctors knew that correcting the perimenopausal lack or shortage of progesterone alleviates many of these symptoms.)

An estimated 40 percent of women experience those soaring estrogen levels—and a companion lack of progesterone—and are miserably symptomatic because of it. Other women have more generally stable levels—that is, not leaping and diving all the time—but those women's levels, too, tend to fluctuate: spike and dive. At the end of perimenopause, close to menopause, all women experience lower levels.

All of this crucial evidence on the actual ways estrogen and progesterone act within us during perimenopause *should* be the foundation of perimenopausal medical care. It is not.

IGNORE THE EVIDENCE AND MAYBE IT'LL GO AWAY

We saw in Chapter Two what an obstacle believing is to seeing. Understanding that is vital for getting our heads around the seemingly *un*believable field-wide myth, believed by researchers and doctors alike, that perimenopause is a time of estrogen *deficiency*.

Never mind the evidence revealing soaring and erratic perimenopausal estrogen—from multiple research teams! Never mind the raging perimenopausal symptoms that Prior points out "cannot be explained by low estrogen levels"—endlessly sore boobs, periods gone crazy heavy, worse migraines, and sudden mysterious weight gain—all of which are instead associated with higher and erratic estrogen.

Bolstering the persistence of this myth of perimenopausal estrogen deficiency is the considerable chunk of time it's been hanging around unquestioned, explains Dr. Prior. From the 1950s through the 1990s, this belief was "so common" that researchers who measured high estrogen levels in some perimenopausal women chased away the inconsistency between the myth and their evidence (visible in tables in the paper!) by leaving their finding unmentioned in the text.

Prior points to a 1995 study of 390 perimenopausal Australian women, ages 46 to 57, by clinical endocrinologist Henry G. Burger, MD, and his colleagues. The Burger team's paper revealed erratic and spiking estrogen levels in these perimenopausal women. Yet the researchers *took no notice* of these elevated estrogen levels, despite at least a quarter of them being *as high or higher* in the 46- to 57-year-old women than the highest they would *ever* be in a woman in her highly-fertile early 20s.

Amazingly, Burger and his team were apparently so hypnotized by the myth that estrogen drops in perimenopause that they summed up their finding of *rising* estrogen levels with the opposite conclusion: "Perimenopause is characterized by dropping estrogen...levels."

Prior was outraged. "These authors had not seen the very high estrogen levels that their data so beautifully showed. They were perhaps unable to see because the data didn't fit their paradigm" (their entrenched beliefs about perimenopause).

In 1996, Prior, with two colleagues, wrote what she described as "a scathing letter" to the journal that published the Burger study, "demanding that the authors 'let the data speak!'"—a call for the authors to have the integrity to report the high estrogen levels they'd found. The Burger team's response, published with Prior's letter, merely conceded that during much of perimenopause, estrogen levels are "preserved" (rather than dropping).

That wasn't good enough for Prior. In 1998, she conducted a meta-analysis, a study that combines and analyzes the results of a group of previous studies—in this case, 12 papers referencing the estrogen levels of 415 women in perimenopause and 292 younger women (women in their more fertile years). The perimenopausal women's estrogen levels were "significantly higher" (30 percent higher, on average) than those in the younger, generally more fertile women!

This is not evidence that we—and, especially, researchers and doctors—should be ignoring. But that's exactly what has happened over the past 25 years—to perimenopausal women's detriment.

Take my experience. About a month after perimenopause started turning me into a one-woman climate crisis, I messaged my Kaiser Permanente gynecologist, asking for a prescription for progesterone to manage my perimenopausal hot flashes. But instead of putting the prescription through, he replied with this:

> Please read more information from our Kaiser resources regarding hormone therapy.

Pasted into his message was a pre-printed fact sheet from Kaiser ("©2006–2016 Healthwise") about hormone therapy for "symptoms of *menopause*" (italics mine), "such as hot flashes, vaginal dryness, and sleep problems." And then there was this:

> It replaces the hormones that drop at menopause...

But remember, *I was not in menopause*—when estrogen levels drop! I was in *perimenopause*—the time when estrogen levels soar and become erratic. The fact that I was in perimenopause was not a secret to my gynecologist. I was emailing him in July, and I had just seen him in February. I was still having periods in February. Raging, horrible, but still-regular, month-apart periods.

A woman is *only* in menopause after she's gone 12 months without periods. He surely knew this. It's truly basic stuff every gynecologist *should* know—and it's all over Kaiser's website: "After 1 year of having no periods, you've reached menopause."

To my horror, I was experiencing firsthand what I'd seen in my reading—that doctors, including gynecologists, don't understand perimenopause for what it actually is: a distinct phase, hormonally different from menopause. The fact sheet continued, "HT" (hormone therapy) "contains two female hormones, estrogen and progestin."

Arrgh! Huge error—akin to describing "two female hormones, estrogen and NyQuil"!

A "progestin" is not a hormone made by our body. It is a drug made in a factory! Incredibly, as you'll see in Chapter Seven, doctors and researchers constantly confuse it with progesterone, the hormone produced by our ovaries during our menstrual cycle. Regarding the inclusion of estrogen, as a woman in perimenopause, the last thing I needed was extra estrogen to top off my body's estrogen tsunami!

This Healthwise "fact sheet" would more accurately be called an "error sheet." Kaiser Permanente, the largest managed-care consortium in the US, with 12.6 million patient-members as of 2022, is just one major institution using Healthwise's write-ups.

Healthwise is a "non-profit"—"non-profit" to the tune of $39 million in revenue in 2015—that develops "health content and patient education" for hospitals and huge healthcare providers like Kaiser. They also sell their content to health websites directed at consumers.

The Healthwise site boasts, "Over 100 team members with medical expertise craft our quality content." "Medical expertise"! That *is* important—except, say, if you're an expert foot doctor expected to wax scientific on the doings of the aorta.

I'm guessing they don't go *that* far, but in December of 2022, I looked up the four doctors they had listed as their ob-gyn experts. *All four* are pregnancy specialists—specializing in baby delivery and pregnancy-related disorders. Not one appeared to have *any* focus or expertise in menopause or perimenopause—in their research or practice.

I was miffed at getting a "fact" sheet instead of the treatment I'd asked for, and I was deeply disturbed—though not surprised—that my gynecologist seemed to believe estrogen therapy was appropriate for a symptomatic newly perimenopausal patient. However, taking a step back—remembering from my office visits that he was not some cavalier jerk practitioner but truly kind, careful, and caring—I realized it wasn't fair to blame him for his less-than-informed response.

Maybe that seems overly generous. It's not.

I used to be quick to condemn doctors who weren't up on the latest evidence in their area as lazy and horrible, willfully endangering their patients—probably so they could get in an extra round of golf. However, a blog post by my friend Michael Eades, MD, a retired nutritional medicine specialist who has consistently immersed himself in dietary science, led me to see things differently.

Eades wrote about a typical packed-to-the-gills day at the Arkansas medical practice he and his wife, Mary Dan Eades, MD, ran together, opening my eyes to the current realities of the business of medicine. Doctors today, especially at an HMO like Kaiser, are slammed all day, every day, seeing one patient after the next—chop, chop, chop—and then completing an electronic medical record novelette for each (often after hours). There's little or no time for even a brief stroll through the medical literature. (Of course, having that time would be pointless if they're among the many doctors who aren't trained in how to read or evaluate it.)

This is probably why doctors rely on prepared "fact" sheets like the one my gynecologist sent me as well as the practice standards their department has adopted. In other words, it's easy to get angry at doctors for all the unscientific advice and treatment they give patients—and I *do* think they have a responsibility to do better—but it's the system, from med school on, that's largely to blame.

OVERCOMING STAGE FRIGHT

Because so many doctors are unaware that menopause and perimenopause are two distinct stages that affect the body in some different ways—hormonally and symptomatically—there's a good chance your doctor, like mine, will lump the two stages together into a single meno-blob.

You need to *diagnose yourself* correctly so you can ask your doctor for the menopause- or perimenopause-appropriate treatment you need.

That probably sounds hard or impossible. I promise you it's not. It just takes going through a short list of the symptoms of perimenopause in the next chapter and seeing whether you're experiencing more than two of them.

But first things first.

Perimenopause is best understood in comparison with menopause.

WHAT IS MENOPAUSE?

Ask a random woman "What is menopause?" and she'll probably answer, "It's when you stop having periods." That's true. She might add, "It's the end of baby-making." That's true, too.

But there's a *physiologically precise* definition that matters—mentioned previously in the chapter:

You're in menopause when you've gone 12 months straight without a period.

You then remain in this menopause phase—no more periods, no more babies—for the rest of your life.

Women, on average, go into menopause at 51. However, menopause can occur between ages 40 and 58. A very small percentage of women (perhaps 1 percent) go into "premature menopause," menopause before the age of 40.

The *12-months-straight* standard for determining a woman is in menopause comes from a University of Minnesota study that followed the menstrual cycles of female college students for decades. In women age 45 and older, after 12 months straight without a period, there's a 90 to 95 percent chance a woman's "last period" really *was* her last. In contrast, after only six months without a period, 28 to 55 percent of women will go on to bloody more underpants.

This 12-month buffer zone thing might seem like meaningless medical trivia; however, when you're on the verge of menopause, counting the months you go through without periods is important. Menstrual bleeding before menopause is normal: an indication that you're still in perimenopause. Bleeding *after* menopause (whether heavy or just spotting) can indicate something's wrong with you—possibly even cancer—and MUST be checked out by a doctor. ASAP.

Though I would hope that *most* gynecologists these days know and go by the *12-months-straight* rule, my friend Susan went to two different doctors who did not apply that standard. In 2020, she told Doctor #1 she was having hot flashes and night sweats. She added that she'd gone three months without a period, and then, in month four, up popped Auntie Flo. Correct diagnosis? Perimenopause. Time to reset the 12-month meno clock! Yet her doctor told her she was "in menopause."

Susan is black, and like other black women who've talked to me about their experiences seeking medical care, she has felt dismissed, ignored, and disrespected by her doctors—including Doctor #1 and Doctor #2. "They didn't listen to me," she said. "I know white women go through that, too, but as a black woman, I'm really sensitive to that." She has had doctors she's appreciated, but her lifetime experience with doctors has been to speak and not be listened to, to be treated like a child, to be spoken to rudely, and to have the strong sense that she was being given a lower quality of care.

Because of that, she's more skeptical of doctors' advice than many women I've spoken to. "It isn't just about the lack of respect," she explained. If a doctor is inattentive, there's a real possibility of harm from a diagnosis and treatment based on incomplete information about what's going on with her—yet they expect her to go along just because they say so. "Like with you and 'Dr. God,'" she said—referring to my former primary care doc who angrily talked over me when I asked him to explain his reasoning and eventually bellowed, "Because I'm the doctor, and it's my clinical judgment!"

When a doctor doesn't listen to Susan, she's understandably reticent to go with the treatment they advise—as was the case in 2022, when Doctor #2 misdiagnosed Susan as "in menopause." The doctor then leapt to the conclusion that Susan's bleeding was not Auntie Flo but Auntie Cancer.

However, Susan had told Doctor #2 loud and clear that she'd gotten her period at the 10-month mark—along with PMS-type symptoms that Dr. Prior explains say "period" (as opposed to "cancer"): for example, sore boobs, bloating, and cramping; clear, stretchy vaginal mucus; and elevated libido.

In other words, Susan's bleeding *was* a sign: No, not that she needed the painful surgical procedure she refused on principle to let this doctor schedule for her at the time—but that she needed to keep doing her part to buy yachts, Aston Martins, and tropical islands for tampon- and pad-company honchos.

BONUS POINT

MEDICAL ERASE-ISM

You'll see in this book that it's deeply important to me to expose the way most women's health research has been conducted on middle-class white women and then applied to all women—ignoring meaningful physiological differences in ways that neglect or harm the health of women of color.

A note on my use of "black" rather than "Black," the current style of some news organizations: Minna Salami, author of *Sensuous Knowledge—A Black Feminist Approach for Everyone,* writes in the *Guardian,* "While the capitalisation of the 'b' assuages race politics, it also validates race politics."

"POSTMENOPAUSE" IS A STUPID TERM IN NEED OF RETIREMENT

The word "menopause," like Socrates, Plato, and Alexander the Great, got its start in ancient Greece, as a combo of *mens* (month) and *pausis* (pause or stop). In the 1800s, Paris was hopping, and it moved to France, becoming *la ménèspausie*—which got shortened to *menopause*.

In the book, I occasionally quote researchers using the annoying term "postmenopause": confusing linguistic overkill, which—if you break it down into its parts, "post" and "menopause"—means "after the after the monthly bleeding stops."

Credit for this mess goes to two panels of researchers—one in the US and one in Europe. They had good intentions: coming up with a consistent term to be used in research. However, the American panel ended up defining "menopause" as the actual day of the final menstrual period itself—which means "menopause" is technically *a single day in a woman's life!*

This created a new problem. They had nothing to call the "no more periods" life phase that starts at that point—the phase the public already knew as "menopause" (or "the change" if your embarrassed grandpa had to mention it).

Well, screw public understanding! The naming team "fixed" the problem by scotch-taping a modifier on "menopause," creating "post-menopause"—not quite putting together that it was already "taken." (A friend of Prior's points out, "after menopause" is an actual stage: death!)

Throughout the book, I use the term "menopause" rather than "postmenopause" because I want to describe what it *is*—the life phase we're in when we're done with periods and baby-making—and not call it "after" that, which is like calling it nothing at all.

WHAT IS PERIMENOPAUSE?

"Peri" is the ancient Greek word for "around," so *peri*menopause is the time around menopause—basically the on-ramp to menopause. It can start as early as a woman's mid-30s and can last from three to 10 years (or more in some women) and ends when a woman goes into menopause.

What marks the start of perimenopause? Well, there's the standard, widely accepted but physiologically incomplete view—leaving out women just starting perimenopause and feeling newly crap-o-ramous—and then there's the more physiologically precise view that reflects what those women actually go through, hormonally and symptomatically.

The standard view is myopically menstrual cycle–focused, and it comes from a collaboration of researchers called STRAW, the "Stages of Reproductive Aging Workshop."

The STRAW panel announced that perimenopause starts when women begin having *persistently irregular menstrual cycles*—or as they call them, "variable." "Variable" means that the number of days one menstrual cycle lasts *varies* from the length of the next by seven or more days. "Persistently" means this fluctuating-length thing repeats itself (at least once within a span of 10 cycles). For example, in May, a woman's period comes just 28 days after her previous one, but in August, she gets her period only 20 days after the one in July.

Now, STRAW's description of irregular menstrual cycles isn't wrong. And healthy women with regular menstrual cycles *do* eventually experience irregular cycles in perimenopause. But STRAW's claim—that *ONLY* upon menstrual cycles getting irregular is a woman in perimenopause—fails to take into account the hormonal changes occurring *before* cycles get irregular, documented by gynecologist Nanette Santoro, Dr. Prior, and other researchers.

These early hormonal changes ignored by the STRAW team trigger a set of symptoms (detailed below) in still-regularly-menstruating women that *should* lead doctors to diagnose the start of perimenopause (and determine the appropriate treatment, if necessary). However, because STRAW ignores the inconvenient evidence that conflicts with their foregone conclusions on timing, and because STRAW is baked into practice standards, the perimenopausal symptoms these changes trigger are a medical no-man's-land—not traceable to any particular cause.

Diagnosis: Inexplicable medical mystery! (Just the thing for emotional tranquility when yoga, meditation, and maniacally raking the sand in your desktop Zen garden aren't doing the job!)

THE EVIDENCE THAT STRAW SNUBBED

Dr. Prior explains that the hormonal shift into perimenopause often starts when a woman's periods "are *still regular* and of *normal lengths*." She may begin experiencing a series of unpleasant perimenopausal symptoms that can include much heavier periods, increased breast tenderness, and new or increased mood swings, plus night sweats and "mid-sleep awakenings."

In the later stages of perimenopause, which could last three to seven years, 15 to 20 percent of women experience intense and sometimes terrifying symptoms. "Terrifying" might sound a bit drama-llama, but unexplained, awful symptoms that women and even doctors don't know to connect to perimenopause are exactly that. Until I started researching this book, I had no idea why, in my mid-40s, I suddenly started getting seriously motion sick if I went more than a few miles by car. I'd throw up and be in bed, all dizzy and nauseated, for a day or more afterward.

I was usually too woozy to read, so I'd pass the hours playing pin the tail on the diagnosis: Did I have a brain tumor? MS? Ménière's disease? In fact, nausea is a perimenopausal symptom—one that only a lucky few of us get hit with—but none of my doctors knew that, nor did I (till I dug into the research on the intersection of migraines and motion sickness).

Learning about this and other more common symptoms of perimenopause gave me both peace of mind and the information I needed to help my doctor buck an unscientific system and give me evidence-based care. Learning the symptoms for *yourself*—the subject of the next chapter—is the start of your empowering yourself in the exact same way.

— 4 —

PERIMENOPAUSE AND MENOPAUSE

Two distinct symptomatic stages, not one big meno-blob

FIGURING OUT WHETHER you're in perimenopause—diagnosing yourself so you can get your symptoms treated appropriately—doesn't take years of med school, a slew of blood tests, or a mini MRI in your she-shed.

In fact, you probably mastered the special diagnostic skill this requires some years back—in nursery school, when you learned to count. That's really all it takes. You skim a quick list of perimenopause symptoms, tally up how many you're experiencing, and see whether you hit three.

We'll get to that list, but first, here's how you *don't* diagnose perimenopause.

RELIABLY UNRELIABLE LAB TESTS

Everlywell is one of the many online companies that offer at-home lab test kits for various medical conditions, including hormone tests for menopause and perimenopause. For $99, you can order their so-called "Perimenopause Test." You prick your finger and pop your blood sample in the mail, and they message you on their app with the results—your levels of three menstrual cycle hormones: estrogen (aka "estradiol"), follicle-stimulating hormone (FSH), and luteinizing hormone (LH).

Their page selling the test explains: "Our perimenopause test will let you know if you are transitioning towards menopause."

Uh, no, it won't.

Estrogen measured in a single sample (whether in blood, urine, or saliva) is not reliable for determining a perimenopausal woman's estrogen level, which is anything but consistent. Estrogen levels not only fluctuate throughout the menstrual cycle, but every 20 minutes or so *throughout the day*. (The same goes for progesterone.)

Follicle-stimulating hormone measurement *can* be useful for women doing in-vitro fertilization. High FSH can indicate diminished "ovarian reserve"—a reduced number of eggs still available for sperm meet-ups. However, FSH is not a reliable indicator of perimenopausal status (nor is luteinizing hormone, which triggers ovulation and stimulates the production of progesterone).

Though FSH levels soar as estrogen and progesterone levels bottom out in menopause, FSH can be elevated way before perimenopause—"sometimes even 10 years before," explains gynecologist Nanette Santoro—for a number of reasons. For example, polycystic ovary syndrome (PCOS), thyroid disorders, rheumatoid arthritis, and various medications can lead to elevated FSH.

Ultimately, as The North American Menopause Society puts it: "There is no simple test to predict or confirm menopause or perimenopause."

Doctors *should* know this—but women keep telling me their doctors did not and ordered blood and saliva tests to determine whether they were in perimenopause. It's tempting to say yes to a lab test, especially if it's covered by your insurance, but these supposed perimenopause or menopause prediction tests are best avoided. Though *you* know the results aren't reliable, your doctor may use them as a basis for treatment that's unwarranted and even harmful.

NINE CLUES YOU ARE IN PERIMENOPAUSE

Detecting whether you're in perimenopause does take a lab, but that lab is *you*. The earliest perimenopause symptoms are mostly forms of menstrual cycle suck gone much suckier: the result of a brewing storm of hormonal unrest in you in the earliest days of perimenopause.

The very simple task at hand? Going through that "quick list" I mentioned and counting up the number of symptoms you're experiencing that make you feel like you need an exorcism instead of an Advil.

Endocrinologist Jerilynn Prior, MD, puts it more technically: "Perimenopause begins with changes in experience" in your body and brain as a woman in your "midlife" years. (Midlife starts around age 40, though there are women who go into perimenopause in their 30s—or in their 50s.)

Take swollen boobs—no stranger to any woman who's ever shopped the period products aisle. Before perimenopause, it's normal for the breasts to swell during the weeks before flow, Prior explains. The changes pointing to perimenopause? Your boobs see no reason to limit this swelling business to PMS time. They might even be swollen most of the time—and *much* more swollen and sore than you're used to. (For a while in perimenopause, I had to sleep in a bra so I wouldn't wake myself screaming when I rolled on my side and had boob-to-sheet contact.)

THE NINE CHANGES

Prior and her colleagues came up with this list of changes you can use to self-diagnose perimenopause. You're in what Prior terms "Very Early Perimenopause"—the symptom-blotched starting gate to perimenopause the STRAW researchers ignored—if you still have regular menstrual cycles about a month apart, yet experience any three of the following:

1. New onset of heavier and/or longer menstrual flow.
2. Shorter menstrual cycle lengths (25 or fewer days between periods).
3. Breasts that are newly more sore, swollen, and/or lumpy.
4. New or markedly increased menstrual cramps.
5. Waking up mid sleep when this was not previously an issue.
6. New onset of night sweats, especially around menstrual flow.
7. New or much more frequent migraine headaches.
8. New or more frequent premenstrual mood swings.
9. Notable weight gain without changes in food intake or exercise habits.

These symptoms can hang around bothering you for several years before there's any change in your menstrual cycle (from regular to irregular), notes Prior.

Unfortunately, your medical institution most likely doesn't use this symptom-checking method for diagnosing the early stages of perimenopause—not because it's inaccurate, but because it's standard practice in the field to go by that timetable the STRAW (Stages of Reproductive Aging Workshop) panel came up with.

The STRAW guidelines underestimate the actual length of perimenopause (suggesting it lasts only two to four years). They come up short due to the STRAW team's physiologically unsupported claim that only when women start experiencing irregular menstrual cycles—seesawing in length from one to the next by seven or more days—are they in perimenopause.

Because women often get hit with the hormonal and symptomatic unrest of perimenopause while they still have regular periods, the STRAW standard that excludes their experience sticks them with looming uncertainty about what might be wrong with them.

Uncertainty—provoking fear of the unknown and what it might hold—is deeply disturbing to us, causing uncomfortable psychological tension. Some women become driven—even desperate—to alleviate it, seeking out what Prior describes as "(disease) diagnoses," such as fibromyalgia and chronic fatigue syndrome, to "explain and legitimize" their suffering. This may cause them to get treatments they don't need that sometimes cause lasting damage.

The damage can also be psychological, Prior explains. To manage the looming uncertainty about the cause of the symptoms, "A perimenopausal woman may start viewing herself as chronically ill." That's a term for feeling persistently sick, which is very much how I felt in perimenopause—though it's a bit institutionally beige to convey my constant undertone of panic at suddenly feeling so swollen, weak, broken-down, and old.

HOW LONG MIGHT THIS PERIMENOPAUSAL HELLSHOW LAST?

It's important that *you* know when you've hit perimenopause and where you might be in the progression to menopause, both so you can tell your doctor in hopes of getting appropriate treatment and so you have an idea of what to expect.

Dr. Prior and her colleagues created a physiologically accurate map of the stages leading to and through perimenopause and menopause—a timeline that, vitally, *includes* the "Very Early Perimenopause" phase STRAW left out, when women with still-regular menstrual cycles start suffering uncomfortable changes.

This led Prior and her team to conclude that perimenopause typically "lasts several years and commonly lasts six or seven." That said, women's experiences vary widely, and a number of us have a much shorter or much longer stint in perimenopause. (Mine was basically a perimenopausal *decade*.)

Accordingly, the Prior team's stages of menopause and perimenopause below are not a template your experiences should conform to but a general idea of how things might play out for you.

Very Early Perimenopause:
The stage you're likely in if you check off three or more symptoms on Prior's nine-item list ("The Nine Changes" above). "This phase may last from two to five years," writes Prior, and "probably lasts longer in those who start it in their 30s" than in those getting started on these changes in their 50s. (Which, yes, happens!)

Early Perimenopause (aka the "Early Menopause Transition"):
"The onset of irregular cycles (varying by 7 days from the start of one flow to the next)" heralds the beginning of this stage, explains Prior.

Late Menopause Transition (taking place in perimenopause):
"The landmark of the first skipped period" on the road to menopause, writes Prior.

Very Late Perimenopause:
"The last count-down year" to menopause, writes Prior—or, in lingerie terms, the year after your last period ruins its last pair of cute underpants. After 12 months straight without flow, you're in menopause. However, if a period pops up in the middle of that year, the clock gets reset—till a whole year without a period goes by.

Menopause:
That year without flow dispatches you into menopause, which goes on for the rest of your life. For a general idea on when you *might* hit menopause, Prior observes that "The average age of menopause in Western countries is approximately 51."

COMMON PERIMENOPAUSE SYMPTOMS

The list of nine changes above is just a tool for figuring out whether you've hit perimenopause. The following are the most common symptoms you might suffer once you're in its clutches—the first six of which (down through "bone loss") are also common menopausal symptoms.

- Hot flashes and night sweats
- Insomnia
- Brain fog
- Mental health issues *(including mood swings and sudden bursts of anger)*
- Weight gain
- Bone loss
- Migraines
- Uterine fibroids
- Period problems *(including weirdly short or long menstrual cycles, skipped periods, and crazy-heavy flow)*

A less common perimenopausal symptom:

- Vaginal dryness

Other perimenopausal symptoms Prior says women may experience:

- Aching knees, ankles, wrists, or shoulders
- A sudden inability to breathe and hunger for air
- Weird dreams (often of being pregnant)
- Inexplicable panic attacks and hyperventilation into breathlessness
- A general, heightened sensitivity—to other people, to sensory stimuli, to perceived slights, and anything else that hits one the wrong way
- The estrogen-driven onset of new allergies or sensitivities
- Dizzy spells, nausea, and vertigo

WHY PERIMENOPAUSE IS BETTER THAN ETERNAL DAMNATION

I managed to find something nice to say about perimenopause. Perimenopause is temporary—as is much of the hormone-induced torment that comes with.

This isn't to say it's all sparkly rainbow unicorns in the land of menopause, which shares a number of distressing symptoms with perimenopause, such as hot flashes and a regular bad night's sleep. However, in menopause, symptoms tend to be less severe and women generally don't feel as ragingly unwell. (Prior describes menopause as a "kinder and calmer phase.")

Being mindful that perimenopause comes with an off-ramp makes you more inclined to question recommendations for invasive treatments with lasting adverse effects. For example, unnecessary hysterectomy surgery is often advised for perimenopausal fibroids that could be left alone: moderately-sized buggers that aren't painful, abdomen-distorting, or organ-squashing and are likely to shrink on their own in menopause.

It is important to reiterate that for many in perimenopause, the symptoms are just an uncomfortable bother, and about 10 percent of women don't notice perimenopause at all. Eventually, they just stop having periods.

You'd find perimenopausal me glowering at them from the other end of the spectrum, all hot and flashy, being roasted like Satan's special marshmallow. For about 10 years, there was no part of my life that was not trashed by perimenopause—from sleep to mental clarity to my long-taken-for-granted ability to get around by car without throwing up into a Rite Aid bag.

BONUS POINT

THE HUMAN RACE
(It's messy)

As I noted in the previous chapter, throughout this book, I've included the distinct risks and symptoms experienced by women in different racial groups—that is, when this research exists.

Scientists are increasingly sensitive to the need to study women of *all* races. A massive dataset collected from American women—from SWAN, the 17-year Study of Women's Health Across the Nation—explored the biological, psychological, and social changes in a diverse group of midlife women.

Of course, we humans don't align neatly into singular Crayola crayon categories of *black, white, Asian, Hispanic, or Native American*. In the study mentioned below, "Hispanic" includes women from 13 countries across the globe! Black women? There are Afro-Caribbean women, Afro-Colombians, and Afro-Asians, just for starters. Many of us are "mutts." Mom's black; Daddy's an Ashkenazi Jew. So...should their daughter expect the intense hot flashes black women tend to suffer—or a more merciful variety?

Though these broad categories—black, Hispanic, Asian, Native American—won't be a custom fit, they're an improvement over the long-unquestioned standard: studying middle-class or upper-class white women and stating the results like they apply to all women—which they might... or might not.

SWAN has other limitations, like Native American women often being left out and a lack of comparisons between racial subsets, like Afro-Caribbeans and Afro-Colombians. However, like newer studies with similar goals, it's a step in the right direction: no longer expecting black, Hispanic, Native American, and Asian women to just hope what goes for white ladies also applies to them.

BAD NEWS: THE "PAUSE" IN MENOPAUSE IS FALSE ADVERTISING
No more periods, but plenty of uncomfortable symptoms

Menopause is supposed to be a relief from perimenopausal hell. And, for me, it has been—a partial relief. My sleep is crap in menopause—crappier than it was in perimenopause. My body temperature regulation in menopause is also crap, meaning I still get hot flashes, though far fewer and much less intense than the ladyfurnace-like ones constantly blasting me in perimenopause.

Unfortunately, I am not alone in either of these crap situations. Clinical psychologist Mary C. Politi and her colleagues report that "nearly 50% of all women" continued to have disturbed sleep and hot flashes four years after their final menstrual period, and "10% of all women reported symptoms as far as 12 years" afterward.

Surely, there's a reprieve when we get up there in age...right? In fact, a study on Australian women found that a third of women ages 65 to 79 *still* suffer these symptoms. For a small but extremely unfortunate group of women, there's never any end. (An American friend told me her mother, currently in her 80s, still has hot flashes, and her late grandma had them until she died.)

Prediction: I'll still be having hot flashes when I'm in an urn.

COMMON MENOPAUSE SYMPTOMS

The top six are also common perimenopausal symptoms:

- Hot flashes and night sweats
- Insomnia

- Brain fog
- Mental health issues *(including feelings of sadness and anxiety)*
- Weight gain
- Bone loss

- Vaginal dryness
  Other pelvic area symptoms include painful intercourse, burning and itching of the vulva (the "lips" outside the vagina), painful urination, incontinence, a frequent need to pee, and recurring urinary tract infections.

Symptoms more common and virulent in menopausal than perimenopausal women:

- Brain drain
  Declines in cognitive performance, including memory, concentration, and the ability to reason.

- Cardiovascular symptoms
  Heart attacks, strokes, high blood pressure, and related conditions like diabetes.

- Skin and hair betrayals
  Dryer, thinner, less elastic skin and hair. Hair loss.

- Sexual issues
  Lowered sexual desire or a lack of interest in sex. Sex can also get painful.

Other menopausal symptoms Prior says women may experience:

- Chest pain
- Nausea
- Inexplicable itching

MENOPAUSE AND PERIMENOPAUSE TURNED INTO MUSHOPAUSE

Many websites that publish so-called "menopausal symptoms" actually list both perimenopausal and menopausal symptoms and wrongly describe them as symptoms of "menopause."

Take perimenopausal symptoms we associate with PMS, like sore breasts. In menopause, when your estrogen and progesterone levels bottom out, you're extremely unlikely to experience sore breasts (of the PMS-y variety) because they are caused by *elevated* estrogen levels! A "feature" of perimenopause!

Depressingly, even respected scientists succumb to this mushing together of perimenopausal and menopausal symptoms, publishing peer-reviewed research papers that refer to the lot of them as "menopausal."

This scientifically incorrect categorization might seem like a small thing. It's very much not, because it perpetuates the physiologically wrong conception of the meno-blob—erasing perimenopause as a singular and unique stage, and with it, the possibility for appropriate diagnosis and treatment for perimenopausal women.

Sure, there *are* a number of symptoms that show up in both perimenopause and menopause; however, the same symptom in one stage can require different treatment in the other. Again, menopause and perimenopause are hormonally very different stages—and we're about to get the details on how and why.

Spoiler: It starts out a little bloody.

— 5 —

PERIOD DRAMA

The vital prequel to understanding perimenopause and menopause

THERE ARE SOME women who have dainty little periods. (*Somebody's* buying those Tampax "light" tampons that look like a toothpick in a tiny white sweater.)

My periods were gushers—at first, when I was in my teens, and then (surprise!), starting in my late 40s. And when I say "gushers," I mean like I was bleeding to death out my vagina. Dismayingly, this got worse before it got worse. Eventually, on bleedy days, I had about 20 minutes between cross-legged runs to the bathroom—despite packing myself with the wildly overpromising "super-plus" tampons and wearing pads so thick they were basically crib-sized futons.

Around the same time, my supposedly "monthly" menstrual cycle decided to go off script timingwise, getting *waaay* shorter. No sooner did one pantyflood end than the next rushed in. The frequency was sick. At one point, somebody asked me what I do, and I was tempted to yell: "Repeatedly plug my vagina!"

But because the timing craziness and my menstrual gush-o-ramas came on somewhat gradually, I simply accepted them as the bummeristic new normal and started shopping for tampons by the crate at Costco so my periods wouldn't land me in bankruptcy court.

Unbeknownst to me, I was in perimenopause, the "menopause transition"—or, in fashion terms, the segue to wearing white without any danger of appearing to be hosting a Civil War reenactment in one's underpants.

MADAME OVARY
The betrayals of our ladyplumbing! Exposed!

Our human reproductive system is truly a marvel—well, okay...save for how giving birth involves screaming for hours while trying to push a bowling ball out a drinking straw.

The star organs in our body's repro factory are our **ovaries**: tiny oval-shaped twin glands on either side of the uterus that are basically our body's egg cartons. They have two jobs: 1) Making the reproductive hormones, estrogen and progesterone—aka "ovarian hormones"; and 2) Prepping eggs to be released for possible fertilization by some determined little spermbro.

Our eggs don't just roll around loose in our ovaries. Each immature egg is encased in "bubble wrap": that is, a protective fluid-filled sac called a *follicle*. One follicle eventually gets to release its egg (called "ovulation") into one of the fallopian tubes for transport to the uterus.

Your **uterus** (aka womb) is essentially an incubator—a hollow, muscular organ waiting for a fertilized egg to move in and grow for nine or so months. Like a classy blazer, the uterus comes with a lining—the **endometrium**: a mucous membrane that menstrual cycle estrogen beefs up and, with progesterone, transforms into hospitable lodgings with a nice nutrient stash for any fertilized egg that happens by.

The uterus keeps the guest-ready endometrial lining hanging around a bunch of days, waiting for a fertilized egg to show. No takers burrowing in? Well, fine! Time to ditch that sad, unused uterine lining in the form of your period.

To understand the ways our menstrual cycle goes off the rails in perimenopause, it helps to see it as a tale in two phases: the first two-ish weeks and the second two-ish weeks of the month on a wall calendar. (The "ish" represents the *range* of days over which these two phases can take place.)

Two hormones are partners in the process:

In the top phase, the first two-ish weeks, the hormone **estrogen** rises—culminating in ovulation, the release of the egg from the ovary.

In the bottom phase, the second two-ish weeks, the hormone **progesterone** rises.

Hormones are messengers in chemical form that travel around the body making things happen: Grow! Digest! Get your period! Hormones on the move are seeking out docking sites in or on cells—protein molecules called "receptors"—that work kind of like door locks. A particular hormone basically has a key, and its receptor has a lock the key fits into. Once the correct lock and key get together (technically, a hormone "binding" with its receptor), chemical changes ensue, causing a physical reaction: a start or stop, an increase or decrease, or a slowing down or speeding up of some process in our body.

Hormones are a product of our ***glands***—organs that "secrete" (meaning "produce and release") hormones into the bloodstream. These include the ovaries, the thyroid gland, and the pancreas, to name a few. They are ***endocrine glands***, which is why doctors like Jerilynn Prior with a focus on these organs and their hormones are called "endocrinologists."

Estrogen is mainly in the business of the development and normal functioning of our reproductive organs and tissues, but it also helps maintain the health of our bones, brain, and cardiovascular system through estrogen receptors that allow estrogen molecules to hook up and get to work.

There are three main kinds of estrogen in adult women. The one we're focused on in this book is estradiol (which I often refer to as "estrogen"). Estradiol is the estrogen of the years from puberty to menopause, produced mainly in the ovaries. In addition to its role in our menstrual cycle, it stimulates "proliferation"—growth through rapid multiplication of cells within our tissues—especially in the breast, uterus, and vagina.

The estrogen phase of your menstrual cycle—that top-of-the-calendar phase from day one of menstruation to the day of ovulation in the middle of your cycle—is called the ***follicular phase***, because it's the prep stage for the release of the egg from the follicle.

The bottom of the menstrual calendar phase is the province of estrogen's partner hormone, ***progesterone.*** Progesterone, taken apart, is "pro" plus "gestation"—named for its important work making our uterine lining, the endometrium, pregnancy friendly. It turns the endometrium "secretory"— nutrient-rich—to feed a (gestating!) embryo and stabilizes the tissue so it won't dump the thing. Progesterone also sends a chemical yoohoo to the immune system to stand down a bit so it won't treat the embryo as an invader to attack.

However, progesterone does much more—acting in every tissue in the body in which estrogen acts. Very importantly, while estrogen is a powerful growth stimulator, progesterone counteracts the cell overgrowth estrogen can lead to in the breasts and endometrium. If there's no pregnancy during a menstrual cycle, progesterone works to break down this uterine lining so it falls away with the menstrual flow. This work by progesterone "is essential," writes Dr. Prior, because the "endometrial thickening" caused by estrogen can run wild—leading to the growth of abnormal or even cancerous cells.

Progesterone also polices generic cells—cells without a special job to do—compelling them to mature from their initial immature state into specialized cells like breast cells. This is called "differentiation," describing the cells being "differentiated" into the type they're supposed to be, which sets them on task so they can't be cellular delinquents, dividing wildly and possibly cancerously.

OVA AND OUT
Ovulation at its normal, healthy best

Estrogen and progesterone have co-workers, dispatcher hormones in the brain. I'll mention just one here, ***follicle-stimulating hormone***, because it's important for understanding Dr. Prior's explanation of the messed-up menstrual cycle of perimenopause.

FSH is the "get the egg out of bed" hormone. It gets released from the pituitary gland in the brain and travels down to the ovaries to kick off (that is, *stimulate*) egg maturation within the follicles.

In a normal menstrual cycle, multiple egg-containing ovarian follicles get stimulated to mature, but one follicle grows bigger and buffer than the rest, becoming the "dominant" follicle. That follicle eventually gets to release the egg upon bursting open (aka "rupturing" and causing ovulation).

Ovulation kicks off the second phase of the menstrual cycle, the progesterone phase. When the egg is sent on its way, the follicular "trash" left behind—the ruptured sac—forms an entirely new (though temporary) gland in the ovary. This is the "corpus luteum," which secretes some estrogen and a lot of progesterone (and gets credited for its work in the official name for the progesterone phase of the menstrual cycle—the ***luteal phase***).

FAILURE TO LAUNCH
Eggs that don't leave make for a nightmarish perimenopause

Perimenopausal women often do not ovulate, despite having a period. Basically, the egg remains in its follicle at check-out time and never leaves. This is called an "anovulatory" (no-ovulation) menstrual cycle, and it's problematic because the post-ovulation progesterone-making part of our cycle is essential for the healthy functioning of our body and mind. Making matters worse, a cycle that's anovulatory seems like any other menstrual cycle; there are no "notifications" that anything's out of order.

But say a perimenopausal woman *does* ovulate during her menstrual cycle. Dr. Prior explains that as perimenopause goes on, women can increasingly experience weakly ovulatory cycles leading to shortened luteal phases (specifically, the time in the second half of the menstrual cycle when progesterone is produced, starting from ovulation to the day before the next menstrual flow).

A normal luteal phase is 10 to 12 days or longer (up to 16 days), and, Prior adds, "The length of the luteal phase is roughly proportional to the amount of progesterone in the cycle." In other words, with a shortened luteal phase, there's "lower total progesterone exposure," meaning less progesterone than in normal cycles.

Too few doctors understand this—or the havoc that anovulatory and weakly ovulatory menstrual cycles can wreak. It's perimenopausal women's lack or undersupply of progesterone to counterbalance the higher than normal and erratically swinging estrogen levels from the first part of their cycle that provokes unpleasant, life-disrupting symptoms, including hot flashes, drenching night sweats, fragmented sleep, weight gain, and mood swings.

This makes it vital for you to figure out whether you're ovulating, and, if you are, whether you're coming up short on progesterone-infused luteal-phase days. The good news: This is easy and even free (if you already have a digital thermometer and maybe $9.99 if you have to buy one). But first, here's the bad news on how ovulation prediction *has* been done—failing vast numbers of women who trusted what they'd been told by the experts.

SHAVE THE DATE
Our 28-day menstrual cycle actually isn't 28 days

Many of us have spent years or even decades hearing that the menstrual cycle is 28 days long. In 2019, data scientist Jonathan Bull and his colleagues tracked more than 600,000 ovulatory menstrual cycles in women across the US, the UK, and Sweden. They found that cycles last *29.3 days*, on average—a seemingly small but actually significant correction, as you'll see below. (The supposedly "typical" 28-day cycle showed up in only 13 percent of women.)

The 29.3-day figure is actually a bit misleading, because it's an *average* including waaaay shorter and waaay longer cycles. Here's the whole spectrum from their paper:

MENSTRUAL CYCLE LENGTH

- 15–20 days: 1% of women
- 21–24 days: 8%
- 25–30 days: 65%
- 31–35 days: 19%
- 36–50 days: 7%

This finding is like a huge flashlight exposing problems in the scientific database. Countless research papers that have shaped the current understanding of our menstrual cycle were based on an error—the *assumption* that women have cycles of approximately 28 days, explains one of Bull's co-researchers, pharmacologist Joyce Harper.

This error has led to the companion erroneous assumption that ovulation happens on day 14, when, for the majority of women, this is not the case. This is no small thing for a woman desperately trying to get pregnant. Calendar-based apps that predict fertility "assume that our historic understanding of the menstrual cycle is correct (ovulation 14 days before the next period)," Bull and his colleagues explain, which could cause many women to "completely miss the fertile window."

However, there *is* a bodily indicator that a woman has just ovulated: a half-degree or one-degree Fahrenheit (or 0.2 to 0.3 degrees Celsius) increase in her daily body temperature—specifically, her "basal" or resting body temperature, taken immediately upon awakening.

Bull and his team suggest that apps that also incorporate basal body temperature (BBT) readings might do a better job of narrowing down an individual woman's fertile days.

Key word: "might."

Not so fast, say Marquette University professors of nursing Mary Lee Barron and Richard Fehring, who wrote in 2005: "Over the last 30 years, the vast majority of researchers have concluded that BBT is not a reliable marker" of the day of ovulation. More recently, a 2017 study led by obstetrician Hsiu-Wei Su only found BBT to be around 22 percent accurate.

The problem? The rise in basal temperature that suggests a woman has just ovulated *can* be due to ovulation—or to other factors, including user measurement errors; the effects of illness, medication, diet, or alcohol consumption; changes in sleeping patterns; and starting or stopping oral contraception.

In light of this, Barron and Fehring lamented that "numerous" doctors and nurses still recommend BBT charting to predict ovulation—"probably because it's inexpensive, easy for women to use, and has wide acceptance by the public."

Again, that was in 2005.

You'd think word of this method's issues would have spread, and healthcare institutions would have stopped advising women to use it. In fact, as of 2022, Kaiser was recommending BBT measurement on their website, as was major health insurer Cigna on theirs—though not in the frank language they both owe the women they're supposed to be serving: "Hey, ladies! Wanna make an unreliable guess at when you'll be ovulating?"

DATA WITH DESTINY
DIY diagnosis of progesterone-gone-missing

Now, I get that most of you reading this book are trying to understand and survive perimenopause and menopause, not hoping for one last hurrah at creating an adorable wee thing that will eventually become a sullen teenager.

I've laid out the BBT info in part because you might have friends trying to conceive who are using these apps. However, an intro to BBT is a helpful stepping stone for understanding a specialized, scientifically validated form of basal temperature-taking—*Quantitative* Basal Temperature readings (QBT, ©CEMCOR). QBT is an easy DIY way to figure out whether you're experiencing anovulatory or weakly ovulatory menstrual cycles in perimenopause. It simply requires taking your temperature right when you wake up and logging it on a calendar—daily, for a few months. *(Detailed how-to, Chapter Twenty-Four—because though it's easy, it's a bit lengthy!)*

Now, QBT has the same problems as BBT—*if you're trying to predict the specific day you've ovulated*. That remains a no-go. However, by logging your first-morning temperature *patterns* over a period of months, QBT predicts whether you're ovulating *at all*—along with the length of your luteal phase—with the patterns you log ruling out temperature rises from an infection, medication, or other factors.

QBT is ultimately a window into the state of your hormones in perimenopause—specifically, whether you're producing little or no progesterone. This is essential to know, both because progesterone is vital for our health and well-being—and because estrogen tends to go a bit feral in perimenopause.

WHY WOMEN'S ESTROGEN LEVELS SOAR IN PERIMENOPAUSE

Estrogen levels spike in perimenopause, often to dangerous levels, because our feedback system between the ovary and the pituitary goes on the fritz, Prior explains. (The "feedback system" is our body's finely tuned sensor apparatus that detects changes in the body outside of normal range and sends messages to the brain to trigger corrective processes.)

For example, the ovary, our body's center of egg production, comes with a brake (in hormone form), called **inhibin B**, that's produced by the developing follicles. As its name suggests, inhibin B's job is to "inhibit": to keep the egg production in check, which it does by keeping one of its co-workers in line.

That co-worker is *follicle-stimulating hormone*—the "get the eggs out of bed" hormone. When inhibin B is doing its job properly, it sees that FSH stimulates only the *normal* number of egg-containing follicles (which is several to a half dozen or more) to compete to be the chosen one.

In a normal ovulatory menstrual cycle, as follicles grow and a single one becomes dominant, a woman's estrogen level spikes. This elevated estrogen level causes inhibin B to message the pituitary, telling it to suppress further release of estrogen (by preventing further release of FSH).

And then, along comes perimenopause to screw things up. In perimenopause, levels of inhibin B begin to drop off. Without sufficient inhibin B, FSH levels rise and run wild, stimulating *a whole bunch* of follicles. This being the last hurrah of a woman's fertile years, these aren't the robust Captain of the Volleyball Team follicles of her fertile prime (the early 20s) but the ones smoking pot behind the dumpster during the biology midterm.

Though these underachiever follicles tend to be on the wimpier side, never rupturing and popping out that egg, *each comes with its own estrogen supply!* So, instead of just one hearty follicle with a reasonable amount of estrogen (and a few other reasonable contenders) that you'd get in a normal menstrual cycle, it's a whole bunch of puny follicles coming up all at once, collectively flooding you with estrogen.

PARTAY!!! Uh, except for the perimenopausal woman whose ovary they're all shooting up in, who's essentially getting overdosed with estrogen: poisoned by her own body. Without ovulation, no progesterone is made. Should an egg manage to emerge, it often does so pretty feebly. Prior explains that the amount of progesterone then produced is simply too low to do its vital job, counterbalancing the effects of estrogen.

YOUR CO-PAY? THAT'LL BE ONE BREAST, PLEASE

So, here you are, a woman in perimenopause, with all of these rotten little runt follicles coming out, each with its own estrogen supply, and you have little or no progesterone for counterbalance. Your body has basically become home to an estrogen prison riot.

The awful symptoms and increased risk of uterine and other cancers from this perimenopause estrogen explosion *could* be eliminated or at least diminished—with a prescription for the progesterone your body isn't making. "Progesterone...should be the first line of therapy for symptomatic perimenopausal women," Prior writes.

It should be—and would be—if only medical practice standards were based not on the longstanding medical fairy tale of dwindling perimenopausal estrogen levels but on the *actual physiology of perimenopause*.

If only.

Instead, there's a scandal in American medicine. Well-meaning doctors often *worsen* perimenopausal patients' suffering and increase their uterine cancer risk through what Prior calls the "illogical" treatment of perimenopausal symptoms: prescribing estrogen therapy when the science tells us a perimenopausal woman's own estrogen levels are abnormally high.

Prior explains that in a normal ovulatory menstrual cycle, this pile-on of prescription estrogen on top of a woman's already-elevated ovarian estrogen would cue her hormonal feedback system, suppressing further release of estrogen. But in perimenopause, without sufficient inhibin B to be all, "Yo, pituitary, we got an estrogen flood here!", the estrogen a doctor prescribes could sharply increase the already problematic imbalance in her body between estrogen and progesterone.

Because so many practice standards for diagnosis and treatment of women in perimenopause are actually institutionalized *malpractice* standards—medical care that harms instead of healing—our prospects for getting evidence-based medical care for perimenopause can seem hopelessly grim. And frankly, they would be—but for how Jerilynn Prior has made it her life's work to change this.

— 6 —

JOAN OF ENDOCRINOLOGY

Dr. Jerilynn Prior's crusade to have perimenopause recognized, studied, and treated appropriately

IT WAS THE 1960s. Women were supposed to be doctors' wives, not doctors, and med school administrators busied themselves rejecting even highly qualified women who applied. (Between 1960 and 1961, only 5 percent of med school graduates were women.)

This dissuaded Jerilynn Prior not at all. She applied to med school—nine times! She was rejected nine times. *Nine times!* Now, we've all heard, "try, try again," and the persistent among us might try a second time or even a third. But it would be *completely reasonable*, on rejection number four, six, or eight, to wave a forlorn goodbye to med school and take up ceramics or accounting.

Prior is not one to give in to what's "reasonable." From grade four on, she and her parents lived in icy, grinding poverty in a desolate part of the Alaskan wilderness, on an island with a population of about 50. Her family's house had no running water or electricity. It sat atop a hill, so at age 10, Prior's chores included hauling water up the incline oxen-style—wearing a yoke her dad made her with a 5-gallon can on either side.

The school on the island had just nine students and taught only the lower grades. The high school was on another island, a two-hour boat ride each way, so Prior had to live away from home to attend, staying "with various people" who took her in and hitching rides on fishing boats to go home on weekends.

Prior's harsh early years—being self-sufficient in a merciless climate without the comforts most Americans take for granted—prepared her for the scientist she'd need to be: a fighter. Accordingly, when Prior opened the envelope with her eighth med school rejection, she saw it as a sign—not to give up but to go get yet another application. On her ninth try, she was wait-listed by the University of Oregon School of Medicine, meaning she might get in if other applicants declined admission. They had an opening, and she became one of just six women in a class of 88 students.

Two years into med school, she got married and moved with her husband to Boston. In 1969, she graduated with honors from Boston University School of Medicine—into a medical world inhospitable to female doctors and doctor-researchers. Residencies in some medical specialties were near impossible for women to obtain, and government agencies offering grants—vital to academic medical research careers from the 1950s on—awarded few to women. Female doctors were refused membership to many medical societies, including, most absurdly, the American Gynecological Society! The he-man gynos keeping the little ladies out admitted just one female member in 1921 and didn't admit the next till 1971!

These days, Jerilynn C. Prior, MD, is a University of British Columbia clinician-scientist ("clinician" meaning doctor who treats patients) and a professor of endocrinology. For decades, she has been leading the charge to have perimenopause and the unique hormonal changes and symptoms of this phase recognized, investigated, and treated according to scientific evidence.

In 2002, she founded CeMCOR, the nonprofit Centre for Menstrual Cycle and Ovulation Research. It is both a research center and a vital informational resource for women (via its website, CeMCOR.ca). She's now in her 80s and no longer sees patients, but she remains a driven researcher, publishing a slew of research on menstrual cycles, perimenopause, menopause, and the causes and treatment of osteoporosis.

She has been honored many times for her scientific contributions. In 2019, she was presented with the Aubrey J. Tingle Prize: a prestigious annual award given to an internationally recognized British Columbia doctor-researcher who has significantly advanced the science in their field and improved the health system and health of patients in BC. The late surgeon and breast cancer expert Susan Love, MD, called Prior "one of the pioneers in actually studying what happens as women transition into menopause."

Disturbingly, the many important scientific findings Prior has produced have not led to the massive reforms in our medical care they should have—and would have, in an *actually* evidence-based medical world.

This is shocking, but not surprising. I'm reminded of a talk I heard investigative science journalist Gary Taubes give back in 2008 at a scientific symposium on childhood obesity. He presented substantial evidence that the current standard of care—the low-fat/high-carb diet prescribed to morbidly obese children—led them to be *more obese* and progressively unhealthier.

The evidence also suggested these kids could be put on very-low-carb diets and lose weight—and maybe have a chance at living normal healthy lives! His talk gave me chills. Change would ensue for these kids—without the medical torment of gastric bypass surgery and drugs with unpleasant and dangerous side effects!

Um...get a clue, Ames.

After his talk, I went out into the crowd milling around outside the auditorium. I asked doctors and doctor-researchers whether they would look into the evidence Taubes laid out and consider revamping the diet they were feeding their child patients.

The answer: a big, resounding NOPE.

I couldn't make sense of this. And not out of any sort of naïveté. I'm mindful that we humans are powerfully driven to cling to our existing beliefs. Sure, Taubes *had* presented compelling evidence, but if the subject had been widgets or car design or even something medical but non-critical, I would've understood (and maybe even expected) their response. However, considering the human stakes in this particular arena—*tragically sick and suffering morbidly obese children*—I found it deeply disturbing that they wouldn't allow any evidence to even *chance* piercing the force field of "What We Have Always Believed."

LET THERE BE FIGHT

It's legitimate—and necessary—to ask whether Prior's findings haven't caught on for good reason, something scientifically lacking. That's not the case, and a story from early on in Prior's career is dismayingly illuminating.

Not long after Prior landed her first job as a junior professor-researcher, she wanted to test what everyone just "knew" at the time: the belief that women who do intense exercise would stop having periods.

It was the 1970s, the age of women's liberation, and women were showing up in all sorts of areas they hadn't before—like the finish line of marathons. "This message" that periods die when women start putting some miles on their Adidas swiftly followed, writes Prior, and "without any proof, it rapidly became fact."

Prior, herself a runner, had done an unfunded study on women who run long distance. Contrary to evidence-free popular belief, she found that healthy, normal-weight post-adolescent women who run regularly maintain "perfectly regular cycles." Her findings did show a difference between women who ran consistently—"regularly," as she puts it—and those who *abruptly began intense training*. The stress of suddenly going all-out did not stop these women from having periods. However, they tended to have anovulatory menstrual cycles or shorter-than-normal luteal phases with too little progesterone made (shorting them on its valuable calming effects and other important benefits and protections).

Prior began to suspect that the missed periods reported in female runners were in women who were "not only dealing with exercise, but with many stressors" or those who were young and just past their first period (a time when the menstrual cycle tends to go through some fits and starts).

She applied for grants to study the effects of exercise on women's menstrual cycles. Her research was not funded. Of course, plenty of research that's proposed is denied funding. There are various reasons for this, and they aren't necessarily "the researcher's a woman" or "it's a woman's issue." However, women's health research has long been hugely underfunded in the US and Canada.

Consider that women make up half the population. Sharlene Rutherford, President of the Alberta Women's Health Foundation, writes: "Logically, one would assume that women's health research also receives roughly half of the funding, correct? Painfully wrong. Women's health research receives no more than eight percent of medical research funding in Canada."

Granted, even if Prior's study had been funded, it's possible the results would've suggested her hypothesis is wrong. However, it's also very plausibly not wrong. If only she—and we—were given the chance to find out.

Instead, this lack of funding affected our public knowledge—and warped my thinking. I've been a runner for much of my life—at one point, hoofing it for seven miles several times a week—and I never, ever stopped having periods. (Admittedly, one person's experience does not count as science.) But despite my experience, I unquestioningly believed the myth that women's periods stop if they exercise "too much"—till the moment I read this skeptical, evidence-based take from Prior.

BATTLE PROD

At the time Prior's menstrual cycle research was repeatedly denied funding, she had no idea what she was up against—and would be up against for the rest of her career: research funders, including the US and Canadian government institutes of health, snubbing studies on female physiology (in contrast with the tsunami of money they shoot out at research on diseases).

Looking back now, she "marvels" at her confidence in pitching this study. It was imperative that she get research published—especially as "a new, part-time academic, shoved from nook to cranny in the hospital and university, a woman in a medical man's world, and just going through a divorce."

"Not daunted" by any of that, Prior dusted herself off and tried again. To make her study sexier to funders, she shifted the subject to bones and bone loss, further sexing up her grant request by proposing to use the nifty new technology of the time—a CT scanner that captured bone mineral density.

The grant was funded. There was an understanding in the field that lowered estrogen levels lead to frail bones. Estrogen alone. Period. End of story. Yet, progesterone's relationship to bone formation was "already well-supported" in research on cells and animals, Prior explains, and it was overdue for investigation in women. Prior sought to test whether "inadequate production of progesterone"—low or missing progesterone (from anovulatory or weakly ovulatory menstrual cycles)—would lead to bone loss.

She found confirmation for her hypothesis: Low progesterone from ovulation on the fritz led to depleted bone—"despite normal production of estradiol and the preservation of normal cycle intervals." Summing up, she explains, "Estrogen levels were fine, whether women were gaining, maintaining, or losing bone. That meant progesterone was important for women's bone" (which, she writes, "was not a thinkable thought in those days").

This was a revolutionary finding, and Prior was ecstatic.

You'd think results like these would be snapped up by a medical journal. In fact, Prior struggled for *three years* to get her paper published, submitting it to journal after journal. Eventually, she had the paper accepted by the *New England Journal of Medicine*. This was huge. *NEJM* is one of the oldest, most widely read, and most influential medical journals.

Prior was over the moon. And then she got the page proofs. The title of her article and her abstract (the summary at the top of a paper) had been altered: rewritten—incorrectly, *entirely contrary to her findings!*—to conform with the dogma in the field that lowered estrogen was the problem.

Prior, as a junior faculty member, *desperately* needed this paper published in order to have the requisite research to get tenure. There's a timetable in which a young researcher needs to show their stuff, and the clock was ticking. Getting the paper bumped from the journal could mean the end of her career as a researcher.

Despite fearing she'd tank her paper's publication, Prior stood firm. She told the editor that the article had to be changed back to her original wording or the journal would not have her permission to publish it.

Prior won. The paper was published in 1990 as she wrote it.

"How I had the courage, I don't know," she writes. "Perhaps because I believe in science—meaning, as it can and should be," she just could not stand for the "perversion of science to maintain the status quo."

ESTROGEN: A MEDICINE IN SEARCH OF A MARKET

To make sense of why progesterone is so ignored, it's important to understand why estrogen gets all the attention.

In the 1930s, a Canadian biochemist, McGill University professor James Bertram Collip, isolated the hormone estrogen from the urine of pregnant women. He'd been courted by pharmaceutical company Ayerst Labs to create estrogen in drug form as a treatment for menopausal symptoms. The drug that came out of this partnership, Emmenin, was pharmaceutical weak tea— low in potency—and had a gross odor. Also, rather obviously, pulling together an assembly line of pregnant ladies to pee into cups is problematic as a source for global drug production.

Next, Collip tried stallion pee. Stallions, despite being male, have almost twice the estrogen in their urine as pregnant mares. But again, a collection issue. Stallions are snorting, bucking, testy mofos. As science journalist Barbara Seaman put it: "Basically, the stallions kicked over the collection buckets."

But Collip stuck around the barn, and, Seaman reports, "The third source of urine proved to be the charm": "the compliant mare," with estrogen-rich urine that's at least two and a half times the potency of human pee.

The drug created from this, conjugated equine (as in horse) estrogen (CEE), is described as "conjugated" because they don't just give you horse pee; it's a cocktail of chemicals that create the drug. There are reasons for doing this, and a biggie is money. You can't patent a naturally occurring substance (progesterone, for example), and without a patent, there's nothing stopping other companies from selling your drug. This means you have all this annoying competition driving down prices, keeping you from making the bajillions you would if you had a patent-protected monopoly.

Collip's creation was tagged with a brand name reflecting its source—Premarin (PREgnant MARes' urINe)—and introduced in 1941 in Canada and in 1942 in the US by Ayerst (merging into Wyeth-Ayerst, which was later bought by Pfizer).

The CEE Premarin, one of the best-selling drugs ever, is a form of estrogen women in the US still take today. Its sales here are in decline—for reasons that will become clear in coming chapters—but, globally, its sales are growing and projected to keep growing on the global market. (Related drugs, Prempro and Premphase, both now sold by Pfizer's Wyeth subsidiary, combine the blended horse estrogens of Premarin with the el cheapo synthetic knockoff of progesterone, medroxyprogesterone acetate.)

Wyeth-Ayerst execs saw that there were massive profits to be made from Premarin. They just had to create a need for their drug. (A sales document prepared for Wyeth-Ayerst called it "a drug in search of a disease.") Though the FDA had approved it for treating menopausal symptoms, menopausal women back then weren't flocking to their doctors to seek out medical help.

In the 1960s, Wyeth-Ayerst launched an aggressive marketing campaign deeming menopause an "estrogen deficiency disease" and pharmaceutical estrogen, the cure: the replacement needed to keep menopausal women looking and feeling young and in the best of health—and to prevent the harms they'd suffer if they didn't take it. This is the origin of the terms "estrogen *replacement* therapy" (ERT) and "hormone *replacement* therapy" (HRT).

Dr. Prior takes issue with the notion that menopause is an "estrogen deficiency disease"—as did the late Susan Love, MD. In 2003, Love voiced her dismay that gynecology textbooks refer to menopause as "reproductive failure" or "ovarian failure," which suggests that women whose bodies can no longer be the vehicle for a baby are "sick" and "failures"—which Love calls a misogynistic notion that "continues to dominate medical thinking."

In a 2021 *Scientific American* essay, Dr. Prior argued that menopause is not a disease state, but "a normal life stage." In menopause, she explains, estrogen isn't dysfunctionally low; estrogen and its companion hormone progesterone are *naturally low*, because they aren't needed for the baby-making process like they were in women's fertility factory years. At the same time, Prior notes that it can make sense to take medicine, including estrogen in menopause, to alleviate disturbing symptoms. However, in place of the "estrogen deficiency" language, she favors deeming the perimenopause-to-menopause years the natural transitional period from a normal reproductive state to a likewise normal non-reproductive one.

Though she's using "reproductive" to mean having the possibility of reproducing, if, like me, you were never "reproductive," my redo of her wording might be more relatable: *Menopause is the life cycle phase in women 35 or older that follows a year without menstrual flow* (which, in my case, probably caused Tampax executives to hold a funeral for their stock price).

ESTROGEN'S SMOOTH BRITISH HUCKSTER

Most of us look down on drug pushers, but it seems we're easily fooled. Give a pusher a British accent, a classy suit, and a crisp white lab coat, and we're in. Ready to listen. Ready to believe. Ready to *buy*.

Wyeth-Ayerst, the pharmaceutical company peddling Premarin, needed a spokesdoctor to sell the public on their horse pee pills. They soon found their man—Dr. Robert A. Wilson, a British-born Brooklyn gynecologist who'd published an article in a prestigious medical journal that enthusiastically and unquestioningly proclaimed estrogen to be a necessity for women "throughout their lives." Wilson could sell the hell out of their Premarin.

Wilson's paper was methodologically outrageous, a leap to utterly unsupported conclusions. However, for Wyeth-Ayerst, shoddy methodology from an estrogen evangelist was not a problem but a plus—a big flashing arrow pointing to a cash cow about to be born.

In 1966, Wilson published the book *Feminine Forever,* which is basically a misogynistic 209-page sales manual for estrogen that he was secretly paid to write by Wyeth-Ayerst. In it, Wilson called menopause a breast- and genital-shriveling "catastrophe" that turned women over 50 into sexually neutered, *dewomanized* women: "prematurely aging castrates"..."the equivalent of a eunuch." He claimed menopause left women not only dried-up and ugly but was a personality killer, making menopausal women horrific to live with. Throughout the book, Wilson's intimation is clear: What husband could be blamed for cheating on such an unsightly, disagreeable old shrew?

Between passages baiting the trap with women's worst fears—about aging, loss of their looks, and losing their husbands to younger women—Wilson repeatedly offers the supposed cure, the magical potion for looking young, sexy, and "feminine forever": Become a customer of pharmaceutical estrogen forever.

You'll see later in the book that estrogen isn't the evil potion it's been made out to be. However, Wilson had no evidence for all of the *fountain of youth/ sexpot from puberty to grave* claims he threw around. Of course, his referencing objective evidence would have unsold Wyeth-Ayerst's estrogen cash cow.

Wyeth-Ayerst had no worries of that happening. They had picked Wilson as their spokes-huckster because he had previously published outright lies about estrogen disguised as science; for example, "There is no convincing proof that estrogen has ever introduced cancer in the human being"—the opening line to his 1962 paper in the *Journal of American Medical Association* (*JAMA*).

In fact, there were plenty of indications that estrogen was carcinogenic, going back to the 1930s and '40s. In 1932, lab rats got breast cancer after being administered estrogen. Research as early as 1936 suggested estrogen caused a dangerous buildup of the endometrial tissue lining the uterus, which can lead to cancer. In 1948, a young cancer researcher, Dr. Saul Gusberg, found a substantial increase in endometrial cancer in women using estrogen—a finding that has been confirmed over and over in the decades since.

However, it turns out the "estrogen equals cancer" conclusion had a missing piece nobody was noticing: a simultaneous lack of progesterone (to counterbalance the estrogen). Recall from Chapter Five that progesterone is needed to inhibit the estrogen-stimulated overgrowth of breast and endometrial tissue that can lead to cancer.

Progesterone had yet to be turned into a drug in oral form that didn't just sail right out of the body in urine. In 1975, two studies were published that showed the addition of a synthetic progesterone imitator—a progestin—was necessary to protect a woman from estrogen-incited endometrial cancer.

Yet, more than 10 years before, in Wilson's 1962 *JAMA* article, he had claimed estrogen not only prevented breast cancer but also "genital" cancer. (I feel sick thinking of all the women who had from 1962 to 1975 to believe him.)

Wilson's work as the Pied Piper for pharmaceutical estrogen had some personal consequences. Following his advice, his wife, Thelma, had been taking estrogen. In 1967, a year after the publication of *Feminine Forever*, she developed breast cancer. "This was not even made known to family members," reports psychologist Timothy Scott (per his 2005 interviews of Wilson's son Ronald, who was deceased by the time I tried to speak with him).

"If word got out, it would have made the papers and newsmagazines. Even the medical records were falsified," writes Scott. "It was years later that Mrs. Wilson told her son the truth—after she was diagnosed with breast cancer again, the disease which took her life."

The tide began to turn for Wilson starting in 1975, when there were widespread news reports of those two studies linking estrogen and endometrial cancer. Afterward, notes Scott, "Robert Wilson was no longer a forerunner and a hero but, in the eyes of many former patients, something of a villain." In 1981, Wilson killed himself.

HOW PHARMA MARKETING DISGUISED AS RESEARCH SNEAKS INTO MEDICAL JOURNALS

Wyeth-Ayerst engaged in the depraved, greed-driven pollution of the medical research base with faked "science": medical journal articles secretly ghostwritten by the pharmaceutical companies or medical communications agencies they hire.

The execs at Wyeth-Ayerst worked with a number of these agencies to hawk their hormone drugs, Premarin and Prempro. Pharmacology and physiology researcher Adriane J. Fugh-Berman, MD, reports that one pharma marketing company alone, DesignWrite, boasted in a 2005 document that from 1997 to 2003, they'd published 50 of these ghostwritten articles for Wyeth-Ayerst in scientific journals.

Researchers are invited to participate in scientific fraud: be the "author" of one of these "studies," which involves no authoring whatsoever. They just sign off on having their name on the article as if it were their work: their write-up of the results of actual research they'd done. This gives them more publications to their name, helping them advance in the "publish or perish" academic world—and oopsy on any patients who suffer the consequences of this "science."

Though these articles, when published, appear to be normal scientific studies, their actual job is advancing a pharma-sales-serving set of "facts" by discrediting legitimate scientific evidence that the company's drug might be useless or harmful, promoting unproven benefits, and casting shade on competing medications.

For example, Fugh-Berman reports that "Wyeth used ghostwritten articles to mitigate the perceived risks of breast cancer" associated with hormone therapy, to defend unsupported benefits, "and to promote off-label unproven uses," such as the prevention of dementia, Parkinson's disease, and vision problems.

The existence of Wyeth-Ayerst's ghostwritten studies was exposed in 2009, but the damage was done. A marketing-based narrative had been created about estrogen and menopause that poisoned and probably continues to poison both the body of research in the field and medical treatment.

DROWNING IN ESTROGEN

It was 1967, the year after Wyeth-Ayerst's huckster-gynecologist Robert Wilson published *Feminine Forever*. Prior was a med student in Oregon about to get married. Desperate to avoid getting pregnant while still in med school, she hit up the local Planned Parenthood for birth control pills. The pill they prescribed, Sequens, contained only estrogen in the first 14 days of the pack, in a *massive* dose (100 micrograms of ethinyl estradiol in contrast with the 20 micrograms typically prescribed today).

She took the Sequens for only five days—until "nausea, depression, fatigue, and swelling" (nine pounds of water weight) and her "first ever migraine headache" forced her to stop. However, the experience was scientifically transformative. The assault on her system from the massive dose of estrogen led to her personal and professional skepticism about all of the credulously "positive estrogen messages" she has read and heard since.

When Prior was 47—a decade before she went into menopause—she began to have terrible symptoms. "My breasts were sore, I was relentlessly hungry, and I was angry.... I dreamed that I was pregnant." She began having migraines—"vomiting, blurred vision, and all"—echoing her toxic time with the massive dose of estrogen in Sequens. These symptoms stuck with her over a hellish 10-year period.

In med school, Prior had been taught the *accepted medical view* of perimenopause: "Midlife women suffer from dropping estrogen levels." In her late 40s, however, experiencing symptoms that seemed like a replay of her time on estrogen-packed Sequens, she had a strong suspicion that the standard paradigm of lowered estrogen in perimenopause was wrong. "What I knew was that my estrogen levels felt sky-high."

Prior then began what has become her life's work: rigorously researching the effects of estrogen and progesterone on women's bodies and health, generating an evidence-driven understanding of perimenopause, and exposing and overturning the unscientific assumptions driving gynecological practice standards.

Since the 1930s, progesterone has been wrongly accused (by researchers, and, in turn, doctors) for the harms estrogen has actually caused—and, since the 1980s, for the adverse effects of the chemically different synthetic, medroxyprogesterone acetate. This "progesterone is evil" myth, as Prior calls it, has been deeply detrimental to women's health and well-being.

The false claims about progesterone are *everywhere*—like on respected medical information websites, including WebMD. On their multi-page entry on progesterone (as of July 2022), they list a slew of awful side effects *supposedly experienced* by taking progesterone—side effects that, correctly labeled, would read: *side effects caused by estrogen and/or the injectable birth control, Depo-Provera.*

These supposedly progesterone-induced side effects include: "Stomach upset, changes in appetite, weight gain, fluid retention and swelling (edema), fatigue, acne, drowsiness or insomnia, allergic skin rashes, hives, fever, headache," and "premenstrual syndrome (PMS)-like symptoms."

Take "fluid retention." Estrogen can lead to water retention and bloating. Progesterone, on the other hand, is a diuretic: a substance that promotes the release of excess bodily fluid in the form of pee! Depo-Provera, not progesterone, is associated with acne and weight gain. And other side effects on the list, like insomnia and PMS, are issues when progesterone is *lacking*.

Coming chapters will show you that the supposed evils of progesterone chronicled by so many "reputable" sources—including massive, multistate medical providers—are basically a list of the types of perimenopausal and menopausal suffering that progesterone alleviates!

— 7 —
IT'S NOT THE MONEY, IT'S THE MONEY

*Women are prescribed a cheap progesterone imitator
with multiple awful side effects—including increased cancer risk*

SOME IMITATIONS OF the original work just fine.

A $40 "Hermès" handbag you buy off a blanket on the sidewalk lacks the quality of the $18K real deal, but it's unlikely to disintegrate as you walk, scattering your lipstick and credit cards like a trail of breadcrumbs.

Other cheap imitations are seriously problematic—like the synthetic knockoff drug you're likely to be prescribed as if it's the same as progesterone.

It's anything but.

This chapter is a story of two drugs—the real deal and the knockoff—and how experts confusing the two have harmed science and women.

I'll lay them out here for quick reference.

REAL-DEAL PROGESTERONE
Oral micronized progesterone (OMP)

Oral micronized progesterone (OMP) is an FDA-approved drug that's chemically the same as the progesterone your ovaries make, and it acts in your body and brain in the exact same beneficial ways.

THE KNOCKOFF DRUG
Medroxyprogesterone acetate (MPA)

This el cheapo synthetic drug, medroxyprogesterone acetate (MPA), is basically pharmaceutical pleather: a progesterone-mimicking concoction called a "progestin."

Though MPA manages to act like progesterone in a few ways, it *isn't* progesterone, so it fails to alleviate many of the symptoms OMP does and sometimes even makes them worse. It also comes with a number of unpleasant, harmful, and even potentially deadly side effects that OMP does not.

YOUR HORMONES AT WORK!

Though you read about hormones and how they act in our bodies back in Chapter Five, it's a lot to remember. Here's a brief refresher (with some added detail) that I hope will serve as a "Huh?" remover as you read this chapter and the rest.

Estrogen and progesterone are ***steroid hormones***, meaning hormones made from cholesterol. Like Samantha from *Bewitched*, they have the power to pass through walls—the membrane walls of cells—though this power comes from their cholesterol base, as opposed to TV witchcraft. (Cell membranes are made of fat molecules, so a cholesterol-derived steroid molecule is enough of a cousin to get through.)

Upon slipping into a cell, these hormones do their work in a few simple steps; basically BAC—Bind, Activate, Change:

1. ***Bind*** with their specific receptor. (Researchers sometimes call this "sitting" on the receptor, which makes me picture a grumpy cartoon hormone molecule on the toilet.)
2. ***Activate*** the receptor—triggering it to send out work orders to parts of the cell.
3. ***Change*** elements of the cell's protein production, which cause functional changes in the cell—and, in turn, lead to changes in the body.

Chemical imitators of steroid hormones like *medroxyprogesterone acetate* work in the same three-step way. However, they get promiscuous in the receptor department, binding not only with the receptor of the hormone they're trying to impersonate but with others—sometimes leading to some nefarious changes.

MEDICAL CARE THAT SACRIFICES WOMEN'S HEALTH FOR FINANCIAL GAIN
OMP gets snubbed and MPA gets prescribed

Since 1980 in France, and since 1998 in the US, there's been a safe, effective form of prescription progesterone on the market. The US version is the FDA-approved drug OMP (the oral micronized progesterone generic for the brand drug, Prometrium).

The starter material for OMP is yams—wild Mexican yams. This doesn't mean you can just eat yams—Mexican or otherwise—as a sneaky-clever way to get progesterone. The progesterone precursor in yams, diosgenin, has to be synthesized in a lab—transformed chemically to have the same structure as the progesterone your body produces. By the time OMP is in capsule form, there might not be even a microscopic trace of the veggie that went into it.

As you'll see in coming chapters, OMP alone alleviates perimenopausal insomnia—without the risks and awful side effects of sleeping pills. In perimenopause, OMP is basically a pharmaceutical lifeboat out of suffering from many other symptoms—and, in menopause, it pairs with estrogen to do the same.

But as I dug deeper into the research, I came to see that it provides more than symptom relief. OMP—filling in for a lack of progesterone in perimenopause and menopause—bolsters, protects, and sustains our health throughout our lives, organ to organ, tissue to tissue, throughout the body (including our brain).

Perimenopausal women are not only wrongly prescribed estrogen for problems likely caused by newly soaring estrogen levels, but it's often paired with what Dr. Prior refers to as the "progesterone-like derivative," MPA: the medroxyprogesterone acetate generic for the long off-patent brand drug, Provera. (Chances are "Provera" rings a bell for you as the tail end of "Depo-Provera," a once-every-three-months birth control injection containing very-high-dose MPA.)

MPA has a different molecular structure from the progesterone in our bodies, which changes how it acts within us in some unhelpful and even harmful ways. As I noted above, it also has some of the same positive effects as progesterone—namely, alleviating hot flashes and night sweats, preventing overgrowth in the endometrial lining of the uterus, and building bone.

In menopause, combined with estrogen therapy, it leads to greater gains in spinal bone density than estrogen alone, per a 2017 meta-analysis by Prior and her colleagues. It does this through its effect on bone-building cells called "osteoblasts." MPA, like progesterone, "sits on" the osteoblast's progesterone receptor, "and therefore, in doses of 10 milligrams a day will increase bone density," Prior told me.

However, MPA's chemical dissimilarities with progesterone cause some problems. It's a drug version of hand-me-downs that kinda-sorta fit—save for how the "adverse effect" of wearing your big sister's old pants was mean teasing on the playground—as opposed to coronary artery damage that hastens your death. (MPA is associated with the "heart goes boom" thing, while progesterone has positive arterial effects.)

In the breast, MPA has what scientists call "a strong affinity" for the wrong receptors, stress hormone receptors called "glucocorticoid receptors." Its stimulation of these stress hormone receptors can increase a woman's risk of breast cancer by causing runaway breast cell proliferation.

OMP, on the other hand, binds "almost exclusively" with the *correct receptor* in the breast, the progesterone receptor, explains cancer researcher Jason Carroll. And just like the progesterone our body makes, OMP provides that essential "counterbalance" or complement to estrogen, preventing what Prior describes as "estrogen-induced" breast cell overgrowth, which can lead to breast cancer.

While MPA has been found guilty of a substantial list of undesirable effects, it has also been falsely accused. Take some of the side effects the FDA lists for MPA: acne, hair loss or hair growing in fun new places, and packing on some extra pounds.

You'd think the FDA would be a reliable source, right?

Think again! It wrongly blames the relatively small dose of MPA given orally in perimenopause and menopause for causing the side effects of the *massive* dose of MPA in an injection of Depo-Provera birth control. Prior, who pointed this out to me, told me the above hairy-zitty-muffin-toppy side effects are actually "rather rare" for women using a perimenopause or menopause-sized dose of MPA. However, weight gain tends to be triggered when the flood of Depo-Provera in birth control "causes estrogen levels to drop to menopausal levels."

To be fair, MPA does provide one form of relief OMP does not: financial relief for healthcare institutions that subsidize drug costs (with patients merely forking over a "co-pay," rather than paying the full price for their medications). As of June 2020, filling a prescription at your local drugstore for 10 milligrams of MPA was about $20 per month compared with around $130 for a comparable dose of OMP. In July of 2022, drugs.com listed the MPA at $27.19 and the OMP at $127.77—prices based on using their discount card. (The full retail price for OMP can be much higher.) The price has been coming down, so I checked again. In July of 2024, drugs.com had MPA at $14.22 and OMP at $44.98.

Obviously, keeping drug costs down is important for keeping medical care affordable for all. However, "cheaper!" can be horrifically costly if you end up getting a double mastectomy because your healthcare provider saved $110 by giving you MPA instead of OMP—which is about the amount mine would've saved back when I started taking it.

OMP VS. MPA IN THE PHARMACY LINE
What's getting prescribed?

Despite all OMP has going for it, in the two-plus decades since its 1998 FDA approval, it was infrequently prescribed in the US—unlike its widely prescribed imposter counterpart, MPA. However, the science that strongly supports the use of OMP over MPA seems to be trickling into medical practice.

Referencing comprehensive US pharmacy dispensing records from April of 2019 to June of 2021, gynecologist Nick Panay and his colleagues found that MPA was prescribed to 29,535 women, while OMP was prescribed to 6,526.

It's likely OMP is now being prescribed to a much greater degree due to the research published since that time, but getting the statistics requires a pricey institutional subscription to a database. To my great *unsurprise*, the database did not respond to my requests to mooch stats from them, good cause notwithstanding. Despite searching obsessively for further studies referencing newer prescribing stats, they were not to be found.

TERM LIMITS
The confusion over the term "bioidentical"

The FDA-approved drug OMP is frequently referred to as a "bioidentical" hormone, a term for a drug that's chemically identical to the substance in the human body it's being taken to replace—in this case, progesterone.

This isn't *wrong*, which is why I use "bioidentical" in the book at times—sometimes to differentiate OMP from synthetic MPA. However, the term "bioidentical" was born not in a scientist's lab but in a marketing department, and it's often used in hopes of duping us into believing a medication or product is safer and healthier than others. This belief—called "the naturalistic fallacy"—involves the erroneous assumption that because something is "natural," it's good: safer, gentler on the body, and better for our health. In fact, plenty of natural substances will kill us—if, say, we don't get our stomach pumped fast enough after we unwittingly blend up a poison ivy smoothie.

Ironically, bioidentical hormones are anything but "natural." They don't pluck them off bushes in the wild like raspberries. They're created in a lab and produced in a factory—whether they're FDA-approved capsules or sketchy potions sold by compounding pharmacies (only a small number of which are inspected and certified for drug consistency and quality by the Pharmacy Compounding Accreditation Board).

Compounded bioidentical hormones are especially problematic. The North American Menopause Society, in its "2022 Hormone Therapy Position Statement," warns that compounded bioidentical hormone therapy "may combine multiple hormones" in untested combinations, delivered in untested forms, such as pellets implanted under the skin. Whether they're safe and effective is anyone's guess. FDA-approved drugs, on the other hand, are subject to rigorous validation of the amount and type of stuff in the capsules or whatever form they come in.

Of course, there are plenty of FDA-approved drugs that never should have been approved and are pulled from the market (like the arthritis drug Vioxx, which was unbelievably effective for tens of thousands of people taking it, in that there's really no cure for arthritis pain like being dead). However, the manufacture of FDA-approved brand and generic drugs is highly regulated (that is, save for generics manufactured in India and China, per investigative journalist Katherine Eban).

Drug manufacturing plants and the drugs themselves are regularly monitored by FDA inspectors, who see to it that the labeled amount of *gonnakillyou*-zine matches the amount in the capsule, and that it is unadulterated by Viagra, horse tranquilizers, and, sorry—so gross...dandruff and other human bodily sheddings.

What *has* been "adulterated" is the language of scientists. Over time, "bioidentical" got so frequently trotted out in magazines, on *Oprah*, and elsewhere that it found its way into medical journals. And not just a little. I see it all the time. Endocrinologist and University of California, San Diego, med school professor Cynthia Stuenkel wrote in 2021, "Although not officially recognized by FDA, the term bio-identical is now used" by mainstream researchers "to describe (hormone therapy) formulations with a biochemical structure identical, or at least very similar to" hormones the body produces. ("Body-identical" is also used, but less frequently.)

PROGESTERONE IS NOT A PROGESTIN
(Contrary to what far too many doctors and researchers believe)

Most of us don't play fast and loose with meanings of words because it's seriously unhelpful.

Say somebody's about to step into an open manhole. We yell, "Stop!" or "Look out!" We don't shout "Potato!"

Likewise, because bioidentical OMP and the synthetic knockoff drug, MPA, are two *chemically different substances* that *do different things in the body*, you'd think scientists would refer to them in a way that makes that clear—especially in research! And the same goes for doctors.

However, for decades, researchers have been scientifically sloppy, referencing these two very different drugs as if they are chemically the same; in other words, chemically interchangeable. Because of this error (which I see *constantly* in the research papers), OMP and MPA are often treated in both research and medicine as if they have the same side effects and benefits—which you've seen from the opening of this chapter is completely not the case!

The scientific sloppiness is not simply a matter of researchers calling progesterone by the wrong name. Nobody means "progesterone" but accidentally says that mouthful "medroxyprogesterone acetate" instead. The problem is with the *category of drugs* each one falls into.

Researchers wrongly use "progestins"—the category for the synthetics—as an umbrella term for both the synthetic drugs and bioidentical progesterone. In fact, as a 2003 North American Menopause Society position statement made clear, "progestins" is the correct term ONLY for the synthetic progesterone imitators—all of which are chemically different from the progesterone in our body. Medroxyprogesterone acetate (MPA) is one of these progestins. Norethindrone acetate is another. (There are about 10 progestins altogether—most of which are used in contraceptives.) MPA is the most commonly prescribed progestin in the US, Australia, and many European countries (though not in France).

Progesterone, in drug form, correctly referenced, is the term ONLY for a substance that is chemically identical to the progesterone produced by our body. Unlike the synthetics, there aren't many. Oral micronized progesterone is a drug in this progesterone category, as is injectable bioidentical progesterone (which you're unlikely to be given unless you're a lab rat or have abnormal uterine bleeding, missing menstrual periods, or fertility issues).

Of course, there are times when scientists *need* an umbrella term—a drug category name to collectively reference the synthetic progestin drugs and bioidentical progesterone drugs. Though these drugs differ in meaningful ways, they are also *chemically similar* because the synthetics were created to mimic progesterone. As a result, the synthetics and OMP have some *shared progesterone-like actions in the body* (on hot flashes, bone, and the endometrium).

Reflecting that, **progestogens** is the umbrella term for "drugs that do progesterone-y things"—a category including both bioidentical OMP and synthetic progestins (MPA and its synthetic compadres).

> **BONUS POINT**
>
> ### DRUG CATEGORY CHEAT SHEET
>
> **Progesterone:** A drug chemically identical to the progesterone produced by your body.
> **Example:** Oral micronized progesterone (OMP).
>
> **Progestins:** Drugs that are synthetic knockoffs of progesterone, chemically different from the progesterone produced by your body.
> **Example:** Medroxyprogesterone acetate (MPA).
>
> **Progestogens:** The umbrella term for "drugs that do progesterone-y things"—a category including both bioidentical OMP and synthetic progestins like MPA.

TRICKLE-DOWN SCIENTIFIC ERRORS
How the progesterone/progestin confusion harms patients

In 2013, perinatologist Roberto Romero, MD, and reproductive endocrinologist Frank Stanczyk, MD, published a paper about a disastrous error some ob-gyns make: the terribly wrong *assumption* that progesterone and an injected progestin, 17α-hydroxyprogesterone caproate (17-OHPC—aka the brand drug Makena), could be used interchangeably in mid-to-late pregnancy to prevent pre-term birth.

"The safety profile of vaginal progesterone and 17-OHPC are different," Romero and Stanczyk explain. Progesterone in vaginal drug form, same as the progesterone in our body, is pregnancy protecting, making the uterine lining nutrient rich and stable and telling the immune system not to attack the developing embryo. In early pregnancy, it's prescribed when there's a concern that a woman's own progesterone levels might be too low, leading to the risk of miscarriage.

In mid-to-late pregnancy, progesterone adds a vital task to its chore chart: keeping the uterine muscles relaxed to prevent premature contractions. (In contrast, in research by ob-gyn Nicole K. Ruddock, MD, 17-OHPC failed to prevent contractions, and, in high doses, stimulated contractions!)

Ob-gyns are well aware of progesterone's benefits for pregnant women, Romero and Stanczyk note, but the widespread incorrect use of "progestins" as an umbrella term that includes progesterone has led to the "misconception that the safety profile of progesterone can be extrapolated to 17-OHPC during pregnancy."

This can have tragic effects. For example, two studies of patients receiving 17-OHPC—women having twins or triplets—"reported significant increases in perinatal adverse events": some women losing their babies and many delivering pre-term.

Makena (the drug sales name for 17-OHPC) is no longer on the market. However, both science and medical understanding continue to be poisoned by the scientific error-gone-viral of progestins and progesterone being used interchangeably.

Because research drives medical practice, uncorrected errors in research get passed on to patients—in the treatments we're given and those that are excluded from consideration (as OMP so often is).

Later in the book, there's a chapter on fibroids—non-cancerous balls of muscle and tissue in or on a woman's uterus that tend to show up in perimenopause. Many scientific studies and research review papers *claim* "progesterone" causes fibroid growth, or worse, uterine cancer—citing previous research as support for their claim.

This claim is, in a word, *insane*—or, more precisely and scientifically put: It makes no physiological sense. There is over a half century of strong evidence that progesterone prevents estrogen-incited cell overgrowth and the cancer that can develop from it. It's especially vital for preventing that overgrowth in the uterus!

I thought I'd have some big horrible mystery on my hands, figuring out the conflict between the strong physiological evidence and their claim. I didn't. After my first read-through of papers with these claims, I'd go back and do as I always do: go to the footnotes at the end of these papers (listing the particular studies behind their claims) and then pull up and read that research they cite.

I was shocked.

I saw—over and over!—that these studies *did not actually test progesterone* but one of its synthetic knockoffs: MPA or another progestin.

You might suspect this is amateur-hour stuff—research by some undersupervised junior scientist overdoing it on the edibles. It's anything but. For example, highly respected ob-gyn researcher and Northwestern University med school professor J. Julie Kim, MD, and her colleagues constantly make this error: using "progesterone" to refer to the effects of research studying the effects of *progestins* in paper after paper.

As such esteemed scientists, their work especially has led to the corruption of the literature in this area. It's possible that, à la "banks too big to fail," other scientists consider them "researchers too respected to double-check." Some assume papers published by important researchers in credible journals have been adequately checked. Others perhaps just prefer to run with that (time- and energy-saving) belief.

Whatever the reason, the damage has been done—and redone. In the wake of the Kim papers in 2012 and 2013, numerous researchers, in their own subsequent papers, engaged in a toxic game of "telephone," referencing these Kim articles to repeat their own unsupported claims that "progesterone" causes fibroids.

Though I happen to cite two examples from Kim and her colleagues, it is no exaggeration to say they have *crowds* of company in making this error. For example, Baylor College of Medicine professor Shailaja Mani, PhD (Shaila Mani in published papers), is respected and serious enough to secure hundreds of thousands of dollars in National Institutes of Health grants. In a 2008 article in the medical journal *Endocrinology*, Mani references "progesterone, the most biologically active progestin of ovarian origin." Of course, over here in biological reality (as I noted in Chapter Three), your ovaries are not little pharmaceutical factories where tiny lab-coated workers mix up a bunch of chemicals to create synthetic drugs like progestins.

The assumption that OMP and MPA are interchangeable has spilled from the research world into the world of medical bean counters—the pharmaceutical boards at medical providers that decide which drugs will be covered through their plan. Because MPA is cheaper than OMP, and institutional drug budgeteers are big on "the same, but cheaper," women who might've had coverage for the superior symptom relief and health benefits of OMP are instead prescribed its supposedly interchangeable counterpart, MPA, with all of its side effects and potential for harm.

The public's ideas about OMP and MPA are likewise misinformation-driven. Even on websites considered legit sources of consumer medical information (like that example from the FDA!), progesterone is *constantly* "falsely accused" of harms it does not cause but that MPA and/or estrogen do. Just google "oral micronized progesterone" or "progesterone." You'll see all sorts of undesirable side effects falsely attributed to it; for example, claims that it causes sleeplessness (when it's actually sleep-promoting, unlike MPA).

Those making these errors are not tinfoil-hatted randos on Facebook and Twitter. They are doctors and researchers—on their websites, in interviews with prestigious publications, and in articles they write for the *New York Times* and other major sites.

For example, in a 2019 *New York Times* op-ed, psychologist and neuroscientist Lisa Feldman Barrett writes, "Women who use contraceptives containing progesterone even have an increased risk of depression and suicide attempts."

Someone needs to tell Lisa that "women who use contraceptives containing progesterone" do not exist, because contraceptives contain synthetic *progestins*, not progesterone. *Never progesterone.*

— 8 —

A BRIEF HISTORY OF A SCIENTIFIC MESS
*Why progesterone got misclassified as a progestin
and how that still misinforms our medical care today*

PROGESTINS ONLY EXIST because progesterone was discovered—but then took its damn time getting into a form that didn't run right through us to become expensive pee.

A BUNNY UTERUS GOES TO LONDON

For a while, there was a rumor circulating that progesterone got its name in a London pub. In fact, that's pretty much what happened. In 1929, six years after the discovery of estrogen, George Corner, MD, and his med student colleague, Willard Allen, discovered what came to be known as progesterone in the follicular bits left behind after the egg makes its exit, called the "corpus luteum."

From the corpus luteum in female pigs, they harvested crude extracts of progesterone: impure but still-usable progesterone. They injected it into rabbits so it would transform their uterine lining into the "secretory phase," a nutrient-rich state necessary for fertilized rabbit eggs to implant. During the course of the pregnancy, it would also stabilize and strengthen the uterine lining (the endometrium) to prevent premature departures and would initiate the immune system suppression needed for the developing embryos to stick around and thrive.

The embryos they implanted in the rabbits did survive—and not just a few days! In 1930, Corner and Allen successfully maintained pregnancies—brought them to term in seven out of their 14 rabbits! A breathtaking scientific breakthrough!

Corner and Allen's experiments and subsequent ones by other scientists showed that even if the body produced no progesterone of its own, injecting the extract would do the job of sustaining a pregnancy. (Vaginal micronized progesterone and other forms are now used to do this in humans.)

Back then, using circa 1920s and '30s technology, the stuff was seriously hard to extract from the corpus luteum of the lab animals in any quantity and quality (that is, purity). Corner and Allen were finally successful at isolating a pure form of it in 1934—as were German biochemists Adolf Butenandt and Karl Slotta.

The Germans brazenly announced that the stuff would be called "luteo-sterone" ("luteo" for the corpus luteum and "sterone" because, like estrogen and testosterone, it's a steroid hormone). Corner and Allen, having discovered it in the first place years earlier, were understandably ticked off—as you'd probably be if you had a kid, and then, four years later, had the babysitter haul off and rename her.

Back in 1930, Corner and Allen had named the stuff "progestin," reflecting its "pro-pregnancy" (aka "pro-gestation") activity. This might make them seem like the source of the current progesterone/progestins confusion; however, "progestin" was a "rough draft" name they agreed to scrap a few years later.

Corner and Allen realized the Germans wouldn't back down easily. In 1935, Allen flew to London for a scientific conference to establish international standards for the newly discovered sex hormones. Over a pre-conference midnight supper at a pub, Allen and two other researchers batted around possible names to propose to the Germans and settled on "progesterone."

They cornered Butenandt and Slotta at a party a few days later, emphasizing that "progesterone had the *'progest'* of progestin and the *'sterone'* of *luteo-sterone*." Butenandt and Slotta were good with the compromise, and the 1935 conference ultimately announced "the adoption, for common use in scientific literature, of the name progesterone" for both the newly discovered corpus luteum hormone produced by the body and any drugs developed that are bioequivalent to it.

The American Medical Association, in 1936, likewise formally adopted the term "progesterone"—and, thinking ahead to the possible development of synthetics, adopted the term "progestin" for any chemically *similar* substances "having similar action, in case any such compounds are subsequently discovered."

Unfortunately, at the time, progesterone as a drug was still five decades away from being viable for more than a few desperate patients. Allen explained that starting around 1934, progesterone in oil could be given in painful daily injections into muscle tissue, but it had "virtually no activity orally." Progesterone taken orally lacked "bioavailability": the ability to be absorbed by the body (in sufficient amounts) so it can have an effect.

Back then, when taken by mouth in a pill or capsule, progesterone would go right through you because it was poorly absorbed by the stomach and small intestine. What little made it through the digestive tract was rapidly deactivated by the liver, so there was little or nothing left to go into the bloodstream and get to work in your body.

There was a way to make it bioavailable: injecting it into a muscle—which tends to be pretty painful due to all the nerve endings there and also requires a big, long, scary needle. People with type 1 diabetes might need to inject insulin *multiple times daily* (subcutaneously, in the fatty layer below their skin). Life or death? They do it. (Also, it's not painful the way muscle injection is.) However, you can probably imagine that a drug requiring menopausal women to become BFFs with a syringe they stab deep into a muscle every day might make all but the most life-stopping hot flashes seem like warm annoyances.

Also, technological limitations at the time made progesterone extremely expensive to produce—costing as much as $1,000 per gram (the equivalent of just ten 100-milligram capsules of OMP).

MEET PRETENDER-RONE
Scientists create progestins

From the mid-'30s on, over the next four decades, various researchers got to work developing progesterone imitators: inexpensive synthetics that could be taken orally. First, they brewed up progestins to help sustain a pregnancy, and later, progestins to prevent it—that is, birth control, first as the pill and now also in other formulations. (The first progestin successfully synthesized for birth control, by Carl Djerassi in 1951, was norethindrone, aka norethisterone: a key component in Enovid, the first oral contraceptive approved in the US, which came on the market in 1960.)

Researchers working on the pregnancy-helping end of things mixed a bunch of chemicals together (including testosterone and other steroid hormones), trying to create a drug with progesterone-like effects. The goal, Prior explains, was for a progestin "to do the uterine things that progesterone normally does": "1) change the uterine lining to allow implantation of a fertilized egg; and 2) support early pregnancy until placental hormones take over in the second trimester."

These two pregnancy-supporting effects were the *only* requirements for a progestin to be considered a viable drug to bring to market—and for the FDA to allow a drug to be classified as a progestin. Progestins are *not required* to have any of myriad other benefits of OMP and the progesterone produced by our bodies.

Ironically, as we saw in Chapter Seven about the pulled-from-the-market progestin Makena (17-OHPC), progestins are not the pregnancy protectors they were intended to be. Progesterone is now the standard of care for protecting and sustaining a pregnancy.

Beyond pregnancy, for a synthetic to be viable as birth control, there were only two requirements, wrote Allen. First, it had to "suppress ovulation when combined with estrogen." Second, it had to have enough mojo to produce "withdrawal bleeding"—meaning that after a woman stops taking it for a week, she gets her period. (In 28-day birth control pill packs, there's a week of placebo pills for the last seven days that fulfill this function.)

It took until the late '70s—almost 50 years after the discovery of progesterone and decades after the birth of the synthetics—for scientists at the French pharma company Besins-Iscovesco to come up with an oral form of bioidentical (aka body-identical) progesterone that could make its way into our bloodstream and cells.

Progesterone had to be micronized—the particles made extremely tiny—and then surrounded by fatty acids to give it a sort of chemical force field around it. This allowed enough of it to get to our small intestine to be absorbed and do its job in our bodies.

Oral micronized progesterone first became available by prescription in France in 1980. It took till 1995 for prescription OMP to be available in Canada and till 1998 for doctors in the US to be able to prescribe it—which isn't to say many did.

And herein lies the source of the mess: As Prior explains it, "Since so many years had passed without access to progesterone, doctors were used to...progestins and had come to think of them *as* progesterone." Researchers likewise slopped the two into one, despite repeated warnings against this by leading scientists.

Willard Allen, all the way back in 1970, explained in a journal article that the substance in "'the pill' is not progesterone" but "a synthetic progestational agent." Decade after decade, year after year, you see these correctives in the scientific literature from highly respected scientists; for example:

In 1980, reproductive toxicologist Anthony Scialli, MD, did his part.

In 2008, it was French reproductive researchers Michael Schumacher and Regine Sitruk-Ware.

And in 2013, reproductive endocrinologist Frank Stanczyk, MD, took a crack at it—reiterating medical practice guidelines from The North American Menopause Society from 2003:

> "To avoid confusion...the term progestogen should be used when referring to progesterone and synthetic progestogens collectively, whereas the name progestin is specific only to synthetic progestogens."

As we've seen, confusion has been anything but "avoided." Prior rightly deems the continuing misclassification of progesterone as a progestin "a mockery of science" that leads to flawed research and "poor medical care."

I saw that for myself as my battle with my healthcare provider continued.

LIKE A BREATH OF FRESH ERROR

The day after my gynecologist sent me Kaiser's menopause fact sheet that applied to me in perimenopause not at all, I emailed him back. I reiterated my request for OMP for my perimenopausal symptoms (emphasizing that I was asking for the generic for the progesterone brand drug *Prometrium*—that is, OMP—*not* a "synthetic"; as in, not MPA). My message:

> I read the Kaiser information; however, I do NOT want to take estrogen; just micronized oral progesterone, in the NON-synthetic version: Prometrium. That is very, very important.

In my email, I pasted in scientific support: a link that included 19 studies reflecting that OMP was the safest, most helpful treatment for my symptoms.

He messaged me back: "You can pick up the medication at the pharmacy today."

Wow. Fantastic.

But a worry kept chipping away at me.

I logged in to Kaiser's website to access my prescriptions, to see whether he'd actually given me the OMP. And there it was...ugh...medroxyprogesterone acetate, 2.5 milligrams. I messaged him again, begging him to correct my prescription.

It turns out he, very kindly, had emailed me despite being on vacation. He probably didn't see my subsequent messages. A nurse in Kaiser's gyno department was my savior: getting the department's on-call gynecologist to correct my prescription—in the nick of time for me to race to the pharmacy before it closed.

Though my Kaiser plan has a $10 co-pay for prescriptions, when the cashier rang up my prescription, I learned it only applies to drugs on Kaiser's "formulary," which Kaiser describes as "a list of covered drugs chosen by" a committee "of Kaiser Permanente physicians and pharmacists."

The drug these pharma oracles had picked for their formulary of covered drugs was the breast cancer risk-increasing progesterone imitator, MPA, that's a big fail at alleviating a bunch of symptoms OMP does. The OMP I was prescribed was not on the formulary.

Rotten.

But I was desperate to get the OMP that might help me sleep through the night again, so I paid $38 for just 30 capsules of the 100-milligram dose. This was just a third of the 300 mg nightly dose I actually needed to help dial down the head-to-toe miseries from my soaring perimenopausal estrogen.

CHASING THE SANDMAN

That evening, I awaited bedtime with the monk-like patience of a three-year-old in line at the DMV. Finally, I took my 100-milligram capsule. (Please, could this be the first night of the rest of my not bolting up in bed every 20 minutes?)

That night, I still woke up—but only twice instead of five or six times. And instead of bolting awake just 20 minutes after dozing off, I first woke up *four whole hours* later! To my relief, it was a drowsy awakeness, and it lasted just briefly. I then scored three more hours. Three *uninterrupted* hours of sleep!

After I'd taken oral micronized progesterone for two weeks, I noticed that I seemed to be having fewer hot flashes during the day. I can't really be more specific. Keeping detailed notes on my daily symptoms would've been the scientific thing to do, but I instead did the slapdash human thing and, every few days, jotted this or that observation on the backs of research papers on my desk.

I couldn't wait to ask my doctor to up my dose.

But there was a problem.

A sudden need for me to pay extra for a prescription was not in my budget. However, because Kaiser deemed my request for OMP some sort of Karl Lagerfeld–like medical excess, they would make me pick up the full tab for it, without their usual subsidy. Though generic OMP has gone down in price since 2017, at the time, 300 milligrams of the stuff could have cost me from $106 to hundreds a month (if I had to get it at a drugstore, via a non-Kaiser doctor) in comparison with my usual $10 co-pay for drugs Kaiser deems medically necessary.

Kaiser, understandably, can't just open the money hydrant for anything a patient wants. As much as I'd love a little complimentary facial rejuvenation, I'm on board with how they require patients to pay for "elective" stuff, like if you want perkier boobs, Botox injections, or lips that double as a flotation device. However, because sleep is shown to be essential for healthy brain function, mental health, and overall physical health, my "electing" to sleep through the night rather than bolting awake every half hour doesn't seem to belong on the list of medical frivolities.

THE SQUEAKY PATIENT

At the time, I'd been going rogue on the amount of progesterone I'd been taking—upping my dose to 300 milligrams a night, thanks to a doctor friend who did me a favor and wrote me a prescription. Since he isn't a Kaiser doc, I had to go to the drugstore to get the scrip filled. I ended up paying $70 for just thirty 100-milligram capsules after the pharmacy rejected the discount coupon I'd found online.

Though the cost made me sick, I told my gynecologist that the 300-milligram dose of OMP—an amount safely prescribed in France since the 1980s—had become my nightly savior: my only hope for "Now I lay me down *to sleep*" instead of "*to convulse like a fish on a dock*." I also zeroed in on the findings that MPA elevates breast cancer risk, pointing out that cancer runs in my family, and I was terrified of taking anything that could fuel it.

On this basis, I asked that he prescribe me the breast-, uterus-, and sleep-protecting 300-milligram dose of OMP, as well as giving me a cost waiver for it so I could get it for my $10 monthly co-pay.

My messages had to be about as welcome as bedbugs checking in at the Hilton, but my gynecologist showed himself to be superhumanly good-natured about the electronic deluge. Even more impressively, he took action on my behalf.

He called and told me he had conferred with his boss, the chief of staff for the department of Obstetrics and Gynecology at the major Kaiser facility near me. She had okayed prescribing me a 200-milligram dose of OMP, and she'd put through a waiver so Kaiser would cover the cost of it, too!

Wow.

Though I wasn't getting the 300 milligrams I had asked for, this was a major victory—and frankly, an unlikely one.

Here I was, this medical diva, trying to order "off menu" at Kaiser: demanding a non-standard drug, in a non-standard amount, and then, best of all, demanding they give it to me at the el cheapo covered drug price. Sure, I'd sent them a bunch of science to back this up, but my timing didn't help. Doctors today are besieged with patients who believe the 20 minutes they spent googling some dubious information on some crackpot's blog is the equivalent of years of medical training.

Like the rest of us, doctors are prone to "confirmation bias": the tendency to favor information that confirms what we already believe and to dismiss conflicting information that suggests our beliefs (and any actions they led to) might've been wrong.

The fact that his boss allowed me the OMP—in effect, saying I was right, or might be—was a tacit admission that they might be wrong. I saw this as a show of character on her part, and the same goes for my gynecologist in sticking his neck out for me: hitting up his boss on my behalf.

It would have been easy for them—in fact, vastly easier—to take refuge in Kaiser's practice and prescription standards: simply ignoring the science I'd snowstormed them with, denying me the drug and refusing to cover the cost. But—to their credit—these two doctors had instead treated me with respect, and in the process, had given me healthcare instead of bureaucracy-care.

MONKEY-SEE/MONKEY-DO MEDICINE

Grateful as I was to my gynecologist and his boss, it didn't make me a more well-behaved patient. I still had another battle to win: getting the entire 300-milligram dose I needed to curb my insomnia and other perimenopausal symptoms.

In mid-August, I again began petitioning (okay, borderline harassing) my doctor and his boss by email. On August 17, 2017, she sent me this reply:

> I actually do not recommend and would not prescribe 300 mg daily of Prometrium as it may be harmful (can cause excessive drowsiness), has not been studied extensively and is not standard practice for menopausal hormone therapy.

Ugh. She was wrong about all of this. I took on each of her claims—starting with progesterone "can cause excessive drowsiness." I acknowledged that this *would* be a problem IF I took progesterone during the day, but I take all 300 milligrams at bedtime:

> At night, progesterone's sleep-promoting effect is not a problem; it's a feature, or as I call "excessive drowsiness"—a good night's sleep. Experiencing that is enormously welcome after my waking up between five and six times a night before I started taking oral micronized progesterone.

Three days later, I sent her an eight-page memo, filled with links to research, including strong randomized controlled trials, refuting each of her claims. She didn't respond. Instead, my ob-gyn messaged me:

> I appreciate the information and research you have provided to our department. I am happy to hear your symptoms have improved. Regarding the approval, we still cannot approve the 300mg dosage. Your research has been reviewed but has not been formally adopted yet within our community here.

I did the adult thing and burst into tears. Then, I remembered something: At one point, his boss had offered to get on the phone with me. I messaged my gynecologist to ask for that phone meeting. His boss emailed me Monday night (August 28, 2017) to tell me she'd call Wednesday afternoon, and rounded out the email by explaining her position:

> I truly do not feel comfortable prescribing the 300 mg nightly of Prometrium. There is no support of that in the literature—we go based on the American College of Obstetrics of Gynecology, and use good evidence to make recommendations and practice medicine-randomized controlled trials.
>
> We practice evidence-based medicine. I surveyed all of my colleagues and none recommend the use of 300 mg nightly.
>
> I have been practicing Obstetrics and Gynecology since 1998. I would happy to discuss with you on the telephone if you would like to discuss further but Prometrium at doses higher than 200 mg could actually be harmful.
>
> What type and dose of Estrogen are you taking (I could not find any in the chart)? Perhaps we can titrate that to improve your menopausal symptoms?
>
> I am happy to work with you but 300 mg of Prometrium is not indicated.

I was disturbed, though not surprised, that my doctor's boss—the head of gynecology—made the error of suggesting estrogen to a perimenopausal woman, which is like prescribing cupcakes to a diabetic. If only she knew the findings Dr. Prior had spotlighted from the research by Santoro, Burger, and others. Again, though estrogen *is* lower in *menopause*, in *perimenopause*, estrogen levels can soar and lead to all sorts of awful symptoms—especially awful symptoms when, due to anovulatory menstrual cycles, there's no progesterone made to counterbalance the estrogen.

Furthermore, the notion that 300 milligrams of OMP might be harmful is ludicrous. As I noted in one of my (2017) messages to her, we've had 37 years to see that this is not the case. "Micronized progesterone has been used widely in Europe since 1980 at dosages ranging from 300 mg/d (taken at bedtime)..." explains French endocrinology specialist Bruno de Lignières, MD.

Next, there's her claim that they practice "evidence-based medicine"—a claim she "supported" by saying she polled her doctor colleagues, asking them what they all do! This is called "prevailing practice," and it is not evidence-based but *hearsay-based* medicine—essentially, "This is what we do because this is what we do."

Finally, her statement, "I have been practicing Obstetrics and Gynecology since 1998" is a well-known logical fallacy: an "argument from authority," meaning an argument that relies on a person's credentials rather than evidence: "We doctors deserve to be believed because we're doctors and you're not!"

Authority-based medicine has a long and tragic history. In the 19th century, Hungarian doctor and scientist Ignaz Semmelweis called for obstetricians to wash and disinfect their hands, pointing out that clinics that mandated this had a dramatic decrease in mortality rates—down to 1 percent or even zero. His recommendation went against the medical establishment's accepted thinking and practices, so he was mocked and his advice ignored—and countless patients died needlessly because doctors continued to stick their bare hands into cadavers and then use those same cadaver-juiced hands to operate and to deliver babies.

The modern shift toward evidence-based medicine came in 1972, when Scottish epidemiologist Archibald Cochrane published a book criticizing the lack of reliable evidence behind many medical interventions that were standard at the time. He called for medical care based on "proven efficacy and efficiency and not on the basis of authority, emotion, politics, fashion (or) fantasy," reports reproductive medicine researcher Jan Gerris, MD.

Though doctors' "clinical experience"—meaning experience from treating patients—is not unimportant, Cochrane fought against what Gerris calls "uncritical copy-and-paste" medicine: doctors simply copying other doctors' care to decide a course of treatment for a patient, as my gyno's boss did by polling her colleagues. In contrast, the practice of evidence-based medicine is an *integration* of individual doctors' expertise with the best available evidence from systematic reviews (comprehensive evaluations of multiple studies comprising a body of evidence).

I was very clear on the sort of medical care I wanted, and it wasn't the "all the doctors are doing it!" kind. I sent the gyno boss three studies reflecting the safety of the 300-milligram dose and re-sent the French endocrinologist's OMP research review with similar findings.

THE SCIENTIFIC ROT STARTS AT THE TOP
58,000 doctors misinformed by the major ob-gyn medical organization, ACOG

My chances of getting Kaiser to give me the additional 100 milligrams I needed to sleep and protect my breasts and uterus didn't seem good. However, the gyno boss had slipped an important piece of information into her email: the source of the practice standards she and her Kaiser gyno colleagues go by, the American College of Obstetricians and Gynecologists (ACOG.org).

ACOG described itself on its website as "the nation's leading group of physicians providing health care for women with more than 58,000 members." In other words, if a woman sees a gynecologist in the US, that gynecologist is most likely an ACOG member.

I contacted ACOG's media relations manager, Maggie McEvoy, on August 28 and 29 of 2017. I asked for two very specific pieces of information: ACOG's position on oral micronized progesterone and their position on the 300-milligram dose of OMP, specifically for "perimenopausal women."

McEvoy consulted with clinicians at ACOG to get answers. Disturbingly, ACOG and scientific accuracy parted company from the start. McEvoy repeatedly emailed me replies that referenced not the oral micronized progesterone I had been so specific in asking about but its synthetic knockoffs, "progestins."

Jaw drop. Yes, even the ACOG's "experts," guiding American gynecological practice, confuse progesterone with pharma pleather, progestins. I wrote back, emphasizing to McEvoy that I was not asking about the synthetics (progestins) but OMP (progesterone). However, she again gave the answer for progestins, and she said that the "Practice Bulletin" she sent (ACOG's published guidelines for their member gynecologists) "has an entire section on progestin—a category that micronized progesterone falls under."

Ugh. No, Ms. McEvoy and you scientifically deficient ACOG "experts" who should know better: Progestins like MPA are *not* the same, nor are they in the same category as progesterone, the human hormone made by women's ovaries and replicated in drug form as OMP!

THE EMPEROR'S NEW GYNECOLOGY

I felt sick.

No wonder my gynecologist had confused progesterone and progestins. ACOG, the organization largely responsible for practice standards for gynecologists across America, leads the way in generating and maintaining doctors' confusion.

ACOG also gives harmful, scientifically unsupported advice for "treating the symptoms of perimenopause": "taking estrogen" (with a progestin if a woman still has her uterus). Of course, in perimenopause, soaring estrogen is *a problem,* so it is most certainly not the solution. Recall how emphatic Dr. Prior is that *no perimenopausal woman should be taking estrogen:* "It is a bad idea to treat symptomatic perimenopause with estrogen in any form!"

Even worse, ACOG's document I read in August of 2017 on treatments for women in perimenopause made no mention of the one medication—OMP—that has been shown to be truly helpful for alleviating sleep disturbances. Yet ACOG spokeslady Maggie McEvoy was quick to lipstick up the scientific pig, characterizing ACOG's "Practice Bulletin" as "evidence-based recommendations." She then summed up ACOG's stance: "We suggest treatments based on symptoms, not by whether someone is in a 'state' of perimenopause or menopause."

Awful. Bad science leading to bad medicine.

Perimenopause is *identified* by the symptoms we begin to experience: for example, with those nine changes Prior lists for determining whether we're in early perimenopause.

However, *treating* based on symptoms, as ACOG advises, rather than looking to underlying causes to determine treatment, is medical malpractice turned into standardized "care." Psychiatrist and evolutionary researcher Randolph Nesse, MD, co-founder of evolutionary medicine, explains that symptoms, while uncomfortable or even painful, are not themselves the problem but reflect "the body's attempt to remedy a problem."

The *source* of the underlying problem—such as low or insufficient progesterone making perimenopausal women feel constantly wired, angry, and sick—is what needs to be understood and treated. When doctors limit themselves to treating its manifestations, the symptoms, the underlying cause gets masked, neglected, or mis-treated—like with antidepressants prescribed for hot flashes. Though they give women who *can't* take hormones an option for symptom relief, antidepressants have a number of adverse effects and, for example, do nothing to fill in for a perimenopausal woman's missing or insufficient levels of progesterone. This means her bones and uterine lining remain progesterone-starved, increasing her risk of fracture and endometrial cancer respectively.

Nesse calls this common medical mistake the "viewing symptoms as diseases" error. It is not only harmful to patients but can even be deadly. Say a patient has had intermittent headaches for two weeks, and she complains to her doctor, asking him to give her something for the throbbing pain.

To her, the pain is the problem to be solved. However, a doctor who limits himself to treating her symptom, pain—like by prescribing medication to block it—may end up killing her. A headache that persists for weeks can be caused by a brain tumor pressing on a nerve, and dimming that pain with meds gives the tumor extra time to grow and invade more brain country.

PLEADING MY CASE

Wednesday afternoon, my phone rang. It was my gynecologist and his boss together on speakerphone. I thanked them for approving the 200-milligram dose of OMP—and then set about dismantling every one of the gyno boss's arguments against giving me the full 300-milligram dose.

ACOG was first on my scientific chopping block. I told them all the ways ACOG's information and standards were at odds with scientific evidence—and that ACOG clinicians had eventually affirmed what I'd written to them: that estrogen levels are actually *elevated* in perimenopause. (What's next on ACOG's agenda, giving somebody OD'ing on heroin more heroin instead of Narcan?)

Finally, in hopes of reassuring them that I didn't just willy-nilly, hazard-a-guess my way to the conclusion that I needed a 300-milligram dose of progesterone, I explained my "conservative approach" to taking any drug: Every medicine has potential costs that come along with its benefits or potential benefits. Unless the benefits sufficiently outweigh the costs—that is, unless you *really* need the drug for your health and/or quality of life—it's best to avoid taking it.

So, I told them, if my only symptom were intermittently feeling like my body'd been colonized by an Easy-Bake Oven, I probably would've toughed out the hot flashes med-free. However, the 300-milligram dose of progesterone had given me back some incredibly precious things—things most of us take for granted, like being able to sleep through the night and get around in cars without upchucking our lunch into a bush.

I begged them not to take these and my other gains away from me, especially in light of all the studies I'd presented them demonstrating progesterone's safety, along with the fact that 300 milligrams had been standard for French women for going on four decades, sans adverse effect. And then, channeling some of our most impassioned legal figures—aiming for Atticus Finch but probably coming off more Judge Judy—I made my closing argument: "I would ask that Kaiser catch up to the evidence rather than asking me to take an insufficient amount of a drug I need to stop life-ruining symptoms."

I took a big gulp of air and sat down.

Silence.

And then the gyno boss spoke. She said she still didn't feel comfortable with the 300-milligram dose.

Ugh.

Silence.

She then asked: Would I accept the risks if anything went wrong?

Absolutely, I told her. Absolutely.

More silence.

And then the gyno boss spoke.

They would prescribe me the 300 milligrams—and cover it, too.

I couldn't believe it. I had won.

I did a little fist-bump crazydance, then lurched back into character, my voice on the phone all coolly professional woman of science: "The risks are on me. I understand them. I *accept* them," I said.

SUBSTANDARDS OF CARE

Though my agreeing to assume the risk had allowed the gyno boss to come through for me, the science I'd sent on the benefits of progesterone was strong and clear, and there really was no evidence of risk in taking a 300-milligram dose. The gyno boss seemed like a smart, sharp lady, so despite her rather depressing grab for "authority"-based defenses for her initial position, I wondered whether she'd been more on board with what I'd been asking for than she'd let on.

About a month after that conference call, I was trying to figure out why a drug called betahistine seemed to diminish my motion sickness. Researchers who study Ménière's disease see that it works for some patients; they just don't know how or why. It's a really interesting mystery, and I ended up talking about it—nerding out for over an hour one night on the phone with the otolaryngologist (ear, nose, and throat doc) and former researcher I'd seen for my motion sickness.

At one point, I vented about the gulf I'd experienced between "evidence-based" and "medicine" in the Kaiser gynecology department—and, most disappointingly, from the clearly smart and accomplished Kaiser gyno boss. The ENT doc said she'd logged into my patient record before calling and skimmed the woman's detailed notes within it. "In her heart of hearts, I think she agrees with you," she told me.

She explained that doctors at an institution like Kaiser *must* go by established practice standards. They can get in a lot of trouble if they ignore or buck them, including possibly getting sued and losing their license if their justification for coloring outside the lines is deemed insufficient by the powers that be.

I hadn't understood this. Back then, to me as a patient, "practice standards" sounded like helpful suggestions for treatment. Her explanation made me understand they can be a *barrier* to evidence-based treatment: keeping doctors from using scientifically informed discretion to make treatment decisions driven by current evidence that conflicts with current dogma (favored in department- and field-wide medical hearsay).

Meanwhile, millions of menopausal and perimenopausal women are trusting their gynecologists to give them evidence-based care. But, just like their doctors, they have no idea that practice standards formulated by the respected American College of Obstetricians and Gynecologists result from their experts' ignorance of the actual hormonal makeup of perimenopause, their succumbing to the "viewing symptoms as diseases" error, and their erroneous belief that progesterone and progestins are interchangeable.

This leads to evidence-*starved* medicine, and it's a serious betrayal of both patients and the doctors who mean to help them. Consider the classic advice for medical practitioners from Greek philosopher-physician Hippocrates, "First, do no harm." That's an impossible goal when practice standards are based in scientific fairy tales and hand-me-down careless errors.

PART 2

SYMPTOMS, SYMPTOMS, GO AWAY

Introduction

SYMPTOMS ARE JUST THE STARTING GATE

Alleviate—and then protect

YOU MIGHT RECALL that this book only exists because I got attacked by a hot flash.

My sole motivation at the time: "Make it go away!" (aka "Alleviate!").

"Alleviate"—stop (or at least diminish!) the hot flashes and other symptoms—has long been the primary focus of researchers and the reason doctors prescribe hormone therapy to women in menopause and perimenopause.

However, as I plowed through the science, I came to see that hormone therapy does more than provide symptomatic rescue. Both OMP in perimenopause and estradiol in menopause (solo or combined with OMP) can be a powerful, health-protecting force.

I first understood this about progesterone for women in perimenopause, thanks to Dr. Prior's research and research reviews showing that progesterone is vital for protecting our bones and cardiovascular health. In fact, it goes a step further: actually *building* bone and improving our cardiovascular health—that is, *in perimenopause.*

In menopause, hormone therapy likewise alleviates our symptoms and protects us from various forms of erosion. However, our building days are largely over. For example, in menopause, you can work on *keeping* the bone you have, but unless you lift barbells with weight plates the size of tires, you're unlikely to build healthy new bone—contrary to the claims by corporate drug pushers hawking rather evil substances called "bisphosphonates."

The depressing menopausal reality? Biologically, all roads lead downhill—and the downhill incline is disturbingly steep.

The thing is, we aren't without brakes. For example, I lay out evidence showing that initiating estradiol *very early in menopause* does a lot to flatten those inclines—seriously slowing our downhill speed and protecting our health.

Great, right?

Well, it's *something*. And, yeah, I get that we age and our brains and bodies don't work like they used to. But this "all-downhill" business really ticked me off. Every part of us, to borrow a Cory Doctorow word, seems subject to *enshittification*. Our fingers hurt from arthritis, and they hurt more when we have the audacity to bend them. Bruises stick around like they're aspiring birthmarks. Even the common cold gets uncommonly long.

Collectively, these "little things" become a bigger thing both physically and psychologically—and a harbinger of big ugly things to come.

I wanted a workaround. For me and for all of us.

A means of maintaining our bodies and brains at their functional best as we age.

Alleviate—and then *protect*.

I came to realize that hormone therapy is a much more powerful protector if it's part of a trifecta—working synergistically with two vital partners: narrowly targeted ways to eat and exercise. "Narrowly targeted" means they do the two crucial things we need—"defend and protect": combat the ways our perimenopausal and menopausal bodies tend to betray us and efficiently and effectively maintain our bodies and brains in top functioning order. *(Details: Chapters Eighteen, Twenty, and Twenty-Two.)*

There's also a third crucial thing I factored in, without which the two above are useless: These diet and exercise measures are doable—and maintainable—by mere mortals, including that lazy, hedonistic pig known as me.

A vital point to keep in mind: *It's all interconnected*. We hear that line from time to time (as "It's all connected"), but I came to understand the above version as a sort of perimenopausal, menopausal, and lifetime health motto—seeing, for example, that strong, healthy muscle bolsters not just the health of our bones but that of our brain. In other words, our health is networked—linked across domains. Each important area is reliant upon and influenced by the others. *Interdependent*.

Accordingly, the ultimate goal of this hormone-diet-exercise trifecta is to actively refuse the natural course of aging—breakdown—by keeping our whole system in top functioning order. Granted, we could get a disease we can't block or stop. And eventually, of course, the erosions of aging and the guy in the black cape and the scythe will get us. But, in the meantime, we'll get to spend our lives living to the fullest instead of frantically trying to stop all the ways we're falling apart.

HOT, SLEEPLESS, AND HURLING

— 9 —
NOW I LAY ME DOWN TO THRASH
Insomnia all night, brain fog all day

SLEEP DEPRIVATION IS a form of torture.

I never gave that much thought—both because my workplace is not a CIA black site and because I'd been extraordinarily lucky. For 40-some years of my life, I hit the pillow like somebody'd clocked me with a cast-iron pan, and—assuming nobody shot a ballistic missile into my living room—I'd remain conked out for eight solid hours.

Then came perimenopause.

I'd get in bed and lie there for an hour, hatefully awake, until I tumbled—ever so briefly—into the sleep trench. Twenty minutes or maybe an hour later, I'd thrash awake. This sleep/thrash-awake funfest would go on all night. Eventually, the stabby knives of sunlight slashed me through the edges of the blinds: my cue to admit sleep defeat and pry myself out of bed—feeling very much like those sheep of counting fame had played soccer all night and used me as the ball.

Growing increasingly desperate to sleep, I banished all light from my bedroom.

I tried breathing exercises and boring myself to sleep with coma-inducingly dull reading.

I ate; I didn't eat; I took a bath before I went to sleep and hot showers when I was stark raving awake at 3:22 a.m.

Nothing helped.

I woke up every day fresh as a stomped daisy.

IT'S ALWAYS FOGGY IN PERIMENOPAUSE-ADELPHIA

If you're like a number of us in perimenopause, you still get eight hours of sleep—it just takes three days.

"Disturbed sleep" afflicts approximately 40 to 60 percent of women in perimenopause and menopause. It plays out in problems getting to sleep ("sleep onset") or staying asleep ("sleep maintenance") or both, with nighttime awakenings the most common sleep-related complaint, reports sleep researcher Fiona Baker. Sleep issues seem to be at their worst in perimenopause and early menopause, save for any women who get to be "special" in the worst possible way.

"Nighttime awakenings" don't just take our sleep; they ravage our waking hours in the form of brain fog. I described mine in perimenopause as "a daily attack of the stupids"—the brain version of paying for turbo broadband but getting staticky dial-up because the neighbors were streaming porn off my Wi-Fi.

"Fog," by the way, is adorable. Fog is mist. Mist is gentle—even the thickest Massachusetts mist. Brain fog, on the other hand, would rightfully be called *brain four wet wool blankets between you and what used to be your ability to reason*.

My murked-up mind really freaked me out—especially since no excess of caffeine would de-murk it. Simple acts of reasoning became hours-long hemming-and-hawing slogs. I once rewrote the opening line of a column 43 times (yes, I counted), and the next morning, went back to my very first version.

It helped not at all that I was well acquainted with the sleep science that explained the congealed swamp that had replaced my previously functional brain. Sleep deprivation dampens brain cell activity, causing neurons to respond more slowly, fire more weakly, and take a longer time sending information around, reports neurosurgeon Itzhak Fried. This erodes memory and concentration and the brain's ability to process visual information. In other words, brain fog is a temporary state of diminished mental capacity: sleep deprivation eating our "cognitive function"—the ability to pay attention, reason, solve problems, make decisions, and remember and use information.

But how we get into that state matters, too.

Though neuroscientists reading MRIs of women with perimeno-mushed or meno-mushed brains have yet to spot a pile-up of gross wet wool blankets within, there actually is a bunch of debris coming between us and mental clarity. Research by neuroscientist Maiken Nedergaard, MD, suggests we need a good night's sleep for the brain's janitor, the glymphatic system, to do its job cleaning out the neural trash we've accumulated during our waking hours.

This janitorial work can't take place during the day because, when we're awake, the brain is too large to allow the cleaning product, cerebrospinal fluid, to get through. During healthy sleep, the brain shrinks enough for the fluid to wash out the dreck. But sleep that's disrupted and deficient in length and sleep cycles leaves the brain a trashed mess—the neural version of a Slurpee cup and Mickey D-wrapper-littered back seat of a teenage boy's car. The neurotoxins that pile up include nasty stuff like beta-amyloid, which has been associated with Alzheimer's disease—which suggests getting enough sleep to let the janitor juice in is pretty vital.

Many people have the occasional trashed-brain day and recover just fine. However, sleep researcher Hans Van Dongen finds that regular sleep deprivation adds up, leading to "significant cumulative...deficits in cognitive performance"—including being too cognitively depleted to grasp the cumulative effects! Van Dongen's research participants "were largely unaware of these increasing cognitive deficits," which, he says, "may explain why the impact of chronic sleep restriction on waking cognitive functions is often assumed to be benign."

MUDDLE WRESTLING
OMP vs. The Insomnia Fairy

Sleep deprivation makes you single-mindedly desperate to sleep. The first night I took OMP, I didn't just hope for relief; I wished for it, kid-style. (If you close your eyes hard and tense up your forehead till it hurts, a passing sorcerer might recognize what a deserving girl you are and grant your wish.)

Well, either that works or OMP did, leading to those gorgeous chunks of sleep I told my doctor about: four whole *unwaking* hours—followed by three more and a few straggling minutes after that.

Only when I sat down at the computer did I understand the sickening level of mental muckage I'd been getting socked with daily. That morning, it was like somebody'd gone in with a shop vac and sucked out the gunk clogging the thinkworks. Though I *had* woken up twice, those nice, long chunks of sleep made me mentally sharp in a way I hadn't been for years.

If only doctors knew what a sleep savior OMP can be for women in perimenopause and menopause. Progesterone—made by our body or as OMP—induces sleep by stimulating the brain to generate sleep-promoting hormones and neurotransmitters. This results in "an ability to fall asleep faster, less disturbed deep sleep, and overall increased total sleep time," explains Dr. Prior.

A major player in this is a chemical messenger called "gamma-aminobutyric acid" (aka GABA), which I remember as Mr. GABA, the delivery dude for calm. Mr. GABA is an "inhibitory neurotransmitter," and what he "inhibits" is the level of "excitement" in our nervous system. When Mr. GABA binds to his receptors, it blocks (or at least diminishes) some "excitatory" signals in our brain—and the activity level on the whole—which allows us to fall asleep and stay asleep... or at least spend less time popping up like breakfast toast.

The GABA-A receptor is particularly important in helping us sleep, which is where OMP comes in—and MPA does not. OMP is a "positive modulator" (basically, a really good influence) on the GABA-A receptor, enhancing its inhibitory effects that promote sleep. MPA, on the other hand, does just the opposite: reducing these sleep-promoting effects!

SAFETY

OMP is "safer than all the sleeping pills currently available" for sleep maintenance, Dr. Prior explains. Common prescription sleep drugs like Ambien (generic: zolpidem) and benzodiazepines like Restoril (temazepam) will conk you out, but they are misnamed as "sleeping pills." They are actually *sedating* rather than sleep-promoting, meaning that they do not foster healthy, restorative sleep but simply slow down activity in the body and brain till you're immobilized into something resembling sleep.

These drugs can dangerously suppress breathing and, in fact, tend to *suppress* vital sleep stages—both "slow-wave" deep sleep and rapid eye movement (REM) sleep. This, in turn, suppresses the absolutely critical effects these sleep stages have on our health and healthy functioning, day-to-day and long-term.

Deep sleep strengthens the immune system, regulates hormone release, and triggers the body to build muscle and do necessary repair work—mending injured muscle, bone, and other tissues. REM sleep, the stage in which most dreaming takes place, is crucial for healthy cognitive function and emotional regulation and helps boost mental flexibility and creative problem-solving.

Both deep sleep and REM are essential for "memory consolidation": sorting through your memories and stabilizing and storing important ones for recall when you need them. Ambien works against this by altering the natural architecture of sleep—the healthy progression of sleep stages. Accordingly, sleep scientist Matthew Walker reports that "Ambien-induced sleep resulted in a 50 percent unwiring of the connections [in the brain] that had been made that day."

These "sedating pills" ("hypnotics" in researcher-ese) are basically blunt instruments—clubbing us with the "artificial sleepiness" of sedation, regardless of whether our sleep is disturbed or not, reports endocrinologist Anne Caufriez.

Progesterone is different. Caufriez and her colleagues find that progesterone has no effect on normal, undisturbed sleep—which is to say, if your sleep "ain't broke," progesterone won't do anything to "fix" it. Progesterone seems to act as a "physiologic regulator," Caufriez explains, meaning that when there are sleep issues, progesterone steps in, inducing and working with the brain and body's mechanisms to restore normal sleep.

For example, Dr. Prior, summing up the findings on OMP for sleep, notes that OMP decreases sleep interruption and induces "deep sleep without risks for addiction, without suppression of breathing control...and with no decrease in restorative rapid eye movement (REM) sleep." In fact, in research on healthy menopausal women, ages 54 to 70, by psychiatrist Petra Schüssler, OMP (in the 300-milligram dose) led to an *increase* in REM sleep as well as a reduction in time spent awake "without impairing cognitive functions during daytime."

Prior adds that OMP "not only doesn't slow down or stop your breathing, but speeds it up!" (MPA, too, stimulates breathing, but it doesn't itself improve sleep—though by decreasing night sweats, it can have an *indirect* sleep-enhancing effect.) And while the "sedating pills" can leave you with a morning-after hangover, this doesn't seem to be a factor with OMP.

OMP, "in a randomized, placebo-controlled trial" was shown to have "no negative effect on morning alertness, cognition, memory, or coordination," reports Prior. Regarding its positive effects, she adds, "After three months of taking progesterone, women's morning responses on a whole battery of memory and other brain tests were unchanged or improved."

EFFECTIVENESS

In multiple studies on *menopausal* women (and even a study on men!), OMP is found to improve sleep. Disturbingly, decade after decade, studies on OMP's effect on women in perimenopause with sleep issues were never funded.

Prior and her team *did* get funding to investigate the effects of OMP on hot flashes and night sweats in perimenopausal women, and part of the study protocol was asking the participants how well they slept. The women, treated with 300 milligrams of progesterone per night, perceived what the researchers describe as "significantly improved sleep quality" compared with those on the placebo.

In light of the gaping hole where research on OMP's effect on perimenopausal women's sleep should be, I'll tell you that it is Prior's clinical experience—her decades-long experience as a doctor treating perimenopausal patients—that *progesterone alone* is effective for alleviating sleep issues in perimenopause.

I emphasize "progesterone alone" as a reminder that doctors tend to prescribe estrogen to perimenopausal women, unaware that many women's estrogen levels soar in perimenopause. These doctors are likely generating overdose levels in some or many patients—or, in practical terms, "giving the gift of turbo PMS."

However, it's important to note that some women seem to do okay on estrogen in perimenopause—even being helped by it (for example, through estrogen alleviating vaginal dryness by keeping vaginal tissue moisturized, thick, and elastic). Beneficial effects from prescription estrogen in some perimenopausal women aren't unexpected. There are individual differences in how any stage or condition affects a person, as well as differences in metabolism. Some women metabolize estrogen more slowly, which can lead to symptomatic misery, while others clear it more quickly from their system. Some of the fast metabolizers might *possibly* do okay taking estrogen.

However, timing probably matters. It's possible the overdose effect might not be experienced till perimenopause is in full swing. Early in perimenopause, if a woman is prescribed estrogen on top of her body's supply, that inhibin-B feedback mechanism you read about might still be functional and do its job: detect when estrogen levels are abnormally high and dispatch messages to have it corrected. ("Yo, pituitary! We're full up with 'E' down here. Don't be sending more!")

Though the breakdown of this hormonal feedback system tends to drag us through a gauntlet of symptoms, it's an important part of the shift from "reproductive" to "non-reproductive": that is, our crossover into menopause. Prior explained to me that "the 'job' of perimenopause is to get rid of responsive ovarian follicles (that could lead to periods in a woman in a nursing home)." This requires disrupting the normal hormonal feedback relationships. Once these mechanisms are disrupted—like with inhibin-B levels plunging till it's pretty much *Anything Goes!*-B—there's "almost nothing" (except a form of chemically induced menopause) that "will reliably suppress the high and erratic estradiol levels of perimenopause."

OPTIMAL DOSE

To help sleep, OMP must be taken in a 300-milligram dose at bedtime, Prior explains. This dose keeps the progesterone in the blood at a level that's optimal for controlling hot flashes and night sweats—which, you'll see in the next chapter, is essential for improving sleep.

In a 2021 review of 10 clinical trials led by endocrinologist Brendan J. Nolan, MD, treatment with 300 milligrams of OMP improved total sleep time—decreasing the time it took to get to sleep and the time spent awake during the night. It also led to improved deep sleep and a sleep stage leading up to it.

The 100-milligram dose of OMP was unfortunately given with estradiol or estrogen while the 300-milligram dose was tested solo (against a placebo). There *were* some improvements in sleep quality from the 100-milligram dose, but in two of the trials using that dose, the effects didn't differ from the group who got no treatment or were given a progestin.

Higher doses—including hugely higher doses—appear to be safe. Endocrinologist Ellen W. Freeman and her colleagues tested the effects of 300-milligram, 600-milligram, and 1,200-milligram doses of OMP in healthy young women, ages 18 to 24. Other than fatigue and drowsiness at the highest dose reported by two of the 24 participants, there were no adverse effects.

FDA-APPROVED CAPSULES, NOT SKETCHY CREAMS

It's vital to take *oral* micronized progesterone—the FDA-approved drug—and not use progesterone lotions or potions from compounding pharmacies or online sellers. Progesterone cream will not restore sleep. It is also inconsistently and insufficiently absorbed, so it does not protect the endometrium against cancer, as do OMP and MPA.

Because OMP's sleep-promoting effects may be unknown by many (or even most) doctors, it's important to take charge of the timing yourself: *Only* take OMP about 20 or 30 minutes before you hit the pillow—even if the prescription instructions printed on the bottle tell you to take it three times daily (as my three-capsule, 300-milligram OMP prescriptions did for the longest time!).

Prior cautions that "In the first nights of taking progesterone, you can feel dizziness or 'drunk' if you are awakened within an hour or two of taking it. And, if you are really behind on rapid-eye-movement sleep, you might feel like sleeping in to catch up," so you might want to take your first dose on a night when you don't need to rocket out of bed the morning after.

Finally, when you're in or near perimenopause, it's easy to slide into the assumption that any new sleep problems you're experiencing are *caused* by the hormonal doings of perimenopause; however, it's important to get checked out by your doctor for other potential causes if you're inappropriately tired. As Prior told me: "What I try to do in someone...in perimenopause with a fatigue concern is to rule out anemia, underactive thyroid problems and depression."

BONUS POINT

A SIDE NOTE ON SLEEP APNEA—POSSIBLY LIFE-SAVING

Sleep apnea, a disorder in which a person's breathing starts and stops many times during sleep, can kill you—or, at the very least, lead to nights of very unsound sleep.

Obesity is associated with an increased risk of sleep apnea. However, people who are slim can also suffer sleep apnea, sometimes caused by the shape of their jaw, neck, palate, or tonsils or a deviated septum in their nose (a curve in the wall between the nostrils that leaves one nasal passage kind of squished).

A major symptom is loud snoring, though not everyone who snores has sleep apnea. Other symptoms include waking up during the night gasping or choking, morning headaches or dry mouth, mood swings, excessive daytime sleepiness, and difficulty concentrating.

If you suspect *you* might have sleep apnea, your primary care doctor can order a sleep study. Getting tested used to require spending the night in a lab. These days, they'll likely send you what looks like a really ugly Playskool "watch" with Bluetooth, along with some electrodes to tape to your chest and directions for uploading the results on your phone the morning after.

ESTROGEN VS. ROASTING BITCHFACE

In menopausal women, estrogen (as prescription estradiol) helps alleviate sleep issues. However, it seems to do this *indirectly*—as a secondary effect of the estradiol diminishing the number and intensity of sleep-interrupting night sweats.

In a study on menopausal women in Finland, six months of transdermal estradiol therapy—delivered by a disposable stick-on skin patch—alleviated sleep problems in a whopping 95 percent of the participants, reports gynecology researcher Risto Erkkola, MD.

Unfortunately, Erkkola's trial wasn't on estrogen alone, but estrogen with MPA. However, the studies that look at estrogen alone likewise find beneficial effects: typically, longer chunks of uninterrupted sleep, along with less thrashing and fewer wakeups throughout the night. These results are similar to those observed with progesterone, such as the increase in REM sleep and the decrease in awake time in menopausal women given 300 milligrams of nightly progesterone in psychiatrist Petra Schüssler's research.

All in all, estrogen (combined with OMP) appears to be a powerful sleep helper for women in menopause who suffer hot flashes and night sweats. However, some women can't or won't take estrogen. Could they take OMP alone not just in perimenopause but in menopause? A 2012 randomized controlled trial by research psychologist Christine Hitchcock and Prior suggests they could. In their study, 300 milligrams of OMP—given alone, sans estrogen—was effective, compared with the placebo, for diminishing severe and frequent hot flashes and improving sleep in 133 healthy menopausal women (ages 44 to 62, one to 10 years since their final menstrual period).

A few notes: Being "effective, compared with the placebo" translates to "was more effective than no treatment at all"; however, that's still something—and it might be enough. Also, in menopause, by taking only OMP, you'll forego the benefits and protections of estrogen (or estrogen plus OMP) for our bones and cardiovascular system that OMP alone cannot provide.

LEAKING BEAUTY
When estrogen goes, so does the plumbing

There's another major menopausal sleep killer—one we don't hear much about: being awakened by the need to pee, aka "nocturia." You know that euphemism, "answering nature's call"? Well, think of nature as an insomniac stalker ringing you throughout the night from an unblockable number.

Nocturia is technically the interruption of sleep *one or more times* by the urge to urinate. Naturally, my body went with "or more," and I spent my nights keeping the toilet seat from getting lonely—sometimes waking up to pee four times. *Or more!*

Nocturia is a symptom of overactive bladder (OAB), along with other fun symptoms like "urinary frequency" (needing to go more than seven times in a day) and randomly leaking pee.

Though nocturia makes it seem like your adult-lady bladder got swapped out for a sparrow's, it isn't that your bladder shrank—just its previous usefulness. It results from the menopausal decline in estrogen and the ensuing erosions of the musculature and connective tissue holding the bladder and other pelvic organs.

When estrogen declines, the bacterial world of the bladder and urinary tract also changes. In premenopausal women with normal estrogen levels, healthy *lactobacilli* overwhelmingly rule the "roost." After estrogen takes its leave in menopause, a more *diverse* bacterial population rises up. "Diversity" might sound good. It's anything but if you happen to be a bladder or would like yours to function properly. "Increased bladder microbiome diversity is associated with overactive bladder," explains microbiologist Krystal Thomas-White.

Thomas-White and her colleagues find that prescription estrogen does some important bacterial population management in menopausal women with OAB symptoms, increasing the amount of helpful *lactobacilli* in both the bladder and their urine. This increase is associated with "modest" improvement in "urgency incontinence symptoms"—which include the sudden urgent need to pee and a renegade bladder that leaks urine, refusing to wait till you get to a toilet.

Based on this and similar findings, menopausal women are prescribed estradiol—dispensed vaginally or throughout the body ("systemically")—for nocturia and other symptoms of OAB. (If systemic estrogen alone doesn't do the job, doctors will often prescribe supplemental vaginal estrogen.)

Personally, my wee-hours pee promiscuity got dialed way down when I started using systemic estrogen: the estradiol patch. I'll wake up once or sometimes twice a night to pee—FAR fewer times than before I started using it. My experience mirrors the evidence on estrogen's helpfulness in alleviating nocturia (along with various other "down there" symptoms)—in addition to diminishing those boil-you-awake alarm clocks, night sweats, which tend to lead to irate, overheated trips to the throne.

DOES YOUR INSOMNIA NEED A CHAT WITH A THERAPIST?

You'll see articles proclaiming cognitive behavioral therapy for insomnia (CBT-i) "the most effective nonpharmacological treatment for chronic insomnia." I'm a fan of cognitive behavioral therapy, and specifically the form called Rational Emotive Behavior Therapy (REBT), founded by the late Dr. Albert Ellis, that involves applying reason to correct counterproductive irrational beliefs and the behavior that results from them. (See his book *A Guide to Rational Living* for a how-to, sans therapist, or google REBT.)

Research on insomnia in menopausal and perimenopausal women *does* report that CBT-i improves sleep: for example, by identifying and challenging negative beliefs about sleep and reducing anxiety about getting to sleep and staying asleep—anxiety that, rather predictably, tends to worsen insomnia. Therapists also suggest limits around time and activities in bed (for example, sleep and sex only) and dispense tips on "sleep hygiene," like wearing a sleep mask and keeping the bedroom cool (information that's valuable, but also plentiful on Google).

But *are* irrational beliefs about sleep issues a problem for you? It is *not* irrational to see your perimenopausal or menopausal insomnia as a seriously suckitudinous state of affairs, nor is it irrational to wish you could sleep through the night (without extraordinary measures like having yourself clocked on the head with a well-seasoned cast-iron pan). If, however, you engage in pointless fretting about not sleeping, which leads to even more fretting, not more sleeping, you might want to give CBT-i a try.

The University of Pennsylvania has an international directory of CBT-i providers (at https://cbti.directory). There are also CBT-i apps—some free—and a slew of CBT-i sleep workbooks for ten, twelve, or twenty bucks. Psychology Today.com and AlbertEllis.org list REBT therapists. (Note that being listed on any of these therapist-finder sites is not synonymous with being good—or even adequate.)

Had *my* perimenopausal sleeplessness resulted or gotten worse from some lapse in reasoning, I would've hopped right on correcting it. However, in perimenopause, it was my body chemistry—estrogen run wild and progesterone gone AWOL—blocking me from getting to sleep and then jacking me awake. Replacing the missing progesterone with OMP not only helped me sleep but also alleviated my other perimenopausal symptoms in a way a therapist-directed chat with my rebellious body chemistry could not.

THE GHOST OF SLEEPLESSNESS FUTURE

A year or so into menopause, I was still taking my nightly 300 milligrams of OMP when my sleep once again turned to crap. It wasn't as terrible as it was before OMP, but I found myself waking up an hour or a couple hours into sleep, struggling to go back to sleep, and repeating the process throughout the night. Eventually, I'd wake up—to a fuzzy brain and a distinct lack of energy to write anything more lengthy and complex than a tweet.

Why did OMP stop being effective? Good question! One that researchers have yet to answer! As experimental psychologist Pauline Maki and her colleagues put it in 2024: "Robust scientific research is needed to...determine the causal mechanisms behind menopause-related sleep complaints."

I take a conservative approach to prescription drugs, and especially sleep drugs, with all their awful ride-along side effects. Supplements also can be harmful, but I started there. I use Consumerlab.com, a fee-based membership site that sends supplements out to independent labs for testing and publishes the results: whether they contain the stuff they claim to, in the amount they claim to, and without any bonus "gift with purchase" stuff, like heavy metals or arsenic.

I tried every supplement with three shreds of scientific validation that it helped improve sleep. None of them improved mine. My writing output again plunged—from productive paragraphs and sections daily to just this side of a haiku. Uh-oh. I had two books to turn in—ideally, before I turned 90. There was a trade-off to be made—sucky sleep vs. sleep drug downsides—and I gave in to the latter.

I have a terrific psychiatrist—wise, kind, and evidence-driven—who prescribes me my meds for ADHD (Attention Deficit Hyperactivity Disorder). I told him I wanted to find a sleeping pill that worked for me with the least awful side effects. He and I came up with about six possible candidates, including the "sedating pill," Ambien (again, zolpidem in generic), which I didn't want to take, and a newer drug, Rozerem (ramelteon in generic), which is basically medical melatonin.

Ramelteon doesn't suppress breathing and washes out of the body quickly (though I do wonder whether it's healthy and safe to take melatonin long-term). I really wanted ramelteon to work. It did—sort of. Because it helps only sleep induction and not sleep maintenance, it got me to sleep—and then left me stranded in my sleep-thrash-sleep-thrash cycle the rest of the night.

Vetting sleep drugs is beyond the scope of this book (that is, making my book deadline), but I'll tell you where I ended up (which absolutely should not be taken as a recommendation and may work for me in a way it doesn't work for others).

My psychiatrist recommended trazodone (the generic for Desyrel), which is classified as an antidepressant. It reduces the levels of arousal-inducing neurotransmitters and only very weakly affects the neurotransmitter serotonin. It has sedative properties (grr... but it's much less potent than Ambien and Restoril, the drugs I've sneered at as "sedation pills"). Because of this, it's associated with less disruption of "sleep architecture"—that healthy, balanced pattern of sleep stages (with sufficient time in each one and sufficient sleep overall).

Trazodone is prescribed off-label for sleep, meaning it is not FDA-approved as a sleep drug. They say they have insufficient data on its effects on sleep, and probably because of that, you'll see warnings here and there online that it should not be used for sleep. However, my psychiatrist had a whole lot of clinical experience with it, and his answers to my questions about it made me feel it was probably the single best drug I could take to get my sleep back.

Even sleep scientist Matthew Walker, a neuroscientist who is a walking encyclopedia of every terrible thing about Ambien and other "sedating pills," has nice things to say about trazodone. Appearing in 2023 on Tim Ferriss's podcast, he said to Ferriss: Trazodone "sounds like a tranquilizer. And it's not like that at all. It's actually very nuanced. And what I like about its profile perhaps is that, from a scientific perspective, . . . it tries to do something more naturalistic. It tries to switch off the volume of the wake-promoting regions and therefore allows sleep, the passage of sleep to be produced and arrive with you in a more naturalistic way."

Though trazodone made me congested at first and continues to give me mild dry-eye (which I manage with preservative-free artificial tears), the major possible adverse effects—like an extended erection!—were not a cause of concern for me. I did get checked out for "angle-closure" in my eyes, as people with it who take trazodone can end up going blind. (My ophthalmologist said this is a very rare condition he sees maybe once a year.)

For me, trazodone ended up being the gentlest and best of the six sleep drugs I tested, so I'm still taking it: 250 milligrams a night (though I started with 50 and then 100—until my insomnia got worse as I progressed further into menopause, and I needed more). The 250-milligram dose is what it takes to give me a full night's sleep—often uninterrupted, which is, lemme tell you, *glorious*. However, I again want to emphasize: If you decide to opt for a sleep drug, you and your doctor need to take your individual health profile into account to decide which, if any, might work for you.

— 10 —

HOT FLASHES AND NIGHT SWEATS

There's a dumpster fire burning and it's inside us

I STARTED CALLING NIGHT sweats "sweats du nuit"—hoping to feel more "slightly overheated Coco Chanel" than "sweat-soaked flophouse wino in late-stage DTs."

It helped not in the slightest.

Hot flashes and night sweats are the most misery-inducing symptoms of menopause and perimenopause. A hot flash is basically a single-serving hellfire—erupting inside you without the slightest courtesy of a warning and blasting you for a minute or two straight (or four or five—or, less commonly, maybe for up to 10 minutes, if you're among the more physiologically cursed).

Hot flashes plague an estimated 80 percent of women in perimenopause and more than 75 percent in menopause. Some women only get them in menopause. A whole lot of us get them in both stages. And for about a third of women, hot flashes are "severely problematic," reports gynecologist Nanette Santoro, wreaking major havoc on their health, mental health, work, and relationships.

Hot flashes come in different intensities—*mild, moderate,* and *severe*—explains Stanford sleep researcher Maurice Ohayon, MD:

- **Mild:** A sensation of heat without sweating.
- **Moderate:** A sensation of heat with sweating, but not enough to prevent the pursuit of an activity.

- **Severe:** A sensation of heat with sweating, causing a woman to stop her activity.

Speaking from personal experience, when you are amongst other humans, "stopping your activity" becomes a mortifying one-woman show.

Pre-pandemic, volunteering as a mediator at LA City Hall, I worked every Wednesday in a low-walled cubicle surrounded by those of my colleagues-slash-audience.

The dreaded beginnings of a perimenopausal hot flash would rise up in me.

I'm frantic. Gotta "get sleeveless"—tear off each of the three layers of clothing (shrug, jacket, scarf) I wear due to City Hall air-conditioning perpetually set on "igloo." I lunge to turn on the tower fan in my cubicle—a "shared" fan for our entire City Hall floor that I share with no one. Final step: a frenzied grope through the paper blizzard on my desk for a crumpled Kleenex or a coffee napkin.

Mop, mop, mop.

More mop—for four or five broiling, runny makeup-faced, drenchingly miserable minutes...

Until... WHOA! I'm FREEZING!

Frantic again! I slam the fan to "off" and fumble my layers on. Layer, layer, layer. Gross sweaty napkins litter my desk. Embarrassment litters me.

In my head, I push past it: "Okay, back to work!"

In my body, "Hah—not for long!"

HOT TIMES—OF UNTOLD LENGTH AND MYSTERIOUS ORIGIN

In Chapter Three, I mentioned my prediction that my hot flashes, still going strong years into menopause, will never end.

As for what the rest of you might expect (from perimenopause on), there's been a myth hanging around medicine that these ladyboilers last only a few years—one or two, or maybe five. However, in 2015, the SWAN researchers found that hot flashes and night sweats last seven years, on average.

(If only that were the bad news!)

The bad news: There are "super flashers" whose hot flashes start before perimenopause or early into it—and persist for *12 years, on average!*

The really bad news: A third of women who had moderate-to-severe hot flashes were still experiencing them *10 or more years after menopause!*

Some still had them *20 or more years later!*

Twenty years—"or more."

"A small proportion of women will never be free of them," notes Santoro.

In light of how pervasive and disturbing hot flashes are for such sick stretches of time, you'd think the causes and underlying mechanisms would be comprehensively mapped out.

They aren't.

Hot flashes are a complex process driven by a combination of chemicals, systems, and different areas of the brain and body, observes gynecologist Nicoletta Biglia, MD. Also playing a role are genetics, diet, medications, and cultural and personal expectations and experiences—especially stressful ones.

So, while researchers have made important advances in recent years, they still have a good deal of work to do. That said, the general understanding we and our doctors have of hot flashes isn't *wrong*: unwanted personal climate change from sudden, intense blasts of heat that surge through our body.

However, this understanding is incomplete.

Hot flashes aren't just uncomfortable. They're harmful.

CENTRAL OVERHEATING
How hot flashes burn down your health

Hot flashes are not just bursts of heat. They are also bursts of "fight-or-flight" chemicals: stress hormones like cortisol and adrenaline (aka epinephrine), preceded by the stress neurotransmitter, norepinephrine, in the brain.

Cortisol is wrongly seen as a "bad guy" hormone, laments neuroscientist Bruce McEwen—dismayed that most mentions of "high cortisol" or "elevated cortisol" paint it as a hormonal Dr. Evil, plotting our physiological ruin. Cortisol is a vital hormone "we would not live very long or well without," he adds. "So let us not blame it for our problems unless it stays elevated when it should not be or is not turned on when we need it!"

McEwen explains that cortisol, elevated here and there on an as-needed basis, boosts our energy level, helps maintain our immune function, keeps our metabolism in check, and is major in helping us cope with stress.

The problem is not elevated cortisol but *chronically elevated cortisol*: cortisol that's endlessly on "blast," which can provoke (or contribute to) a cascade of harmful inflammatory conditions and effects—many of which are also chronically cortisol elevating!

Chronically elevated cortisol chemically vandalizes our health all the way from our brain to the muscles in our big toe; for example, suppressing our immune response and accelerating bone loss. Persistently high cortisol puts us at risk of weight gain, type 2 diabetes, and other metabolic diseases, reports gynecologist Angelo Cagnacci, MD, "thereby increasing the risk" for cardiovascular disease.

Now, a single hot flash does not turn on an endless fire hose of cortisol. However, in women who suffer *frequent* hot flashes and night sweats, Cagnacci and other researchers are increasingly finding cumulative effects: chronically elevated levels of cortisol.

Hot flashes and night sweats are associated with a host of inflammatory symptoms and chronic inflammatory conditions that echo those associated with elevated cortisol; for example, the eroded bone quality and fracture risk of osteoporosis and an increased risk of cardiovascular disease.

And this is scary: *As a group*, women like me who suffer *severe* hot flashes—the sort so ragingly awful we have to stop whatever we're doing—are more than *twice as likely* to suffer a "non-fatal cardiovascular event": a heart attack, stroke, or angina (chest pain from reduced blood flow to the heart). We are also almost twice as likely to have a hip fracture.

Before we go on, it's important to note three words above: *As a group*.

Remember "relative risk" from Chapter Two? That "more than twice as likely!" statistic *is not our personal, individual risk* but the risk of our *group*—in this case, women who suffer severe hot flashes—relative to the group of women whose bodies remain temperate like a beautiful, breezy spring day. So despite my being in the group of women whose bodies seem to be inhabited by a tiny but determined arsonist, my individual "cardiometabolic" health metrics—low triglyceride level, normal blood sugar, very healthy blood pressure, and very low bodily inflammation—suggest my risk of heart disease is *extremely low*.

If your risk is moderate to high, then being told you're a member of this group could be an important wake-up call: Better hop to it on getting "heart healthy" (and the same goes for doing more than ignoring your bones).

The negative health effects from both chronically elevated cortisol and chronically elevated inflammation are major players in a hot-flash- and night-sweat-afflicted vicious circle. Severe hot flashes and night sweats in menopausal and perimenopausal women are "strongly associated" with chronic insomnia. Insomnia is not only linked with brain fog but weight gain and irritability, which can lead to relationship clashes, tanking job performance, and a big gloomy slump in life satisfaction: the sort of stuff that can keep us awake—even more than the insomnia already doing a number on us!

The weight gain is an especially pernicious symptom. In menopausal and perimenopausal women, being overweight or obese is associated with suffering more intense and life-torching hot flashes. The more overweight a woman is, the worse the hot flashes. Female smokers who are overweight or obese have *the* most horrible hot flashes of all.

Finally, hot flashes and night sweats that torment us for long stretches of time are particularly concerning. Research on menopausal women found that 10 or more years of hot flashes and night sweats was associated with an increased risk of breast cancer. Lest you suspect hormone therapy might've been a factor, study participants were women who'd *never used hormone therapy*: 25,499 menopausal women, ages 50 to 79 (from a 2018 WHI follow-up analysis, comparing women with persistent hot flashes to women who'd never had them).

YOUR BODY'S HVAC SYSTEM
Pretty amazing till the thermostat breaks

Hot flashes actually have a function: cooling us off by releasing our body heat through the surface of our skin.

Hot flashes and night sweats are "neurovascular"—brain- and artery-driven attempts at "thermoregulation": the *process* of maintaining a steady internal (core) temperature—within healthy boundaries.

Your brain tells your body to adjust your temperature by altering the flow of blood to your skin. Say you're cold. Constricting your blood vessels reduces the blood flow to your skin, decreasing the amount of heat that can escape from it. If you're overheated, the blood vessels near the surface of your skin "dilate," increasing blood flow to your skin to dissipate heat. ("Perspiration"—aka sweating like a plowhorse—is often a partner in "facilitating heat loss.")

It's that increased blood flow to your skin that makes you feel hot—or if you're like me, on the verge of self-incineration—leading you to tear off every article of clothing you can without arrest for public indecency... while seated amongst your completely chill co-workers in a climate-controlled conference room.

Welcome to Dante's Humiliating Inferno. Population: You.

Dress! Undress! Dress! Undress!

(Boil with hate.)

Our body's temperature control center is the hypothalamus. It's a tiny structure in the middle of our brain in charge of maintaining the body in its normal, stable state (called "homeostasis"): not too hot, not too cold, and not keeling over from hunger or thirst—to name a few.

The hypothalamus monitors our internal environment by taking readings of our hydration and nutrient levels, blood pressure, temperature, hormone levels, and our stress level (which it tracks by keeping tabs on the doings of cortisol and other stress chemicals). Additionally, it monitors the external temperature, as it affects us, through thermoreceptors in our skin. ("As it affects us" reflects that it doesn't "care" that it's a breezy day; it just gets to work on temperature adjustment if it's so breezy we're freezing cold.)

If any adjustments *are* needed to maintain homeostasis, the hypothalamus puts the word out to get 'er done: sending out calls to action in hormone form—to our body and to its junior exec, the pituitary. The pituitary then signals our other glands and organs to take necessary action.

Say the hypothalamus notices that our blood is low on water. It tells the pituitary, "Dude, get on this!" The pituitary releases antidiuretic hormone, which signals the kidneys to reabsorb water while they're filtering waste from your blood, which minimizes the amount of water that gets sent out in pee. We, the person with this amazing process going on inside us, also get a work summons—in the form of being pinged with the sense that we're thirsty, which motivates us to grab a drink.

The same process can trigger hot flashes. We're flipping through a magazine in the air-conditioned waiting room at the dentist when the hypothalamus notices something out of whack—some apparent temperature irregularity.

It sounds the alarm: "Help! Help! HEAT POLICING TIME!"

But... *is it?* Sitting there in that chilly waiting room, is our internal temperature *really* at some health-impairing, scary-deadly level and in need of correction?

In fact... IT ISN'T! False alarm!

One that triggers the hypothalamus to send the cool-down crew in the form of a hot flash to expel the supposed heat supposedly boiling our guts out.

Unfortunately, the "Hot or Not?" metric it uses has parted company with reality—reality being our normal "thermoneutral zone": the rather broad range of temperatures in our external environment that allow our body to maintain its core temperature without needing to instigate heat-up or cool-down processes.

The "neutral" in "thermoneutral" effectively means "no conflict." (*No emergency. Nothing to be done here; please move along.*)

In women who are hot flash sufferers, this "neutral" range shrinks bigtime—narrowing to the point that even a tiny bump in temperature sets off the hypothalamic fire alarm.

But is it just narrowed—or might it even be *gone*? The notion that it was merely narrowed was the prevailing belief in the field—till endocrinologist Robert R. Freedman, MD, in the 1990s, had female research participants swallow a data-transmitting pill thermometer. Some participants were hot flash sufferers; some were not. Freedman found that in women with hot flashes, "the thermoneutral zone, within which sweating and other heat-decreasing processes are not triggered, is virtually nonexistent." Meanwhile, in asymptomatic women, it remained normal, with the usual broad range of temperatures.

In menopause, prescription estrogen significantly reduces the number of hot flashes women experience through its effects on the thermoneutral zone. Freedman's pill thermometer research found that estrogen raises the "core body temperature sweating threshold"—the temperature at which the hypothalamus triggers the body to sweat to cool down. Ultimately, estrogen makes the hypothalamus more tolerant of minor ups and downs in temperature, which translates to fewer hot flashes.

YOUR BRAIN IS AN ESTROGEN JUNKIE
It's estrogen withdrawal, not low estrogen, overheating us

There's been an entrenched assumption in research and medicine that hot flashes and night sweats are caused by *low* estrogen levels. Period. Case closed. But low estrogen alone as an explanation is contradicted by readily available inconvenient facts—like how children, with their low estrogen levels, are not overheating like crazy (though a good many will grow up to be women who suffer hot flashes).

Women with low estrogen levels *do* experience hot flashes—but not *all* women with low levels. Take menopausal women. "All menopausal women have low estrogen levels," Prior notes, yet only some have hot flashes. Meanwhile, the often-elevated estrogen levels of perimenopause are associated with *more* hot flashes, as well as *more severe* hot flashes, than the low estrogen levels of menopause.

Freedman's research on both women and animals suggests hot flashes are triggered not by *low* estrogen levels but by precipitously *dropping* estrogen levels—like we see with estrogen spikes and dives in perimenopause, with the dive suddenly leaving the estrogen "cupboard" way understocked or bare. Other studies likewise find fluctuating estrogen (rather than the mere presence or lack of it) to be a hot flash trigger.

Additionally, Freedman notes that in animals, elevated levels of the stress neurotransmitter norepinephrine ("brain norepinephrine") trigger the narrowing of the thermoneutral zone, inciting hot flashes. He hypothesized that it would do the same in women. To investigate, he dispensed the tree-bark-derived supplement yohimbe, which elevates brain norepinephrine, to women with hot flashes. As he'd suspected, it "led to an increase in the frequency and severity" of their hot flashes. His finding adds to the evidence that elevations in norepinephrine join lowered estrogen and estrogen fluctuations in provoking hot flashes and night sweats.

The stage is set for this estrogen/stress hormone tumult decades before perimenopause and menopause. When we start having periods, our brain—and specifically, the hypothalamus—becomes "habituated" to the high estrogen levels that accompany our monthly cycle, Dr. Prior explains.

This habituation continues throughout our 20s and 30s. Then, after all this month-after-month consistency, rebellious perimenopausal estrogen comes on the scene, soaring and then diving erratically. This sudden drop, temporarily cutting off the expected estrogen supply, causes our body to have a "Hey, where's my 'E'?!"-driven stress chemical freakout, the ignition point for hot flashes.

We can also experience this "Where's my 'E'?!" freakout in menopause. Though, in menopause, our estrogen levels are not jumping around but low, our hypothalamus has spent a long time during our menstruating years getting used to (and thus expecting) a consistently high supply of "E." The fact that it's our own body cutting off our supply is immaterial.

The same habituation takes place with prescription estrogen that gets cut off. Some menopausal women who start taking estrogen and then stop get clobbered with "rebound" hot flashes and night sweats—more intense than those they had before initiating estrogen therapy.

This "rebound" effect might sound a bit familiar—maybe in a *Drugstore Cowboy*/*Panic in Needle Park* kind of way.

In the 1970s, pioneering reproductive endocrinologist Samuel Yen, MD, likened going cold turkey on estrogen to going cold turkey on drugs. Hot flashes, he writes, seem to be a "manifestation" of "estrogen withdrawal"—a sort of jonesing for estrogen—brought about by "estrogen-sensitive neurons within the brain, which are linked to thermoregulation."

Yen offers the example of women with a genetic disorder called "Turner Syndrome." Because these women's ovaries produce very little estrogen, they don't experience hot flashes—that is, not until they are administered prescription estrogen and then have it stopped. Their bodies are used to a certain level of estrogen, and then it's suddenly gone—and for the first time, they experience what Yen refers to as "classic menopausal hot flashes."

Yen sees striking similarities between estrogen withdrawal and opiate withdrawal (from trying to kick drugs like heroin or oxycodone). In each case, there's a surge in stress neurotransmitters and hormones, triggering a slew of the same symptoms: hot flashes, a flushed face and neck, intense sweating followed by chills, and, at night, extremely disturbed sleep with drenching night sweats.

Withdrawal is a form of chemical panic—that WHERE THE HELL IS IT?!! internal frenzy I wrote about above—when a substance our body has grown dependent on suddenly gets cut off. Though the internal commotion comes from our body jonesing for its regular fix of oxy or "E," our brain and body's ancient threat detection apparatus reads this chemical ruckus as a warning that we're under attack. The hypothalamus triggers our threat defense system, our "fight-or-flight" response, and the release of norepinephrine and cortisol, which amp up our alertness and blast us with energy to do battle or run like hell.

The turbocharge provided by these and other fight-or-flight chemicals is an important protective force on the rare occasion we're in danger. On less perilous occasions, it can be problematic. Hot-flash-provokingly problematic.

Elevations in norepinephrine and the various stress hormones that get triggered can also provoke anxiety, which might explain why night sweats make me bolt awake—night terrors-style. My head seems to be in a clamp; I'm breathing in stabs, hard and fast; and I feel like I've been poisoned—every cell of my body toxified—due to the fight-or-flight chemical army mobilizing in me, rendering me right and ready to take on those vicious bedcovers.

Prior experienced something similar: "I know that I felt angry (in fact, furious) when I suddenly wakened in what was my first night sweat, and those emotions occurred before I even started to sweat!"

A PRESCRIPTION FOR CLIMATE CHANGE

OMP—prescribed on its own—appears to alleviate hot flashes and night sweats in both perimenopause and menopause, as does MPA (though MPA always brings along some ugly baggage in the form of side effects).

"Progesterone, produced by our body or as OMP, raises the temperature [threshold] at which sweating starts, and therefore corrects the narrowed thermoneutral zone that is the key problem" in hot flashes, Prior explains. The same goes for MPA.

However, only OMP—"full-dose" OMP of 300 milligrams nightly—suppresses estrogen's stimulation of norepinephrine levels, likely by "decreasing or stabilizing" norepinephrine and its partner stress hormones, speculates ob-gyn Rong Chen, MD (with Prior and other co-authors). By suppressing estrogen's effects, it decreases the boomeranging of estrogen and stress neurotransmitters and hormones: estrogen elevating these stress chemicals and the stress chemicals elevating estrogen, making for a fiery hot-flash-apalooza.

In menopause, when your own internal estrogen levels are low, "treatment with estrogen alone or in combination with MPA or OMP is found to be the most effective therapy for hot flashes and night sweats," explains Prior.

"Interestingly, and something rarely mentioned, is that estrogen-progestin therapy" [estrogen plus MPA] "was statistically more effective than estrogen-alone" therapy," the Chen-led study reports. Extended use of this combo "brings women relief" from persistent hot flashes and night sweats, "and may also have positive bone mineral density (BMD) effects and prevent fracture."

Not surprisingly, the merits of OMP as a stand-alone treatment for hot flashes and night sweats have been heartily ignored by the research community. The same goes for MPA as a treatment for hot flashes and night sweats. (MPA and other progestins mainly show up in research as a uterine cancer–preventing add-on given with estrogen-alone therapy.)

Over a 40-year period, from January 1980 to January 2020, there were only seven randomized controlled trials on MPA or OMP for alleviating menopausal symptoms, report ob-gyn Shelley Dolitsky and her colleagues. Prior and her colleagues tried to get funding from the Medical Research Council of Canada to run a comparison of the effects of low-dose oral contraceptives (which contain MPA) and progesterone therapy on menopausal symptoms.

The funding request was a no-go. Three times. The funding entity that rejected each version of these three submissions claimed that testing progesterone was unnecessary. They based their determination on a trial that deemed oral contraceptives successful in alleviating menopausal symptoms (and never mind the trial's methodological problems—which meant the results could be due to mere chance). Of course, oral contraceptives are not designed to treat menopausal symptoms or typically prescribed for that purpose, while OMP is.

The lack of funding to even *consider* scientific questions means we patients continue to be treated based on fossilized beliefs rather than well-validated testing. But Prior is beyond dogged, and in the 25 years since she tried to get this study funded, her research and that of a small circle of other researchers have found both OMP and MPA to be effective treatments for hot flashes and night sweats in menopause and perimenopause.

We've known this about MPA for quite some time. "Since the 1970s," Prior explains, "many progestins...especially medroxyprogesterone have proven to be effective treatment" for hot flashes—when paired with estrogen and on their own. For example, "One progestin called megestrol (Megace) that is used in women with advanced breast cancer decreased hot [flashes] by 83% over only one month."

OMP is likewise powerful for alleviating hot flashes and night sweats in menopause. The North American Menopause Society (NAMS) endorsed it in their 2022 practice guidelines for treating menopausal women, explaining that oral "micronized progesterone 300 mg nightly significantly decreases" hot flashes and night sweats "compared with placebo and improves sleep."

As support for this recommendation, the NAMS researchers cite a study referenced in Chapter Nine: Christine Hitchcock and Dr. Prior's 133-participant randomized controlled trial on OMP for menopausal women's hot flashes and night sweats—research deemed "high-quality evidence" per a methodology assessment tool called GRADE.

SORRY, PERIMENOPAUSAL LADIES FRYING ON THE INSIDE

It's like perimenopausal women don't even exist!

"There is almost no evidence" informing treatment of hot flashes in perimenopause—the very stage in which they begin, Prior complains. "This is astonishing!" The lack of evidence is decidedly not for lack of effort—for three whole decades!—on Prior's part.

There's ONE STUDY! One lone study researching OMP's effects on these symptoms suffered by 80 percent of women in perimenopause!

At the 2018 Endocrine Society conference, Prior and her colleagues presented their data from that study: "the first ever" randomized controlled trial investigating OMP as a treatment for perimenopausal hot flashes and night sweats.

The participants were 189 perimenopausal women, given 300 milligrams of OMP nightly. OMP significantly decreased both the number and intensity of the women's hot flashes and night sweats, with a reported 55 percent decrease in the number suffered. The reduction was even greater in the 46 women in the trial with severe symptoms (defined as more than 50 hot flashes and/or night sweats a week). None of the participants reported adverse effects during the treatment or rebound hot flashes or night sweats upon its discontinuation.

Unfortunately, the study ended up being "underpowered" (a statistical term indicating the sample size—i.e., the number of participants—was too small, meaning there were not enough participants to determine whether the results were from the treatment rather than random chance).

However!...

They researchers did find a *"clinically important benefit"*: a clinical research term describing improvements in a patient's health and/or quality of life perceived by a doctor or patient. Though this doesn't have the same weight as evidence from a scientific study, it's considered a meaningful outcome, reflecting enhanced well-being from the patient's perspective. In this case, the clinically important benefit was the OMP-treated participants' perception that they had fewer night sweats, significantly better-quality sleep, and, consequently, "less perimenopause-related life interference."

In the wake of the study, Carol Herbert, MD, professor emeritus and former Dean of the University of Western Ontario's School of Medicine & Dentistry, told the medical news service Medical Xpress, "Given the evidence and urgent need for effective treatment of perimenopausal [hot flashes and night sweats], a physician can reasonably prescribe a trial of 300 mg of oral micronized progesterone for a menstruating woman having night sweats waking her twice a week or more frequently."

Clinical experience—individual experiences of patients observed by doctors—lacks the protective measures of experimental studies, like controlling for bias. However, due to the giant empty crater where the slew of randomized controlled trials on OMP *specifically for perimenopausal hot flashes* should be, it's what we've got.

Back when I decided to try progesterone, the possibility it might rescue me from the whirling vat of fiery perimenopausal torture, combined with its safety record in the decades it's been prescribed in France, led me to take the plunge. Dr. Prior, before me, arrived at the same calculation.

She writes, "When I began jolting awake every night in a wringing sweat, taking oral micronized progesterone (bio-identical and sold as FDA-approved Prometrium) saved me." As she saw it, "It made sense—if estrogen's too high and progesterone's too low—take what's deficient."

My experience mirrored Prior's. OMP didn't make my hot flashes and night sweats go away entirely, either in perimenopause or menopause, but they were fewer and much less intense—making me feel like a person who gets inexplicably overheated instead of like Satan's 24-hour, remote-controlled ladyfurnace.

WHEN "ALTERNATIVE MEDICINE" MEANS ALTERNATIVE TO MEDICINE PROVEN TO WORK

Big Pharma gets all the sneers while Big Vitamin gets a pass.

It shouldn't.

I searched for the magic supplement that could beat out or at least come close to the effectiveness of drug therapy for alleviating hot flashes and other menopausal symptoms. Summing up what I discovered, gynecologist David Archer, MD, writes: "Substantial funding from the National Institutes of Health" and other non-pharma sources "has failed to show any benefit of over-the-counter therapies compared to placebo for hot flashes."

Consider oft-recommended plant extracts, such as red clover isoflavones and black cohosh, which have estrogen-like effects. Large randomized controlled trials have found these supplements are no better than a placebo.

Hormone therapy via regulated FDA-approved prescription drugs—for example, OMP and transdermal estradiol—is backed by extensive research showing its effectiveness for alleviating hot flashes and other symptoms. More importantly, we don't have to cross our fingers that the contents of the OMP capsules will be powerful enough to counterbalance estrogen and protect our endometrium.

Standards for supplements ideally would be as rigorous as those for pharmaceuticals, but, for example, nobody'll make megabucks funding a trial on the vitamin B12 that anybody with a vitamin factory can throw into a bottle. In the absence of scientifically acceptable evidence that a particular supplement can stand in for hormone therapy or come close, opting for it amounts to opting out of protecting your health and alleviating your symptoms.

The same applies to scientifically unproven concoctions prescribed by "naturopaths," who typically hawk them as safer and more bodily harmonious: claims which are, in a word, *hooey*. Naturopaths tend to favor estrogen lozenges called "troches" and compounded estrogen mixes like "Bi-est" and "Tri-est." Outrageously, the Bi-est and Tri-est formulas are not based on the potency or bioavailability of each estrogen in the combo, "but simply on the milligram quantity of the different agents added together," explains clinical endocrinologist Walter P. Borg, MD.

So, yes, this stuff is technically hormone therapy—in a potion your eight-year-old nerdbro baby brother might've whipped up for you in the garage. As Borg puts it: "There is no scientific evidence" for the improved safety or efficacy of these "bi" and "tri" cocktails "compared to FDA-approved pharmaceutical products in treatment of menopausal women."

LISTENING TO PROZAC—OR TELLING IT TO SHUT UP?

Antidepressants *do* diminish hot flashes—but at what price?

Certain antidepressants, including fluoxetine (Prozac), paroxetine (Paxil), desvenlafaxine (Khedezla and Pristiq), and citalopram (Celexa), can reduce hot flashes by 50 percent or more. *(More on these in Chapter Fifteen.)*

However, side effects from these drugs include sleepiness, weight gain, and sexual issues, such as a decreased libido and delayed orgasms—or an inability to orgasm altogether. There's also an emotionally numbing effect. So, yay, fewer hot flashes, but you're maybe heavier, sex is a dull chore, and you feel dead inside.

Should all of this start to wear on you, you might get to experience "discontinuation syndrome": the slew of persistent, debilitating symptoms like dizziness, nausea, fatigue, vomiting, and insomnia that hit many people when they try to get off an antidepressant. Breaking up with an antidepressant *requires* very gradually tapering off the drug—taking progressively less and less, as directed and monitored by a doctor. Even then, some patients find it near impossible to pry themselves out of its chemical clutches.

Additional non-hormonal drugs that can help with hot flashes include gabapentin (Neurontin), pregabalin (Lyrica), and clonidine (a drug primarily used to lower blood pressure).

KISS AND COOL DOWN
Looking forward to possible treatments

Other chemical hooligans inciting hot flashes may be three signaling molecules—collectively called KNDY (pronounced "candy"). These include kisspeptin, named for Hershey's Kisses. (The others, sadly, lack cute chocolate snack names.) This KNDY trio acts as a sort of switch to turn on the hormonal and other changes associated with puberty. In perimenopause and menopause, their feedback mechanisms can go on the blink. This can muck up our thermoregulation and react to estrogen withdrawal or other changes in us by triggering hot flashes. This area of research is in its infancy, but it's possible that kisspeptin-influencing drugs could provide symptom relief to women who cannot use estrogen to manage hot flashes and night sweats.

THE CALMER SUTRA
Drug-free ways to temper the hormonal stressfest

Because stress and the stress hormones it gives rise to are two of the perps behind hot flashes, Prior advises making a serious effort to reduce social and emotional stress in our lives. Wise as this advice is, it's not like you can just up and quit your job and wait for the mortgage to be paid by a benevolent genie. However, some of these measures below might help reduce stress, and with it, the stress-hormone fuel supply for hot flashes and their nasty nighttime siblings.

COGNITIVE BEHAVIORAL THERAPY

As I explained in brief in the previous chapter, CBT involves identifying and challenging negative thought patterns and behaviors. It can help us improve our ability to regulate our emotions and cope with what life throws us—leaving us less stressed.

In a randomized controlled trial, cognitive behavioral therapy (CBT) was found to decrease menopausal women's hot flashes and night sweats. Maybe it would decrease yours. However, as with CBT-i (CBT for insomnia), I'm skeptical about its power for change if you, like me, suffer that special estro-stressfest combo pack—intense hot flashes and meth-head-like wired anxiety—making it feel like your life's been relocated into that crazed crows attack scene from Hitchcock's *The Birds*.

DEEP BREATHING

I use slow deep breathing to quickly calm down and fall asleep so I can nap between writing jags. I inhale for about five seconds, hold the breath in for maybe five more, and then very slowly exhale. Slow, deep breathing like this engages the body's Department of Chillaxing, the parasympathetic nervous system.

Again, because my hot flashes and night sweats were so searingly intense in perimenopause, the claim in a few studies I skimmed that a little huff 'n' puff would help alleviate them seemed ludicrous—akin to shooting harsh words at an advancing army: "Take that, you meanies!"

As for you, sure, regular deep breathing *could* knock back your stress a bit. It won't hurt, and I'm guessing we can all use a little calm-down time to take the edge off. However, diving deeper into the science, research on "paced respiration" at the time of a hot flash suggests slow exhales in the moment will not be your heat-beating savior.

EXERCISE

While there's no evidence you can exorcise your demons, exercising them might help. "There is accumulating evidence that physical activity can decrease levels of stress biomarkers, specifically cortisol," in healthy menopausal women, notes epidemiologist Christine Friedenreich in 2019. She mentions some conflicting evidence: "Conversely, several studies of physical activity interventions did not have any effect on resting cortisol levels measured in urine, saliva or blood."

Chances are the type and intensity of exercise are a factor in the contradictory results. In menopausal women, consistently performed resistance training—lifting weights heavy enough to stress your muscles in 10 reps—and cardiovascular exercise (of jogging, running, or aerobic dance intensity) are associated with more time asleep and better-quality sleep, along with myriad other health benefits, including improved mood. (The same goes for perimenopausal women—in the few studies where researchers bothered to look at them.)

People who run Ironman Triathlons tend to be smug about how much healthier they are than we mere mortal exercisers. In fact, when it comes to exercise, more is not necessarily more. "Too much exercise causes inflammation...as does too little," explains Dr. Michael Eades. Overdoing it on vigorous exercise can also release high levels of stress hormones (just like my perimenopausal body managed to do when I wasn't moving at all).

— 11 —

BLOW UP AND THROW UP

Nausea, migraines, bloating, and inflammation run wild

I STARTED CALLING MY cute little Honda hatchback "The Vomit Comet." In my mid-40s, out of nowhere, I began suffering debilitating motion sickness from car travel. Eventually, I couldn't go by car from Venice to downtown Santa Monica—about three miles on flat, pin-straight, grid-style streets—without getting queasy. And no—not even if I were driving. Going even a few miles farther made me so dizzy and nauseated that I'd throw up—which typically led to *days* of being so dizzy, nauseated, and pukey that I was unable to get out of bed.

Inevitably, someone would suggest I take Dramamine before driving. They meant well, so I'd thank them instead of yelling in their face, "WOW...THAT NEVER OCCURRED TO ME!" I likewise resisted the urge to mention that the drowsiness it causes is *just the thing* for an impromptu nap behind the wheel—ending in a flaming head-on collision with the church youth-group minivan.

Even the hardcore motion-sickness med, the scopolamine patch, couldn't cut all the queasy—plus, it gave me intense dry mouth and made me woozy for days.

HURL, INTERRUPTED

A few days after I started taking OMP, my boyfriend at the time had to drive me to the Kaiser pharmacy to pick up some prescription eye stuff. We zigged and zagged through side streets—the only way we might beat the unusually ugly Friday rush-hour traffic and get there before they closed. I was so busy calculating and recalculating the exact best streets to take, I never got around to being all afraid and bummed out that I would for sure throw up when we got there (or maybe before).

We arrived just in time, and ... whoa. Holy crap. I wasn't sick. Not at all. This was especially noteworthy because my former boyfriend, who has many merits, drives with the plodding, lurching finesse of a drunk grandmother.

We still had to get home. Surely I'd get queasy on the way back.

Nope!

As I continued taking OMP, I chanced going longer distances in cars. I mostly did okay, meaning not throwing up unless we took winding roads, made a lot of turns, or got stuck in miles of smoggy stop-and-go traffic. (I hate you, 134 Freeway!)

I'm aware that the drop-off in car sickness I experienced while taking OMP could be a wild coincidence. However, it was so remarkable to me to do the *unremarkable*—travel by car without getting out to throw up into a bush— that I ended up connecting some dots I otherwise might've blown past.

WELCOME TO PERIMENOPUKE

When my motion sickness first started kicking up, I emailed a researcher in the field, Thomas Stoffregen, a University of Minnesota kinesiology professor, hoping his work would help me claw my way to some answers.

Stoffregen had published a paper that caught my attention. Citing research showing that women are especially prone to motion sickness, he and his colleagues ran an experiment comparing the reactions of male and female research participants to a dizzying, oscillating visual. In line with prior research findings, only 9 percent of the males suffered motion sickness—in contrast with 38 percent of the women.

Scientists are like cats. Give them catnip—novel, exciting, scientifically informed questions—and they'll pounce. My email was 50 percent catnip and 50 percent pitiful desperation, and Stoffregen, being a generous guy, called me from an airport somewhere shortly after I sent it.

Unfortunately, the results from the women in his study didn't apply to women in perimenopause, like me. College-age women (19, 20, 23) have different hormonal circumstances from women in their mid-40s. For example, though anovulatory menstrual cycles occur in menstruating women of all ages, in our 40s, as perimenopause starts rising up in us, these progesterone-starved cycles tend to increase in frequency—as do their unpleasant effects.

In line with this, across social media and web forums, in conversation and in research papers, you'll discover that one group of women disproportionately develops motion sickness in adulthood: women in their 40s, suddenly and mysteriously getting struck with it, just as I did.

Sure, that could be a coincidence—or it could be more.

MIGRAINES
("Excuse me, sir, but did you leave your ice pick in my left temple?")

In addition to the motion sickness that tyrannized me in my 40s, I started having vicious migraines. Migraines are classified as "headaches"—probably because the person who tossed them on the pile with the rest of the headaches never had one. They are excruciatingly painful, throbbing head *attacks* that can pulverize their victims for hours or even days—with their savage accomplices: nausea, vomiting, blurred vision, and intense sensitivity to light, sound, and the slightest smell.

Women are three times as likely to suffer migraines as men. Though some women are afflicted from puberty on, for a number of women, they strike in perimenopause. Mercifully, for many women, migraines are no more in menopause (or become infrequent compared with perimenopause and years prior). However, women who go through "surgical menopause" (the removal of their ovaries) face an increased risk of migraines.

Further research is needed to determine why women get migraines (and how we might inhibit or stop them). The science that has been published is a vat of dueling findings—leaving us pretty much nowhere...with a red-hot iron bar stabbing us through our left temple keeping us company.

IS ESTROGEN THE PERP BEHIND MIGRAINES AND MOTION SICKNESS?

Some studies suggest that taking prescription estrogen leads to migraines or more migraines. Some studies suggest otherwise. These conflicting conclusions seemed inexplicable—till I went deep into the pharmacology of estrogen:

specifically, the *pharmacokinetics*, the science on how the body absorbs, distributes, and excretes a particular drug.

One study's results suddenly made a lot of sense. This study found that women taking oral estrogen had an increase in migraines while women using the skin patch form of estrogen did not.

All forms of estrogen are not equal. While transdermal estradiol is delivered through our skin straight into our bloodstream, oral estrogen or estradiol has to take a big detour. It gets sent through our digestive tract to our liver. Our liver does a really good job of neutering chemicals we ingest, breaking them down and diminishing their effects. This means we need a dose of oral estrogen or estradiol that's 10 or 20 times higher than the dose of transdermal estradiol for it to achieve the same protective and symptom-alleviating effects.

As you'll see in Chapter Nineteen, oral estrogen is associated with a number of harms not seen with transdermal, most of which are likely due to the massive dose required. A high dose of estrogen can cause the spike-'n'-dive of estrogen withdrawal—the dive taking place when the liver metabolizes much of the dose. Might some migraine-suffering women be extra sensitive to the high dose required with oral estrogen? In fact, this is a hypothesis there's some evidence to support: estrogen spiking and then diving, with the drop in estrogen triggering a migraine, just as it triggers hot flashes.

There's another potential factor. When estrogen drops, serotonin, a neurotransmitter (aka chemical messenger in the brain), takes a dive, and excess glutamate—an excitatory (aka "stimulating") neurotransmitter—hangs around in the brain instead of being removed. Its hobbies include overstimulating nerve cells to death, provoking anxiety and irritability, cognitive impairment, and DING! DING! DING! ... migraines!

Luckily, there's a way to bust up its fun. Progesterone inhibits excess levels of glutamate through its conversion to good ole Mr. GABA and other calming chemicals in the brain. *(For special dosage instructions for OMP for women with migraines, see Chapter Twenty-Six.)*

It's helpful to understand migraines and motion sickness as a pair of sorts. A number of women experience a middle-aged onset of both. In fact, they "become more prone to motion sickness as their migraine tendency increases," observes motion sickness researcher Timothy Hain, MD, about women seeking treatment at his medical practice.

Research investigating whether motion sickness susceptibility corresponds with a woman's menstrual cycle hormones shows ragingly inconsistent results. This is not surprising, given the ragingly inconsistent methodology from study to study.

Additionally, motion sickness researchers are often so endocrinologically unversed that their results are simply meaningless—like when a rocket scientist (not a euphemism!) decided to investigate the influence of different phases of the menstrual cycle on motion sickness susceptibility in women.

He and his colleagues assembled a subject pool of 16 healthy menstruating women, ages 18 to 36—justifying this choice (most absurdly!) by citing a study by a Royal Air Force pilot-turned-doctor that supposedly found that women's greater motion sickness susceptibility does not vary significantly with age. The participants in that study? Children ages nine to 18 and young adults of college age!

The rocket scientist's study had numerous methodological shortcomings. However, the biggest and most disqualifying was the failure to account for the hormonal differences in women of varying ages—most notably, the increased likelihood of anovulatory menstrual cycles in the 40-something perimenopausal women they'd neglected to include. (Of course, the possibility of anovulatory cycles occuring in *any* women should have been taken into account.)

One way to get an idea of estrogen's effect on motion sickness and migraines is to study what happens when estrogen gets yanked from the picture. Estrogen can be blocked by certain breast cancer drugs. Two Italian sisters who were breast cancer patients "experienced a striking reduction of their intense seasickness after receiving tamoxifen," observed oncologist Lorenzo Gianni and motion sickness researcher John Golding.

Tamoxifen, the most widely prescribed drug for breast cancer worldwide, is an estrogen-blocking SERM (selective estrogen receptor modulator). A SERM acts like that sneaky jerk driver who zips into the parking space you'd been waiting for—except it attaches to estrogen receptors. This prevents estrogen from docking there, which stops it from triggering migraines or motion sickness.

THE INFLAMMATION SUPERHIGHWAY

The more research I read, the more it seemed estrogen plays a role in motion sickness. Elevated perimenopausal estrogen, sans progesterone, leads to swelling and fluid retention—to the point where you suspect you'll show up on Google Maps as a body of water. Spiking estrogen also jacks up a chemical called "histamine," which returns the favor—most charmingly!—by boosting our already-elevated estrogen levels. This can set off a false alarm in the body: a massive *ongoing* false alarm.

Histamine, part of our immune-response team, is tasked with neutralizing and evicting undesirable elements that sneak into our body, such as bacteria, infectious diseases, pollen and other allergens, and toxins from food way past its "eat-by" date.

Histamine is dispatched to the invaded area from specialized white blood cells: immune-system defender cells called "mast cells" and "basophils." The histamine release from these cells causes what we recognize as an allergic reaction: inflammation, swelling, itching, mucus production, and other miseries. As unpleasant as that is—especially when snot production levels lead us to contemplate emergency rowboat purchase—the purpose isn't to torment us or to keep the Nasal Spray Industrial Complex in the black.

Take the swelling and inflammation. These effects are caused by one of the vital roles of histamine: widening our blood vessels so our immuno-soldier white blood cells have open roads to rush down to find and fight the invaders. So, yay histamine—that is, when there's an actual intruder.

But if histamine goes soaring when there's no danger—like when that bitch, turbulent, elevated perimenopausal estrogen, pushes histamine up for no good reason—it leaves you constantly and needlessly inflamed and swollen. Damagingly inflamed and swollen.

We think of inflammation as redness, which it is, but it's also much more. Inflammation is a *process*—a protective response run by our immune system, our body's Department of Defense. It works much like the one in the Pentagon: recognizing foreign invaders, removing or killing them, and then repairing any destruction left behind. In its repair work, it also acts on injuries to the body, with the goal of fixing whatever's harming our health.

However, though the underlying goal is good, there's healthy inflammation and then there's inflammation gone rogue. Healthy inflammation, called "acute inflammation," is temporary—right-now, one-and-done inflammation. Say you get a cut. Your immune system dispatches the white blood cell soldiers to fight infection and get your tissue on the mend. Once that work is done, your immuno-warriors depart, going back to bed till there's another battle to fight.

Inflammation gone rogue, "chronic inflammation," is dysregulated endless inflammation—the immune soldiers in forever-war mode: going to battle and staying in battle when there's no actual injury or disease to fight. This plays out like actual soldiers gone rogue, ravaging the land (your healthy organs and tissues). Over time, this can cause serious harm to your immune system, impairing normal immune function, eroding your health, and elevating your risk of disease and even premature death.

In perimenopause and menopause and as we age, inflammation is pretty much out to get us at every turn. (Most age-related diseases are inflammatory diseases.) Immunologist Claudio Franceschi, MD, coined the term "inflammaging" for the low-grade, chronic inflammation throughout our body that develops and increases as we age—leading to an always-on immune system releasing toxic inflammatory chemicals (in the absence of any disease, bug, or injury that acute inflammation would be part of addressing).

Inflammaging significantly raises the risk of disease and premature death in elderly people. It's a perp in *pretty much everything that goes wrong in us in old age*, increasing the risk of—to name a few—osteoporosis, arthritis, type 2 diabetes, gastrointestinal disorders, depression, kidney disease, and especially, cardiovascular disease. All of the above-mentioned conditions also increase chronic inflammation within us—as do poor sleep, being sedentary, chronic stress, an altered gut microbiome, and being overweight or obese, just for starters.

Perimenopause and menopause also play a major role in increasing our inflammatory load. Most of the symptoms and negative health effects of menopause and perimenopause are both *provoked* by dysregulated inflammation and are *provokers* of it—which brings me to a bit of good news. By diminishing these symptoms and the accompanying health issues—the focus of these chapters on symptoms as well as those on long-term health—there's a ride-along decrease in chronic inflammation. For example, it comes with improving your sleep, cutting down on the chronic expression of stress hormones, maintaining brain health, and especially, through protecting and maintaining your cardiovascular health. (Once pernicious inflammation takes off in your cardiovascular system, you might as well be on a bobsled to the grave.)

THE POWER OF POSITIVE SHRINKING

Progesterone is anti-inflammatory—an inflammation-fighting police force in hormone form. It inhibits inflammation by downregulating inflammatory substances, thus preventing the destruction they can cause. Personally, in perimenopause, I especially appreciated its work as a diuretic—a substance that makes you pee—releasing the fluid buildup caused by estrogen that made me feel like a giant water balloon with legs.

In contrast, *abnormal* progesterone levels—either no progesterone or very little on duty—can lead to a "pro-inflammatory" state: raging unmitigated inflammation. When inflammation is chronic—like from anovulatory cycles month after month—it can contribute to tissue damage; for example, in parts of our body we really need to avoid trashing, like the lining of our arteries. (We can't just tell our blood supply to find other means of transportation.)

Reflecting on my sudden inability to travel by car without hurling, I wondered: Had I just been bloated in the head—and specifically, in the brain's balance center, the inner ear? If so, was the bloatage relieved by progesterone going "Nuh-uh!" to inflammation—or did its diuretic effect reduce swelling in my inner ear?

There were no clear-cut answers, but pulling all the findings together, it seemed I might be on to something. If progesterone *were* curtailing the swelling and inflammation, it might explain some positive physical changes—a bit of *reclamation* I'd experienced—since I began taking OMP.

One of the affected territories was my osteoarthritic knee, which, in my 40s, became searingly painful. In lieu of the "pointless" arthroscopic surgery I was offered, I decided to try dietary supplements said to decrease inflammation—those for which the collective scientific findings didn't amount to "Send in the clowns!" I ended up taking krill oil (a kind of fish oil) and a few others.

Well, good news! A few months of supplementation—or, let's be honest, mere coincidence and/or the placebo effect!—led to my pain level decreasing.

Somewhat. Maybe 20 percent, if I hazard a perhaps overgenerous guess. That's not nothing, but it's also not "Yahoo! No more searing pain!"

A few years later, I started taking OMP. Maybe two months afterward, it occurred to me that my knee didn't hurt—*at all*. I also realized I'd been migraine-free for two months, while I'd previously gotten hit by two or so migraines a month. Full disclosure: Writing those two *OMG/jeezo/peezo/amazeballs!* sentences above grosses me out. My apparent physiological good fortune could have been due to complete coincidence—for example, perhaps some hidden knee injury (unseen on the original X-ray) that had finally healed. Other highly plausible explanations include a stew of poor memory, wishful thinking, and/or the placebo effect.

Even so, I can't help but notice a distinct difference between my experience with my knee and a prior scare with my toe. Earlier in my 40s, after a lifetime of speedy healing from cuts and bruises, I stubbed my big toe super hard on the vacuum cleaner. I expected Toesie to be back to normal in about a week. Instead, it turned varying scary shades of maroon and deep purple, with a touch of green—getting darker and scarier every day. ("Greetings, gangrene, amputation, and death!")

My toe remained purple and swollen for two months. Weirdly, it was also both painful and relatively numb. Worried that I might have nerve damage, I got an X-ray. No nerve damage, the doc said. Great! But why was I suddenly so unable to heal?

He had no answer. Looking back, I suspect that soaring estrogen was on an inflammatory rampage in me, with little or no progesterone to balance it out. This is just my opinion based on my experience; it doesn't count as evidence. However, as unscientific as it is to leap to the conclusion that "correlation is causation"—believing *apparent* cause-and-effect relationships are *actual* cause-and-effect relationships—it's equally unscientific to shrug off correlations as meaningless. Additionally, the slowed healing I experienced is one of the effects of inflammaging that Franceschi and his colleagues lay out.

Clearly, progesterone's effects on tissue and wound healing join migraines and motion sickness as subject areas begging for comprehensive investigation. At the very least, I hope this chapter leads perimenopausal women who are being hammered by motion sickness and/or migraines to consider consulting their doctor about trying progesterone to see whether it might help.

DRUG-FREE FIRE PREVENTION

Non-prescription ways to decrease inflammation include: exercise (without overdoing it), avoiding cigarettes and alcohol, getting sufficient sleep, and decreasing the bite of emotional stress through improved coping. Additionally, it seems you "are" not just *what* you eat but *how often you do it*.

NO SUCH THING AS A FREE MUNCH

You know those experts who told us to eat small meals throughout the day? Adorably, they based this on scientific assumption rather than evidence.

It's important to avoid spending your entire day el muncho—especially if you're feeding a sweet tooth. Sweet snacks, and particularly those containing fructose, the simple sugar that makes up 50 percent of table sugar, are the worst for your health. Dr. Michael Eades explains, "Fructose specifically causes the most rapid and intense inflammatory response of all."

However, Eades notes that eating itself is an inflammation-provoking process. "Food coming into the body is a foreign substance that fires up the innate immune system"—though just briefly, till the various nutrients are broken down and absorbed into the bloodstream. "When the average American noshes along throughout the day...the inflammatory response becomes chronic."

Conversely, some research finds that intermittent fasting—going without eating for part of the day or a few days—reduces inflammation. And inflammation isn't all that's reduced. My former boyfriend lopped off (and kept off) 90 pounds by eating breakfast and then going food-free till dinnertime, maybe 10 or 12 hours later. Of course, this is not a trade-off everyone's willing to make. Personally, as a plate-licking hedonist and a complete baby about discomfort, my idea of intermittent fasting is waiting till lunchtime to hoover down lunch.

SMOKING AND VAPING: SLOW, SMELLY INFLAMMATORY SUICIDE

Smoking is one of the most inflammatory things you can do to your body, short of setting your hair on fire with your blowdryer. It leads to chronic inflammation, contributes to insulin resistance (a broken insulin response), "oxidizes" LDL cholesterol (turns it into a more harmful form that damages arteries), is ruinous to your lungs in every possible way (from compromising your ability to breathe to highly increased risk of respiratory diseases and lung cancer), and increases your risk of a slew of other cancers, along with type 2 diabetes. Just for starters.

It's also a major instigator of suffering and death from cardiovascular disease. For example, smoking irritates your blood vessels, causing the body to incite an immune response. This response leads to pernicious "oxidative stress" (harmful molecules damaging your cells), resulting in tissue damage, chronic inflammation, and the impaired functioning of your entire cardiovascular system.

Sadly, puffing out candy clouds instead of cigarette smoke is not a health measure. Though e-cigarettes (aka vapes) don't wreak ruin on the level of the OG cigs, use of e-cigarettes is associated with a higher risk of atherosclerosis, strokes, and heart attacks. The compounds within them provoke inflammation and give rise to oxidative stress, cellular harm, and chronic inflammation, damaging your arteries and other tissues.

E-cigarettes are found to increase blood pressure and the risk of abdominal obesity. When they contain nicotine, e-cigarettes erode the function of the interior lining of your arteries, the endothelium, which is actually an organ that works to maintain the health of your entire cardiovascular system.

There are surely additional adverse effects from e-cigs, but because they're relatively new, research on them is just picking up.

PSYCHOLOGICAL RESILIENCE: THE TRIUMPH OF COPE OVER EXPERIENCE

Because emotional, social, and workplace stress play out in physically stressful ways—with elevated cortisol and inflammation—it's important to decrease or eliminate sources of chronic stress in your life. However, as previously noted, because you can't always *banish* the stress (without banishing the source of your mortgage payment), what you can do is foster psychological resilience: your ability to cope.

Psychological resilience involves "the ability to rally after adversity and to experience positive emotions," writes happiness researcher Sonja Lyubomirsky. "This is accomplished primarily by managing negative emotion" and taking meaningful action to "improve the stressful circumstance." For example, Lyubomirsky observes that we have "the capacity to turn traumas into assets and bad experiences into growth experiences—for example, to bounce back from a divorce and even emerge from it stronger than before."

Emotional upset often comes from irrational expectations, so a few sessions of Rational Emotive Behavior Therapy (REBT, the powerful type of cognitive behavioral therapy I mentioned in a previous chapter) may be helpful for training you to use reasoning to put stressful situations in perspective. However, the late Dr. Albert Ellis, who created REBT, was a firm believer that you could train yourself, and a terrific resource for this is his inexpensive paperback *How to Stubbornly Refuse to Make Yourself Miserable About Anything—Yes, Anything!* (My suggestion: Highlight the hell out of it and use it as a workbook.)

Lyubomirsky's research suggests you can build or increase your resilience through the use of "happiness-enhancing interventions"—such as taking stock of what you have to appreciate in your life and expressing gratitude (in a journal, recorded on your phone, or to others). Practicing optimistic thinking (looking to the future in positive ways), doing kind acts for others, and social connection are other happiness enhancers her research and others' has found effective.

The increased resilience from these interventions seems to come through three mechanisms, Lyubomirsky explains. "First, emotions like joy, satisfaction, and interest marshaled by positive interventions provide individuals with a sort of 'psychological time-out' in the face of stress and help them perceive the 'big picture' of their situations. Hence, a negative or even traumatic circumstance can become less overwhelming and less impactful on all life domains."

Second, happiness-enhancing activities can "counteract negative, dysfunctional thoughts and, instead, bolster positive thinking. For example, hopeful expectations produced by the optimism strategy can replace thoughts of hopelessness and powerlessness." And lastly, "happiness activities often bring about positive experiences. For example, practicing acts of kindness produces moments in which people feel efficacious and appreciated and can even generate new friendships."

Ultimately, though our level of resilience is partially shaped by our genetics, there's an important idea packed into Lyubomirsky's "we have the capacity" and the advice she offers, and it's that we can *choose* resilience. My friend

Leslie Gray Streeter, newspaper columnist and author of *Black Widow*, shows this so beautifully with her words in this tweet:

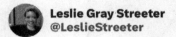 **Leslie Gray Streeter**
@LeslieStreeter

I choose joy. I am the descendant of the enslaved and the survivors of Jim Crow. I choose joy. I am a widowed single mother. I choose joy. I am the daughter of a father who died before he met my son. I choose joy.

8:27 PM · 8/9/24 · 39 Views

THE "DOWN UNDER"
*Fibroidzillas, Desert Vagina,
and Clitty-Clitty Dead Zone*

— 12 —

NEEDLESS GUTTING

*Countless unnecessary hysterectomies
for fibroids and heavy menstrual bleeding*

WHEN I WAS in perimenopause, I went in for a Pap smear—a quick swab of my cervix to make sure it wasn't becoming a cancergarden. Afterward, my gynecologist revved up his ultrasound wand and went for a look-see in my uterus.

"You have a fibroid," he announced. "About the size of a tennis ball."

I pictured a cartoon boulder blowing up balloon-style and exploding my uterus. He said it wasn't at a size where I'd need surgery, but we'd watch to see if it got bigger. (I was already picturing it not only bigger but with teeth—like that thing in *Alien* that busts out of John Hurt.)

Though I couldn't shrink this creepy invader, I had some control over the stuff colonizing my head. I named my uterus-crasher "Freddie the Fibroid"—the tubby, bumbling antithesis of "Invasive Ladycancer Leading to Horrible Suffering and Death."

FIBROIDS: THE BALLS IN AND ON THE WALLS
Misunderstood and overtreated

Fibroids are technically tumors, but they're almost always benign—non-cancerous. They are hard, dense balls of muscle cells and fibrous tissue that grow in or on the uterus. Size-wise, the smaller variety range from about 1 to 5 millimeters (the size of a pencil lead to the size of a pea), but some fibroids grow to 10 to even 30 centimeters (grapefruit-sized to watermelon-sized).

Fibroids mostly start showing up in women in their 30s or 40s. By age 49, more than 70 percent of white women and 84 percent of black women are diagnosed with them. Black women tend to have more fibroids, as well as more fibroids "of size," and experience more fibroid-related symptoms and suffering. They also tend to grow fibroids at an earlier age—in their 20s (which is relatively uncommon in other populations). This, unfortunately, gives the fibroids a head start on developing into the big organ-squashing uglies that can require surgical intervention.

Researchers understand relatively little about how and why fibroids develop, explain reproductive endocrinologist Erica Marsh, MD, and gynecologist Serdar Bulun, MD, though "it is widely accepted" that the growth of fibroids is stimulated by estrogen.

Fibroids, in fact, are pretty much estrogen theme parks. They contain high estrogen concentrations and have many estrogen receptors, allowing more estrogen to bind to them, reports the journal *Contemporary OB/GYN*. Fibroids also do their best to hang on to the estradiol they have by messing with estrogen metabolism. Estrogen is broken down much more slowly than it would be in a uterus that's fibroid-free. This could potentially lead to more fibroids popping up or contribute to the staying power of the uterus-squatters already there.

You might recall from Chapter Seven that progesterone gets blamed for causing fibroids, in large part due to all those research papers that confuse progesterone and progestins. Of course, it's *possible* progesterone could play a role—perhaps through triggering production of tissue-regulating substances called "growth factors" that send signals to cells to grow and repair tissue. However, a strong argument against progesterone causing fibroids is the fact that perimenopause, with often-spiking estrogen levels and low or absent progesterone, is prime time for fibroids to crop up—and blow up in number and size.

Estrogen as a principal stimulator of fibroids also makes sense in light of how estrogen is "proliferative," kicking off cell growth that can run wild—and at its worst, can morph into cell overgrowth and even lead to cancer. In contrast, we've seen that progesterone is basically the estrogen wrangler in the breasts and endometrium.

Not only does progesterone keep cells from going wild making of copies of themselves, but it is also Dr. Death to would-be cancer cells, telling unnecessary, abnormal, or otherwise past-their-prime cells to kill themselves (through that programmed cell-death process called "apoptosis"). Estrogen, on the other hand, can impede apoptosis, allowing cells that should've been served their death warrant to stick around—and what better way to pass the time than by dividing uncontrollably into tumors!

THE UNFABULOUS FOUR
Know your enemy

There are four kinds of fibroids, named for where they grow.

The most common kind are those like my guy, Freddie the Fibroid, that grow sandwiched between the inner and outer walls of the uterus, in the muscular middle layer. These are "intramural" fibroids—making it sound like your uterus is hosting a junior-high sports fair—but it's just Latin: "intra" plus "muros," meaning "within walls."

Intramural fibroids are typically asymptomatic unless they're seriously large ("Moby the Fibroid"). My only symptoms were fear and horror—and those only rose up when my gynecologist told me he'd spotted the thing on his vagina cam.

The three less common fibroids are those I call "The Protruders," because they jut out from the exterior or into the interior of the uterus:

- **Subserosal fibroids** grow just under the outer wall of the uterus (the "serosa"). Most remain small, but some can become pretty big and cause some problems.
- **Submucosal fibroids**, the least common kind, grow inside the uterus, just below the inner "wall," the endometrial lining, and stick out into your uterine cavity.
- **Pedunculated fibroids** are the *horror movie-meets-biology textbook* version of the fibroids above: subserosal or submucosal fibroids that, like super-creepy cauliflower, grow on a "stalk."

WELL-INTENTIONED MEDICAL MUTILATION
Unnecessary surgery for fibroids and heavy menstrual bleeding

Because fibroids and "menorrhagia"—crazy-heavy menstrual flow—often show up around the same time, researchers have leapt to the evidence-free conclusion that fibroids *cause* the crazy-heavy flow. This scientific fairy tale has been baked into medical understanding and practice, leading unwitting doctors to subject vast numbers of women to harmful, unnecessary medical intervention—including fibroid surgery and even hysterectomies (the surgical removal of the uterus).

However, the belief that fibroids *cause* el-floodo periods *makes no physiological sense.*

Dr. Prior explains that only one relatively rare type of fibroid "could cause flow problems": the uncommon submucosal fibroid. That's the type that grows into the uterine cavity from just beneath the inner uterine "wall" (technically, the mucous membrane of the endometrial lining—the part that sheds with each menstrual period).

Fewer than 10 percent of fibroids are submucosal, and *only* submucosal fibroids have any contact with the uterine lining, Prior adds. In other words, "about 90%" of fibroids are nowhere near anything that bleeds and sheds at period time, which means they *could not possibly influence flow!*

Submucosal fibroids, like other fibroids, *could* become problematic if they get so huge or numerous that they cause you pain, protrude from your body baby-bump-style, or impede normal organ function. Horrifying as all of that sounds, Prior notes that "It is very rare that fibroids become so big that they push on the bladder or the bowel" or "cause pain or change the shape of the abdomen." Prior is emphatic: These "are the only (acceptable) reasons for surgery for fibroids."

Reassuringly, she adds that in her 40 years of clinical practice, only one of her perimenopausal patients with fibroids required surgery. "It was because the fibroids were so large that she looked six months pregnant and the fibroids were pressing on her bladder."

I *was* reassured—and then I remembered that Prior, now retired from medical practice and focused on research, did her doctoring in British Columbia. There, in the 2016 Canadian census, a whopping 1 percent of the population was black. Again, fibroids tend to be particularly rotten to black women—bigger, more numerous, and more suffering-inducing. Chances are another doctor in, say, Columbia, South Carolina (with a 39 percent black population in the most recent US census), is likely to come upon the battleship-sized buggers with a bit more frequency.

If you have fibroids, you're likely to encounter some pressure to have them surgically removed. Unless they are painful, organ-crushing, or abdomen-distorting, Prior says: "Don't worry about the fibroids and don't DO anything. Except exercise. Keep your weight normal and don't have more than one alcohol drink a day," which will help keep your estrogen levels lower. Remember: In general, "Fibroids shrink when women become menopausal."

If only giving this advice were standard medical practice. "About 40–50% of North American women" are given hysterectomies due to the presence of fibroids and/or crazy-heavy menstrual bleeding, reveals Prior. These surgeries are "performed primarily" on perimenopausal women between ages 45 and 47—for conditions that are temporary! (Consider that the average age at menopause in North America is 51, which means a 47-year-old woman is pretty much standing on the doormat to it—meaning it's likely her fibroids will soon shrink or disappear on their own.)

All surgical procedures, necessary or unnecessary, involve the risk of accidental harm—whether you get three stitches in your pinkie finger or an unwarranted hysterectomy. Hysterectomies, however, impose a number of major costs. In addition to the financial bite for women with less-than-royal health coverage, Prior notes that an abdominal hysterectomy involves at least six weeks of post-op recovery. Abdominal hysterectomy requires a large abdominal incision, while vaginal, laparoscopic, and robotic-assisted hysterectomies require smaller incisions and are associated with less tissue trauma and shorter healing times. They also tend to be lower cost.

However, all forms of hysterectomy are associated with long-term health risks, even if the ovaries get to stick around. For example, an observational study by endocrinologist Elizabeth Stewart, MD, found a 33 percent higher risk of coronary artery disease, along with an increased risk of high blood pressure and obesity, in women who had hysterectomies.

With or without a hysterectomy, when both ovaries are cut out (called a "bilateral oophorectomy"), shoving a woman into "surgical menopause," the associated health risks are far worse. They include increased risk of heart attacks, strokes, and bone fracture—all of which are associated with an increase in the health-risk biggie, premature death.

SLASH AND BURN

Other often-unnecessary surgical procedures performed on women with fibroids

Dr. Prior's admonition, "Don't do anything" (unless you've got abdomen-distorting, organ-choking, and/or painful fibroids), extends to "less invasive" (and equally unnecessary) surgical procedures often offered to women with heavy bleeding or fibroids. These procedures—detailed below—include: embolization, focused ultrasound surgery, myolysis, endometrial ablation, and morcellation.

With these techniques, all a doctor can do is shrink or remove your existing fibroids and block the blood supply that feeds them. There's no spigot you can turn to dial down your spiking perimenopausal estrogen levels and no way to put the brakes on genetic propensities or other possible factors in fibroid growth. In other words, soon after the procedure, you could start growing a whole new crop of uterine baseballs or regrowing the shrunken ones. Additionally, as with every medical procedure, each of these supposedly kinder, gentler alternatives to a hysterectomy comes with potential adverse effects.

UTERINE FIBROID EMBOLIZATION (UFE)

The surgeon (guided by a real-time X-ray machine called a fluoroscope) uses a catheter to inject the arteries leading to your fibroids with tiny bead-like particles. These block blood flow, which causes fibroids to shrink. (The technical term for this blood vessel blockage is "embolization," and another name for this surgery is uterine artery embolization, UAE.)

"This procedure has a shorter recovery time than surgery, because no incision is made," notes health policy analyst Diana Zuckerman. "However, interrupting the blood supply to your ovaries or to other organs can cause the ovaries to stop working for a short time or permanently. This can cause menopause" or affect fertility, so "it may not be a good choice for women who may want to have children in the future."

FOCUSED ULTRASOUND SURGERY (FUS)

This MRI-guided surgery uses targeted, high-energy sound waves to heat up and destroy fibroids. The peer-into-your-guts imaging of the MRI machine allows the surgeon to clearly discern between fibroids and healthy tissue so only the nasty bits get burned to hell.

"No incisions are made and the uterus is preserved," reports Zuckerman. "The advantage is that it does not cause menopause. However, the long-term effectiveness or the risk of recurrence is not yet known. This procedure is also not recommended for women who want to become pregnant."

MYOLYSIS

This procedure destroys fibroids' blood supply by cauterizing the blood-delivering arteries: burning them closed. This is done with a tube called a resectoscope, with either a laser fiber or an electricity-generating electrode on the end that is inserted *laparoscopically*: through a tiny incision.

When a doctor suggests myolysis, patients assume they're being offered a safe, effective procedure. Zuckerman reports that "the safety, effectiveness, and risk of recurrence" from myolysis has yet to be determined. "Women who are planning to have children should not have this procedure because it can increase the risk of uterine rupture, a serious emergency, during the birth of a baby."

ENDOMETRIAL ABLATION

Endometrial ablation is typically done only to address heavy menstrual flow and to remove small submucosal fibroids that are three centimeters or less. The surgeon goes through the vagina to the uterus with a laser or a hysteroscope (a thin tube with a light and camera at the end and a channel for slim surgical tools). She then uses heat to destroy ("ablate") the top layer of the endometrium—the part that gets shed in menstruation.

MORCELLATION

Morcellation is a technique used to cut fibroids or other pieces of tissue into fragments for easier extraction. The surgeon inserts a morcellator—a tiny device with rotating blades—into the uterus through a hysteroscope to chop the fibroids into pieces. In laparoscopic morcellation, used for larger fibroids, the morcellator may be inserted through small incisions in the abdomen.

Morcellation can be deadly for a woman with undiagnosed uterine cancer because it can disperse the cancerous tissue fragments into the uterus and the abdominal cavity. Though it's estimated that fewer than 1 in 1,000 fibroids are cancerous—uterine sarcomas—they are very hard to differentiate from the merely annoying but *benign* fibroids. (Women often experience no symptoms till the cancer is in a late stage.)

Dr. Amy Reed, an anesthesiologist and mother of six, was one of these women whose fibroid morcellation turned deadly. "A biopsy after the operation found that Dr. Reed had a hidden leiomyosarcoma, an aggressive type of cancer," writes Denise Grady in *The New York Times* in 2017.

"A biopsy *after* the operation." Whoa.

Reading this, I thought, "Hello? Wouldn't a biopsy—*before* surgery rather than after!—offer the best chances of differentiating between benign fibroids and the evil cancerous ones that led to Reed's terminal leiomyosarcoma?" In fact, pre-surgical biopsies of fibroids are, as a rule, not done—for good reason. Fibroids are densely packed with blood vessels, making biopsies unsafe due to risk of hemorrhage—uncontrolled torrent-like bleeding that can turn into a serious medical emergency.

During the time Reed had left, she and her husband, cardiothoracic surgeon Hooman Noorchashm, MD, turned their family's devastating impending loss into a crusade to ban the use of morcellators, reports Grady. "Because of their efforts, the Food and Drug Administration reviewed morcellation" and, in 2014, advised against using morcellators for fibroid removal in "'the vast majority' of women undergoing surgery for uterine fibroids."

The FDA has since backed off that stance—likely due to pressure from both manufacturers and some members of the medical community prioritizing profit over patient safety. Their current suggested restrictions sound pretty *unrestrictive* to me. The FDA's 2023 guidance—with the obligatory veneer of concern for the increasing risk of uterine sarcoma with age—states that morcellation "should only be used in women who have fibroids if they are premenopausal and under 50 years old."

In other words, the watchdog-gone-lapdog FDA suggests "restricting" morcellation to *every woman under 50*—save for the few who hit the menopause finish line a bit early.

In the FDA's 2020 report (cited in their 2023 update), they do advise that the manufacturers of these morcellating devices should include *labeling* on the machine to warn surgeons, such as: "Laparoscopic power morcellators should only be used with a containment system" to catch tissue. (Well, okay—but we patients are supposed to just cross our fingers and hope our doctors read all the labels on their equipment?)

The "containment system" they're referring to is a bag to catch tissue, approved by the FDA in 2016. ACOG (the American College of Obstetricians and Gynecologists) and two gynecologic surgery societies recommend bag-contained morcellation procedures "as potential solutions" to keep potentially cancerous chunks of flesh from flying around inside a woman, reports gynecological surgeon Brooke Winner, MD, in a 2017 article in *Missouri Medicine*. However, these organizations "also warn that these techniques require advanced laparoscopic skill and that appropriate training and credentialing are important considerations."

Well, sure. And we're all for advanced surgical skill, and all the rest. But here in the unfortunately imperfect real world, even highly skilled surgeons can make mistakes—which brings us to the bottom line from the FDA: "A tissue containment system cannot prevent all cases of tissue spread."

BONUS POINT

GYNECOLOGICAL EXAM ROOM OR MEDIEVAL TORTURE CHAMBER?
Women forced to endure painful procedures without anesthesia

If you have a penis and testicles and a doctor is going to hack a chunk of flesh out of them (formally known as a biopsy), they will give you anesthesia. Because not doing so is monstrous.

Disgustingly, monstrous tends to be business as usual in gynecological biopsies, *diagnostic* hysteroscopies, and other gynecological interventions—all typically performed on women without anesthesia. These procedures can be excruciatingly painful—to the point some women pass out from the pain—as can be IUD insertion or removal for some women.

Very often, women are not informed about the potential for extreme pain—which, conveniently, prevents them from asking for anesthesia. The lack of anesthesia saves providers money and makes the procedures less complicated for them. Insurance companies may also refuse to cover anesthesia.

However, patients have a *right* to have pain from a procedure minimized. To put this differently, *we women deserve equal treatment*—the same pain relief men are given for painful genitourinary procedures.

Don't just *ask* for pain relief. Demand it. And have your provider advocate for you with the insurance company, if necessary.

Please spread the word on this. All women need to know.

SICCING THE PHARMACY ON FIBROIDS
Loads of ugly side effects, modest shrinkage

There are a few drugs commonly used to shrink fibroids, though they don't eliminate them, and they sock women with some awful side effects. These drugs include: gonadotropin-releasing hormone agonists, androgens, ulipristal acetate, and Depo-Provera.

GONADOTROPIN-RELEASING HORMONE AGONISTS (GNRHA)

These drugs (such as Lupron and Synarel) "work by 'switching off' the ovaries, meaning that they reduce the production of estrogen and progesterone," explain ob-gyn researcher Ruth Hodgson and her colleagues. This usually stops a woman's periods and puts her into a menopause-like state—complete with hot flashes and other menopausal symptoms. (This typically reverses after stopping the treatment.)

These treatments have been found to shrink fibroids by almost 35 percent, and are typically prescribed to reduce fibroid size before surgery. However, they come with a major downside: They can cause and accelerate bone loss. Due to this, doctors are advised against prescribing them to a woman for more than six months. Unfortunately, stopping the drug tends to cause any fibroids that initially shrunk to "immediately" grow back—"to their original size or beyond," note reproductive medicine specialist Vikram Sinai Talaulikar and his colleagues.

ANDROGENS

Androgens are male hormones—though women's bodies also produce them (in lesser amounts than men's). The androgen drug Danazol, a derivative of synthetic testosterone, may shrink fibroids by approximately 23 percent. It also may give a woman a little more in common than she'd like with 'roid-bros at the gym. Side effects include acne, oily skin, voice changes, hirsutism (hair popping up in all the wrong places), weight gain, and liver damage.

A "review of the use of danazol for uterine fibroids concluded that the benefits of danazol do not outweigh its risks," report ob-gyn researcher Mohammad Ebrahim Parsanezhad, MD, and his colleagues.

ULIPRISTAL ACETATE

Ulipristal acetate, an emergency contraceptive, is shown to reduce heavy menstrual bleeding by approximately 50 to 60 percent and shrink fibroids by approximately 25 to 40 percent. It has fewer and less awful adverse effects than these other drugs above—for most women, as you'll see below. The most commonly reported side effects are headaches, nausea, abdominal pain, and painful periods. Some women experience hot flashes.

However, an *uncommon* side effect associated with ulipristal is liver damage—serious liver injury, including liver failure, leading to a need for a liver transplant. (This occurred in under 1 percent of ulipristal users.)

The European Medicines Agency (EMA) recommended avoiding the medication in women with known liver problems and restricting patients to one course of treatment, except for women who were ineligible for fibroid surgery. Additionally, because not all liver problems are known, the EMA called for doctors to test liver enzymes in patients before prescribing the drug, as well as during and after stopping treatment.

In case that's not off-putting enough, ulipristal can block progesterone, keeping it from doing its vital work to thin the lining of the endometrium.

Without progesterone in action, "an unopposed estrogen effect could occur which could cause (pre-)malignant lesions in the endometrium," reports ob-gyn Inge de Milliano, MD, in a 2017 research review. Accordingly, it's prescribed intermittently for the treatment of fibroids and heavy bleeding: on and off in three-month stints.

Granted, the studies included in the review "did not report any non-reversible (pre-) malignant lesions of the endometrium," the researchers note. However, these studies had limitations: Most "focused on short-term use," and follow-up was limited. De Milliano calls for more research on the long-term intermittent use of ulipristal for fibroids before its use can be deemed safe.

DEPO-PROVERA

This injectable birth control drug is another that's shown promise—both for shrinking and preventing fibroids—but it brings an entourage: the "slew of awful side effects" listed in Chapter Seven, including acne, weight gain, fluid retention, and the smorgasbord of fun that comes with PMS.

WHEN THE JONESTOWN FLOOD IS RED AND HAPPENING IN YOUR PANTS
Signs you've got crazy-heavy periods

I'm pretty sure women like me who have "HELP! I THINK I'M BLEEDING OUT!" type periods don't need a list of bullet-point items to tell us our flow is "heavy."

During late perimenopause, I had such apocalyptically floody, "better-call-FEMA!" periods that I had to change my super-extra-plus-plus-plus tampon and massive diaper-like pad every 19 minutes. (And yes, 19 minutes. I know because I got so angry, I timed it with a stopwatch.)

However, to assuage the curiosity of those of you who use those cute little tampons the size of baby carrots, the American College of Obstetricians and Gynecologists notes that any of the following can be a sign of abnormally heavy menstrual bleeding. Quoting from their website:

- Bleeding that lasts more than seven days.
- Bleeding that soaks through one or more tampons or pads every hour for several hours in a row.

- Needing to wear more than one pad at a time to control menstrual flow.
- Needing to change pads or tampons during the night.
- Menstrual flow with blood clots that are as big as a quarter or larger.

BETTER LIVING THROUGH AVOIDING SURGERY
No-knife solutions for the blood flood and its effects

IBUPROFEN

Prior advises that whenever your period is super heavy, you should start taking ibuprofen (like Advil, Motrin, or their generic versions). She recommends "a dose of one 200-milligram tablet with breakfast, lunch, and dinner on every heavy flow day," explaining, "This therapy decreases flow by 20-40% and will also help with menstrual cycle-like cramps." (When I looked up the papers on this, I saw that naproxen was associated with a similar decrease.)

Ibuprofen's most common adverse effect is heartburn, she says, which is why it should be taken with food. I will tell you that ibuprofen can also cause constipation. If this happens to you, magnesium ("nature's laxative") will be your BFF. Magnesium is safe and healthy and a vital mineral many people are deficient in. It helps maintain muscle and nerve function, your immune system, a stable heart rhythm, and healthy bones.

If you get constipated, you could take one magnesium tablet or capsule per ibuprofen or naproxen and see how it goes. There's no standard amount of magnesium in the capsules and tablets from brand to brand, so you could go by this guideline: Take as much as you need to remain intestinally unblocked. (You will not overdose on magnesium.) If you've taken too much, you'll get diarrhea, and you can pull back on the amount. The current RDA for magnesium for women is 320 milligrams, but there's a strong possibility this amount is incorrectly low. Also (per testing by Consumerlab.com and others), it's likely that the amount of listed on various bottles of magnesium is mineralized fiction.

Nephrologist (kidney expert) Judith Blaine, MD, observes that healthy kidneys filter "approximately 2,000–2,400 mg of magnesium per day." If you have impaired kidney or liver function, any other serious health conditions, or are taking any prescription drugs, you should get your doctor's okay before taking ibuprofen, naproxen, or magnesium. It is also vital to read and follow the per-day dosage limits on the naproxen or ibuprofen bottle so you don't trash your kidneys or liver or both.

EXTRA FLUID AND SALT FOR BLOOD LOSS

"In the context of heavy flow, any time you feel dizzy or your heart pounds when you get up from lying down it is evidence that the amount of blood volume in your system is too low," Prior advises. "You will likely need at least four to six cups (1–1.5 liters) of extra liquid that day." You should also drink more salty fluids, like salty broths, she adds. Increasing fluid and salt intake together can help increase your blood volume.

Of course, if you have or might have a medical condition in which additional salt could be a problem, consult your doctor to see whether this might help you—or kill you.

IRON

We menstrual floodsters are prone to iron deficiency—which puts us at risk for iron-deficiency anemia, a condition in which blood is short on the healthy red blood cells it needs to carry oxygen to the body's tissues. Eighty percent of women whose periods are gushers—with a flow of more than 80 milliliters per period (in case you've got your measuring cup out!)—"will have one or more" lab tests revealing an iron deficiency, explains Prior.

If you've got flood-like periods, ask your doctor to test your iron level. Which tests should you be getting? The American Society of Hematology (specializing in the study of blood and blood disorders) explains that "Iron-deficiency anemia is diagnosed by blood tests that should include a complete blood count (CBC). Additional tests may be ordered to evaluate the levels of serum ferritin, iron, total iron-binding capacity, and/or transferrin."

If you are low on iron or if the CBC finds low hematocrit and hemoglobin, your doctor may want you to take a daily over-the-counter iron tablet (like 35 mg of ferrous gluconate). You can also increase the iron you get from foods. Oysters, beef liver, beef, spinach, lentils, dark chocolate, tofu, sardines, and cashews are some of the foods high in iron.

The US Recommended Daily Allowance (RDA) for iron for women prior to menopause—from age 18 to age 50—is 18 milligrams a day, taking into account blood loss from menstruation. For menopausal women, the RDA is 8 milligrams.

VITAMIN D

Low levels of vitamin D are associated with menstrual disorders of various kinds—including symptoms of PMS and PCOS, adverse effects in pregnancy, and floody bleeding.

Your doctor can test your level or you can use an online lab, such as the non-profit ownyourlabs.com. *(Details, Chapter Twenty.)* The Endocrine Society's 2011 guidelines call for a level of between 40 to 60 ng/mL.

Vitamin D3 (cholecalciferol) is the type to take. I'm a redhead with skin the color of fresh Wite-Out, and I take 5,000 IU daily, which in me, tests out at 50 ng/mL. I started with a lower dose (1,000 or 2,000 IU) and after taking it for three months, I got tested again and upped the dose. Black women and dark-skinned people from other populations might need different amounts—and let's hope somebody gets on researching that soon so we know what those amounts might be.

Because vitamin D is distributed in body fat, Prior advises that "heavier people need more" (and notes that because menopausal weight gain is common, menopausal women may also need more).

TRANEXAMIC ACID

Tranexamic acid, a prescription drug used in patients with bleeding disorders, was approved in 2009 to treat heavy menstrual bleeding. It works by blocking or slowing the breakdown of blood clots. In a randomized controlled trial, it reduced menstrual blood loss by 40 percent (compared with a placebo). Other research has found it to reduce bleeding by 26 to 60 percent. Putting this in perspective, naproxen showed a 34.58 percent reduction and lacks the adverse effects associated with tranexamic acid—the most common of which are fatigue, bone and muscle pain, joint pain, nasal congestion, and a viral upper respiratory infection.

Tranexamic acid *could* be dangerous or deadly for women with blood clot disorders, due to a risk of deep vein thrombosis or pulmonary embolism (a clot blocking blood flow to the lung). However, the research results are conflicting, inadequate, and inconclusive.

THE MIRENA PROGESTIN-ONLY IUD

The most powerful drug treatment for reducing heavy bleeding is the one IUD (intrauterine device) approved by the FDA to treat it: the Mirena, a long-acting contraceptive IUD that continuously releases the progestin levonorgestrel. In a 2019 study, nearly 75 percent of the women with a Mirena reported no longer experiencing the blood flood by the end of a single menstrual cycle. After the second cycle, it was 83 percent of the women. (Some women end up having no period at all.)

The Mirena (and the various progestin-only pills below) decrease the amount of bleeding by thinning the source: the lining of the uterus. The Mirena also thins the wallet. If you don't have medical insurance, you could pay between $500 and $1,300 for it. Softening that bite somewhat, the FDA recently announced that the Mirena is effective for eight years.

Of course, in addition to the high ticket price for the IUD, side effects from this treatment include irregular or painful periods (with increased menstrual cramps). Relatively rare side effects include migraines and other headaches, nausea, breast tenderness, vaginal infections, and ovarian cysts. As with any IUD, there's a risk of organ perforation on insertion ("very rare," per Prior), and, afterward, a risk of expulsion—or, most horribly, the thing could get stuck in the uterine wall and need surgical extraction.

Levonorgestrel has "androgenic" side effects (related to male sex hormones like testosterone) that can lead to hair loss, hair growth in places you don't want it (the "Mirena mustache"), greasy skin, and acne. The levonorgestrel and other progestin formulations—including combined oral contraceptives—are also associated with a slightly increased risk of breast cancer.

Unlike other hormonal contraceptives, the Mirena doesn't completely quash ovulation—though the evidence typically given to support this claim is beyond pathetic: a study on only seven women, back in 1980. In the first year, 85 percent of this tiny group didn't ovulate. In the second, only 15 percent did. I don't trust those numbers. However, for the most part, the Mirena appears to act "locally"—just in the uterus—with only perhaps 10 percent of the levonorgestrel it releases absorbed into the bloodstream: a level that might be enough to mustachio you up, but is too low to suppress ovulation.

ORAL PROGESTINS

Oral progestins prescribed to reduce heavy menstrual bleeding include medroxyprogesterone acetate and norethisterone. MPA is inexpensive, as is norethisterone (as low as $15 per month with one of the easy-to-google online coupons). However, in decreasing heavy bleeding, a 2019 systematic review from the Cochrane Collaboration finds them "inferior" to the progestin-releasing IUD (though Cochrane notes the quality of the evidence was "low or very low"). Additionally, they didn't even beat out OTC ibuprofen! The studies found "No clear evidence of difference in menstrual blood loss"!

COMBINED ORAL CONTRACEPTIVES

Combined oral contraceptives are estrogen and progestin combo pills—formerly the most commonly prescribed treatment for heavy menstrual bleeding. However, they are much less effective than the Mirena IUD, which reduced major bleeding by 83 percent by the second menstrual cycle in the study referenced above. In contrast, a 2019 Cochrane review suggests that the estrogen/progestin combo pill, taken over a six-month period, reduces heavy menstrual bleeding by 12 to 77 percent according to "moderate-quality evidence."

Side effects of the combined pill include nausea, headaches, abdominal cramping, breast tenderness, increased vaginal discharge, decreased libido, and breakthrough bleeding (spotting between periods). These drugs can also cause high blood pressure in some women or make it worse in those who already have it.

Women who smoke or have cardiovascular conditions (and related metabolic diseases like diabetes) are at increased risk from these drugs. For example, women with diabetes may experience impaired blood sugar metabolism for the first six months on the pill, possibly requiring adjustments to their blood sugar medications or insulin intake—or necessitating the consideration of alternative contraceptive methods.

ORAL MICRONIZED PROGESTERONE

Though—of course!—there's a dearth of clinical research on OMP for heavy bleeding, Prior offers her clinical *experience* in decades she was treating patients: "Full-dose progesterone exposure (oral micronized progesterone in a [daily] dose of 300 mg at bedtime for three months continuously)" diminishes the estrogen-driven crazy-heavy menstrual flow. After one month, "If flow is still sometimes heavy," Prior advises adding ibuprofen on every heavy flow day. "If any heavy flow is present after two months, the bleeding needs expert investigation."

Women in the US tend to be prescribed doses of progesterone—100 to 200 milligrams per day—that are insufficient for managing heavy flow. Prior explains that low doses—given cyclically (for two weeks or less per cycle)—"are not effective." Basically they're too wimpy and there for too little time to do the job.

She adds that for heavy flow in perimenopause, the daily 300-milligram dose of OMP is sometimes required for three months, paired with ibuprofen on every heavy flow day. Your flow will become irregular at first but will decrease over time. After three months of daily OMP, your doctor can switch you to the "cyclic" dosing mentioned above. *(Dosing details, Chapter Twenty-Six.)*

In Prior's medical practice, the ibuprofen/OMP combo almost always decreases flow to "something manageable," she says. However, if it doesn't, "vaginal or rectal progesterone capsules can be added as a morning dose." Prior again cautions that "it will take a few cycles before balance is restored." In other words, give the stuff a chance—instead of figuring it isn't working if the raging Red Sea doesn't immediately become The Red Puddle.

— 13 —

MENOPAUSE BY SCALPEL
*Side-effect-laden gyno cancer protection
for high-risk women promiscuously applied to all*

THE "JUST ANOTHER day at the scalpel factory" blandness of the term "surgical menopause" makes it sound like natural menopause with a slightly different neck treatment—the medical version of a knockoff Halston dress that comes in both T-neck and V-neck.

It's anything but.

Natural menopause involves an easing into menopause over a period of years, a gradual transition to the menopausally low levels of estrogen and progesterone. Surgical menopause—from the surgical removal of both of a woman's ovaries—is like being shot out of a cannon into menopause: abrupt, instant menopause with extra-severe effects, immediately and long-term.

The surgical procedure leading to immediate menopause is a "bilateral oophorectomy." Bilateral means "both sides," referring to the removal of ovaries on both sides of the uterus. The "ooph" part comes from *oophoros*, the Greek word for "egg bearing," the job description of the ovaries. In contrast, a "unilateral oophorectomy"—removal of only one of the two ovaries—does not lead to the same abrupt onset of menopause. Retaining one ovary when possible, called "organ sparing," helps preserve fertility, makes for a less symptomatic perimenopause and menopause (compared with surgical menopause), and maintains the health benefits and protections provided by the ovaries—even in menopause.

Surgical menopause is health demolishing in multiple ways natural menopause is not, even if the surgery is done close to the age of natural menopause. Gynecologist Cristina Secosan, MD, cites an "increased overall mortality rate" associated with surgical menopause—3.5 more women dying (per 1,000 women per year) compared with women who hang on to their ovaries. That increased risk can be reduced by starting hormone therapy immediately after surgery, which also serves to mitigate some of the other negative health effects from surgical menopause.

We saw in the previous chapter that surgical menopause increases the risk of coronary heart disease (both fatal and non-fatal), strokes, and bone fracture. It also increases the risk of lung and colon cancer, and in women who have the surgery before age 50, there's an elevated risk of cognitive impairment or dementia—one that is even more elevated in women who undergo the procedure at age 45 or younger.

Now, we all get that natural menopause is not exactly a festival of feel-good and robust health. And in the transition years to natural menopause, due to the ups and downs of perimenopausal estrogen, many of us may suffer estrogen withdrawal and the stress-hormone-related symptoms that come with. But estrogen is going in and out, diving and then coming up again. It generally maintains a presence.

The sudden removal of the ovaries, on the other hand, triggers estrogen withdrawal of the most extreme kind: ovarian estrogen just GONE. (Other parts of our body *do* produce estrogen but in minuscule supply.) Not surprisingly, surgical menopause is associated with particularly harsh symptoms when estrogen treatment is not initiated. These include extra-boilacious hot flashes, an increased (and even doubled) incidence of insomnia, and a heightened risk of mental health symptoms, as well as sexual problems—caused by vaginal dryness and decreased libido.

It isn't just the surgical removal of our ovaries that causes us problems. For example, a hysterectomy—*just* the removal of the uterus—can damage pelvic nerves integral to women's sexual response. Gynecology researcher Risa Lonnée-Hoffmann, MD, reports that about 10 to 20 percent of hysterectomy patients experience "deteriorated sexual function" due to painful intercourse or "altered orgasmic experience" (for example, decreased sensation making orgasm elusive, near impossible, or simply unattainable). A friend of mine was one of these women. Despite being no pushover, she came out of her surgery feeling she'd had all the informed say of a roast chicken on a carving board:

> My menopause was surgical based on the fact that I had fibroids, was 48 and therefore close to natural menopause anyway, and had some markers in my bloodwork that were red flags for ovarian cancer. More tests were done, I didn't have cancer (phew) but a hysterectomy was recommended. I didn't realize the doc was gonna take my ovaries too (plus the cervix)—so I was basically gutted and surprised.
>
> She's a lady doc, and a woman friend of mine who's also a doc and who was my general practitioner at the time (she's since retired) was in on it too: I trust their medical judgement, but wish I'd been clearly informed on what exactly was going to happen. I could have asked more questions too, but oh well. It's done, so whatever.
>
> I lost my libido pretty much overnight, but even when I had sex (which I did attempt, after I healed from surgery), not having any more natural lube was a real bummer. It just wasn't much fun anymore... so we just gave it up.

Beyond the nerves for sexual function that can be damaged in a hysterectomy, the surgical removal of the uterus and the cervix, independently or along with the ovaries, can also damage nerves that are vital in bladder and bowel function. A nerve-sparing hysterectomy technique was pioneered in Japan, but it is intricate, and doctors require special training to perform it. It is typically referred to as a "nerve-sparing radical hysterectomy" or a "nerve-sparing surgical technique."

Some gynecological oncologists at major cancer centers may be trained in it, but it is not widely offered in the US. Not all women are candidates for it; for example, wider surgical margins may be required in women with cancer to ensure no diseased tissue is left behind.

Nerve damage is just one factor in the loss of sexual function. For example, the cervix produces mucus that acts as a natural lubricant during sex. Remove the cervix; remove the lube. With the loss of estrogen at menopause or from an oophorectomy, there's a decrease in vaginal elasticity. This unfortunate duo alone makes for a very unhappy sexual combo.

PREVENTION VS. PROMISCUOUS OVERTREATMENT

Hysterectomy is one of the most frequently performed surgical procedures for women in the US. Approximately 80 percent of the 400,000 to 500,000 hysterectomies performed every year are for non-cancerous conditions such as pelvic pain or fibroids. Within this group of women, *40 to 50 percent* were persuaded by their doctors to have their ovaries cut out along with their uterus, explains gynecological surgeon William Parker, MD.

Tacking on removal of their ovaries to their hysterectomy surgery when they show no disease—called "prophylactic oophorectomy when hysterectomy is performed"—is usually done in hopes of reducing a woman's risk of ovarian cancer.

Ovarian cancer, the fifth deadliest cancer among women, tends to be asymptomatic. Heartbreakingly, this leads to frequent late-stage diagnosis.

Proactive removal of the ovaries with a hysterectomy allows an estimated 1,000 women a year to avoid ovarian cancer, resulting in a 12 percent reduction in the total cases diagnosed, reports urogynecologist Elisabeth Erekson, MD. The procedure also decreases the risk of breast cancer, likely due to the loss of estrogen with the loss of the ovaries.

Picturing this invisible killer disease hiding in us—undetectable on medical imaging—the natural response is a hyperventilating, "Excuse me, nurse—can you point me to the line for oophorectomies?" But let's give another look at what that translates to: "Excuse me, nurse—can you point me to the line for surgical menopause and the heart attacks, crumbling bones, lung cancer, and premature death that come with?"

In other words, by having prophylactic ovary removal within the cutoff period, you'll decrease your risk of dying of breast and ovarian cancer, but you'll likely die faster while suffering horribly.

Due to the substantial health harms associated with surgical menopause, proactively removing the ovaries during a hysterectomy to reduce ovarian cancer risk appears to "unintentionally cause more deaths from all causes by age 80 than the number of lives saved from ovarian cancer," concludes Erekson.

Parker concurs—in multiple papers. With his colleagues, he homed in on exactly what "more deaths" from adding a bilateral oophorectomy to a hysterectomy mean. They created a powerful risk-benefit calculation tool and plugged in large datasets from studies on ovarian hormone-related disease and death. Let's lay out their model and their results.

Meet the women: 10,000 women ages 50 to 54 undergoing hysterectomy who also choose to get their ovaries removed (and don't use estrogen therapy).

Next, we check in on them at age 80: Fewer women have died from ovarian cancer—47 fewer than if they *hadn't* had their ovaries removed with their hysterectomy.

However, this benefit came at a price: 838 more women died of coronary heart disease and 158 more died from hip fracture!

In sum, tacking on ovarian removal with a hysterectomy, while saving the lives of 47 women who would otherwise have died of ovarian cancer, causes 949 more women to die from heart attacks and hip fracture than would have if they'd hung on to their ovaries!

Parker sums up: "The risk of ovarian cancer has been overemphasized by physicians to the exclusion of other long-term risks," which has led to "preventive surgery" in women who are not at high risk of ovarian cancer. "At no age" was this associated with a survival benefit.

There *are* ways to mitigate ovarian cancer risk without ovary removal, Parker points out. Hysterectomy alone is shown to reduce the risk of ovarian cancer "by an average of 46%." And though hysterectomies are neither risk- nor cost-free, their effects are vastly less severe than the loss of the ovaries.

But the most significant way to mitigate ovarian cancer risk is recognizing that the ovaries are actually not the source of *most* ovarian cancer. They're just a landing pad for it. A cancer hotel.

A REVOLUTIONARY FINDING: MOST OVARIAN CANCER IS FALLOPIAN TUBE CANCER

Because the removal of the ovaries decreases the incidence of ovarian cancer, there was a long-standing assumption that the ovaries were the source of the problem. However, we've been missing a vital bit of detail that Dr. Parker pointed out to me: Pretty much whenever an oophorectomy is done, they don't just take out the ovaries. The fallopian tubes get cut out, too, technically making the procedure not just an oophorectomy but a "salpingo-oophorectomy"—a tubes-plus-ovaries removal. ("Salpingo" comes from the Greek *salpinx*, a long, straight, tube-like trumpet.)

The fallopian tubes—twin tubes, one by each ovary—are basically the Interstate for egg transportation from the ovaries to the uterus, though they aren't directly *connected* to the ovaries. Each has what look like funny little cartoon fingers called "fimbriae" extending on the end by the ovary. When the dominant ovarian follicle ruptures, allowing the egg to make its exit from the ovary, the fingery things sweep over to the ovary and pick up the egg—and then, with the help of muscle contractions, send it on its way to the uterus.

Pathologist and ovarian cancer biologist Louis Dubeau, MD, proposed in 1999 that many "ovarian" cancers actually originate in the fallopian tubes and subsequently spread to the ovaries. Extensive research has been conducted since then, supporting his hypothesis. As gynecologic oncologist Kara Long Roche puts it, "The fallopian tube is now well established as the site of origin for most ovarian cancers, particularly high-grade serous carcinomas."

There isn't a single type of ovarian cancer; however, 60 to 80 percent of all ovarian cancers are high-grade serous carcinomas (HGSC). They are both the most common and most lethal kind, often showing themselves only at an advanced stage, and these are the ones that start in the fallopian tubes—in the finger-like end projections near the ovaries, the fimbriae—and migrate to the ovaries. This is thought to happen through cell shedding and the close proximity to the ovary of the fimbriae.

Prophylactic removal of the fallopian tubes is now being used as a protective measure to reduce the risk of ovarian cancer. By taking out the fallopian tubes alone—without removing the ovaries, uterus, and cervix—women maintain their hormonal, sexual, bladder, and bowel function, which can be compromised when pelvic nerves are severed during a hysterectomy or other surgery.

After bilateral salpingectomy (both fallopian tubes surgically removed), there is an estimated 35 to 65 percent reduction in the risk of ovarian cancer, according to a large observational study led by gynecology researcher Gillian

E. Hanley in Canada. Two other large observational studies in North America and Sweden reported similar results.

The findings from these studies and other research are strong enough that major North American medical societies (ACOG and its Canadian counterpart, SOGC, the Society of Obstetricians and Gynecologists of Canada) recommend what's called "opportunistic salpingectomy" for "average-risk women who have completed childbearing and who are undergoing pelvic surgery for benign disease," reports experimental surgery researcher Kevin Verhoeff. This is the removal of the fallopian tubes during surgery that's being done for another reason.

By "benign disease," he means surgeries in the pelvic area that are not being done to remove cancer. Examples include an appendectomy, a cesarean section, or laparoscopic hernia repair. In 2013, the Society of Gynecological Oncology announced that in "Women at average risk of ovarian cancer, salpingectomy should be discussed and considered prior to abdominal or pelvic surgery."

The procedure appears safe, with safety data from three studies (140 patients total) reporting no post-op complications. However, there *could* be "complications such as bleeding or inadvertent injury to the ovarian blood supply." Additionally, he notes, "surgeons should also discuss the continued risk of ovarian cancer following [opportunistic salpingectomy] since certain types of epithelial ovarian cancer do originate from the ovary itself."

DON'T LET CANCER TELL YOU IT'S PMS

If your body's a crap carnival of symptoms in perimenopause or menopause, it's easy to jump to the conclusion that any new discomfort that rises up in you is part of it—which can leave you shrugging off symptoms of ladyparts cancers (officially called "gynecologic cancer").

"The five main types of gynecologic cancer are: cervical, ovarian, uterine, vaginal, and vulvar," according to the Centers for Disease Control and Prevention. The following are common symptoms, adapted from the CDC's website:

- Abnormal vaginal bleeding or discharge. (Common for all gynecologic cancers except vulvar cancer.)
- Feeling full too quickly, having difficulty eating, or experiencing bloating or abdominal or back pain. (Common for ovarian cancer.)

- Pelvic pain or pressure. (Common for ovarian and uterine cancers.)
- Increased urinary frequency or urgency and/or the onset of constipation. (Common for ovarian and uterine cancers.)
- Itching, burning, pain, or tenderness of the vulva (those vaginal "lips"); changes in vulva color; and skin issues, such as sores, warts, or a rash. (Indications of vulvar cancer.)

According to CDC data from 2012 to 2016, the most common gynecologic cancer overall was uterine cancer (which is usually endometrial cancer, cancer of the uterine lining), and the least common was vaginal cancer.

Uterine cancer diagnoses are generally on the rise, but this is especially true for black women. Black women are more likely than white women to have uterine cancer and are *twice as likely* as white women to die from it.

Hispanic women are less likely to have uterine cancer but more likely to have cervical cancer. White women are prone to uterine, ovarian, and vulvar cancer. Asian women may be less prone than white women to have uterine cancer—or may be equally prone (according to different studies from 2003 on with annoyingly conflicting findings). Native American women (American Indian and Alaska Native) appear to have lower rates of uterine cancer than other groups.

These differences are *general*, meaning *individuals* in these groups may not fit the usual pattern. So, for example, if you are a Native American or Hispanic woman, don't shrug off symptoms of uterine cancer because your group tends to have a lower occurrence.

Again, *any* bleeding after menopause MUST be checked out pronto by a doctor—and I mean *pronto*, like, make a doctor appointment within the hour after you notice it, unless it's 3 a.m. The same goes if you're experiencing any of these other symptoms. (If you don't currently have healthcare or much money, look for free clinics like the wonderful Venice Family Clinic, here in LA.)

We've all lost too many friends to cancer, and that long, terribly sad list of all their names should remain free of yours.

— 14 —

SEX, LIBIDO, AND DESERT VAGINA

WE'RE A COUNTRY of people embarrassed about sex. We'll give a doctor encyclopedic detail about our ugly divorce, but talk about our sexual functioning or any of the parts involved? We'll just pretend we're like Barbie, with a small stretch of flat plastic between our legs.

Because doctors are also people, many are no less embarrassed and uncomfortable talking about sex than the rest of us. Including doctors who spend their working hours prospecting in vaginas with a speculum and a flashlight!

This is a problem, because there are a host of genital, sexual, and urinary symptoms that frequently arise in menopause (and, for some women, in perimenopause). The official umbrella term for this funpack is the "genitourinary syndrome of menopause" (GSM). We'll get into the "urogenital" details, but, in short: Everything in or on your pelvis that you've long relied on may decide to stop working or just sort of work and itch or hurt or both. ("Hurt" encompassing the full spectrum from mild throb-'n'-ache to feeling like you're being stabbed in the vagina.)

Surveys of women in menopause find that doctors "seldom ask about GSM symptoms," reports gynecologist Kimberly K. Vesco, MD. "As a result, symptoms are often unaddressed"—that is, often allowed to rampage on, untreated.

"Often unaddressed" is something of an understatement.

An estimated 84% of menopausal women experience symptoms of GSM: among them, dry, suddenly sandpaperish vaginal tissue; painful sex; painful urination; recurrent urinary tract infections; and leaky pee.

Yet, in the US, only 6 to 7 % of menopausal women are diagnosed with these issues! And not necessarily because their doctors asked anything about The Department of Down There. Chances are some women got so desperate that they flung embarrassment out their car window while speeding to their doctor's office, where they murmur something tactfully ladylike to the receptionist, such as, "MY VAGINA FEELS LIKE IT'S BEING EATEN BY FIRE ANTS!"

There is a way to get women to open up. In 2016, Italian gynecologist Angelo Cagnacci, MD, and his colleagues published the AGATA study (an acronym extracted from letters here and there in "Atrofia Genitale Associata all'Età della Menopausa"—in English, "Genital Atrophy Associated with Menopause").

Gynecologists performing vaginal exams on menopausal women were instructed to tell each woman exactly what they were seeing during the exam: the physical signs of vaginal erosion and other issues. No sooner did they do this than they got an earful from many of the women, who complained about these symptoms and their effects. Ultimately, this conversation-prompt method led the gynecologists to diagnose GSM in 64.7 to 84.2% of the women—allowing all of these women to understand what's going on in their body and opt for treatment.

Let's look at the effects of the AGATA method on a major GSM problem, vaginal dryness—or as I (ugh!) came to call it, "desert vagina." Compare the 6 or 7% of women in the US who are diagnosed with various symptoms of GSM with the huge percent of women in the AGATA study who opened up about *their* vaginal dryness—along with their other symptoms.

Below, I give you AGATA data points two ways. On top, there are the symptoms the doctors told women they observed (Speculum Says!) and below that, the symptoms the women reported in response (Survey Says!):

SEX, LIBIDO, AND DESERT VAGINA

SPECULUM SAYS!

The physical signs of GSM that doctors observed in vaginal exams

- 99% of the women had evidence of vaginal dryness.
- 92.1% had thinning of vaginal tissue.
- 71.9% showed vaginal tissue fragility.
- 46.7% had burst capillaries under their vaginal skin, a sign of tissue trauma.
- 90.7% had tissue pallor: vaginal tissue that appeared an unhealthily pale shade.

SURVEY SAYS!

The related GSM symptoms women revealed upon hearing their doctor's observations

- 100% of these women reported vaginal dryness.
- 77% found intercourse painful.
- 57% experienced vaginal burning.
- 57% experienced vaginal itching.
- 36% had pain in urination.

Vesco and her team note that we women spend a third of our lives in menopause, so urinary, vaginal, vulval, and sexual symptoms that are ignored and left untreated can gnaw away at our quality of life for a substantial chunk of time.

That's an important considerati   because your US doctor is unlikely to give you the symptom prompts of   GATA-style exam. To motivate yourself to speak up so you can have an   M symptoms you're experiencing diagnosed and treated, you might   yourself of two things:

1. "Dying of embarrassm   " is just a figure of speech.
2. The ongoing misery of untreated GSM far exceeds any momentary discomfort from disclosing GSM symptoms.

To overcome the embarrassment, accept reality: It'll be uncomfortable. Then tell yourself that you don't *need* to feel comfortable; you just need to do it: Rip the band-aid off. Make yourself say the words: "I have a lot of vaginal dryness" (or whatever).

Like four seconds, and it's over—and it should get your doctor to examine you, ask you some questions, and diagnose you, which should give you potential treatment options you wouldn't have heard about if you'd kept that band-aid taped over your lips like a gag.

THE GENITOURINARY FAMILY
The sex and peeing pack of organs that give out on us

Anybody who lived in New York in the 1980s and '90s probably remembers the 1-900-PEEE ads that ran on late-night cuckoo public access TV: "1-900-PEEE! The extra E is for extra PEEEEEEEE!"

There was apparently enough of a market of pee fetishists in the tri-state area to make this profitable—for a decade or more!

I was not among them. However, I was a long way from menopause back then. There's little that turns a woman pee-obsessed like the urinary effects of menopause: a bladder and urethra and the muscles thereabouts suddenly going, "Look, we're tired. We're kinda done here." This means she suddenly has, among other things, a tendency to *leak pee*—or blow out a bunch of it if she does something ill-advised, such as sneeze.

Urinary issues are just one of the collection of joys that pop up in our genitourinary system, which includes the vagina, the bladder and its urine-transporting tubing (the urethra), the clitoris, the pelvic floor muscles and tissue, and the vulva (the lippy entranceway to the vagina).

Take the vagina, the highway to and from our uterus. It's an elastic, muscular tube inside us, three to six inches long and an inch to just over an inch wide, on average. It's highly elastic and resilient—at least during our menstruating years, thanks to estrogen. Along with providing elasticity, estrogen helps keep our vaginal tissue thick and moist, with a healthy pH (low enough and acidic enough)—all of which help prevent tissue damage from traffic in our vagina (babies being born...sex toys...penises).

With the loss of estrogen at menopause, there's a loss of its benefits for vaginal tissue, which thins out, loses folds that gave it flexibility, and becomes less elastic.

Oscar-winning actress Halle Berry got unexpectedly introduced to this tissue thinning, reported Yahoo and BuzzFeed. "I finally meet the man of my dreams," said Berry, referring to her boyfriend, Van Hunt. "We're having sex and everything is great."

Out of the blue, Berry, who had yet to hit menopause, experiences pain afterward—"terrible" pain. "I feel like I have razor blades in my vagina." She drives straight to her gynecologist, who goes for a vaginal look-see. "He says, 'Halle, you have a new guy right?' I said, 'I do, I'm really excited.' He said, 'You messed up again... You have the worst case of herpes I have ever seen.'"

From the doctor's office, Berry calls Hunt, who is shocked and says he does *not* have herpes.

They both get tested.

Diagnosis?

No, not herpes! Just a gynecologist breathtakingly ignorant about perimenopause—and especially late perimenopause when estrogen levels tend to be lower, progressively declining while on final approach to petering out to a trickle.

It isn't just the tissue thinning that turns sex into a scrapefest. Bottomed-out estrogen levels in menopause make for reduced blood flow to the vagina, explains gynecologist Nanette Santoro. This leads to reduced "vaginal secretions"—stingy amounts of what's basically vagina sweat: the natural lubrication produced in the wake of sexual arousal. So, for example, make-out sessions that previously got a woman "wet" so her boyfriend's penis could slide in no longer do the job, and El Peeno makes its entrance like an oversized beater car scraping the walls of a narrow garage. (I know—where do we all sign up?)

The vagina can also narrow (and in very rare, severe cases, close up). The vulval lips may thin out, and the clitoris can shrink (or as one deeply dismayed woman on Menopause Reddit put it, "my clitoris has all but disappeared"). Not to be left out, the bladder and pelvic floor muscles tend to weaken, potentially leading to a more frequent need to urinate (including that annoying nocturia waking us up), as well as incontinence (uncontrolled urinary leakage) and urinary tract infections.

Dunno about you, but I can't help but look back fondly on my days of PMS, immobilizing menstrual cramps, and Tampax the size of pool noodles.

WHY SO DRY—AND YET SO LEAKY?
Potential causes beyond estrogen decline

The widely accepted reason for genitourinary symptoms, from leaky pee to sex that feels like you're getting it on with a belt sander, is the menopausal decline in estrogen. This does make sense as *a* reason. We see that the physical and functional declines driving these and other indignities are led by estrogen decline, while replacing estrogen diminishes or reverses the physical and functional issues—alleviating or even preventing many symptoms. However, there *is* an "it's complicated" to estrogen's benefits. "Estrogen replacement has been shown to alleviate most GSM symptoms except for UI" (urinary incontinence), explains Santoro.

Actually, there *is* one form of urinary incontinence that estrogen is shown to alleviate, but only "local" vaginal estrogen (in contrast with "systemic" full-system estrogen, which is probably what Santoro had in mind). Vaginal estrogen reduces "urge incontinence"—marked by a sudden strong need to pee and by pee sometimes sneaking out before you can make it to the throne. Vaginal estrogen can also be helpful for decreasing nocturia and other forms of overactive bladder (OAB).

Estrogen, whether vaginal or systemic, *doesn't* seem to alleviate "stress incontinence": abdominal pressure from a cough, a sneeze, or a jog that causes you to leak pee. In fact, there were claims that estrogen—from systemic hormone therapy—made it worse!

Not so fast, says urogynecologist Eleonora Russo, MD. Because stress incontinence investigations were tacked on to studies primarily looking at other conditions, the researchers lacked the instruments needed to assess the type or severity of urinary incontinence. "Therefore, these data need to be interpreted with caution," she concludes—collegial researcher-ese for "Shame on you, you methodological slobs!" Echoing Santoro, she emphasized in a 2021 paper: "To date, there is no evidence for the efficacy of systemic estrogen treatment for any form of incontinence."

There *are* a bunch of ways UI is managed. These include inserting little rings and tiny dishes made of soft silicone to help support your pelvic organs and reduce urinary leakage. But the ideal way to *start* managing UI or other urinary issues is to see a urogynecologist—a specialist in women's urinary and pelvic floor disorders—who is likely to give you the most expert, up-to-date diagnosis and treatment.

Conflicting with the notion of low estrogen as the *cause* of vaginal dryness and other menopausal symptoms is the fact that some perimenopausal women whose bodies are still making estrogen experience vaginal dryness—as do some estrogen-producing women in their late teens and early 20s. In fact, about 17 percent of *pre*menopausal women—women from 18 to 50 years of age who are *not yet in menopause*—struggle with this issue, according to the British Menopause Society. The reason, Dr. Prior writes, is "unknown."

Other potential causes of vaginal dryness and the rest of the symptoms remain disturbingly uninvestigated. These include flattened menopausal progesterone levels and muscles gone to seed from being sedentary. The latter one might seem odd: muscle erosion from sitting around too much that travels to your vagina?! In fact, muscle weakness from disuse eventually has chronic systemic effects, meaning it becomes a full-body thing.

We *do* know estrogen can soar in perimenopause (conflicting with the "It's deficient estrogen!" diagnosis perimenopausal women are given for vaginal dryness), and estrogen levels are lower close to menopause. But yoo-hoo, researchers! Which hormone is low in both perimenopause and menopause? (That would be progesterone!)

In a randomized controlled trial led by dermatologist Gregor Holzer, MD, a 2% progesterone cream applied to the skin of perimenopausal and menopausal women increased both elasticity and firmness. This was the "upstairs" skin—the face—the subject of a slowly growing area of study.

However, I found only a *planned* study—a randomized controlled trial on vaginal progesterone for "atrophic vaginitis," the medical term for the thinning, drying, and inflammation of vaginal tissues. It was registered in 2015 at clinicaltrials.gov by gynecologist and menopause researcher Wendy Wolfman, MD.

I emailed Wolfman about when her results might be coming out, and she responded: "Unfortunately we never completed the study due to lack of funding." There could be a number of reasons her study wasn't funded, but I'll place my bet on the belief that estrogen is *the* treatment for vaginal tissue erosion playing a major role. Prescription estrogen *is* a major savior for menopausal women suffering genital, sexual, and urinary symptoms. It's just that other potential causes and solutions should be investigated, too.

For example, a potential contributor to vaginal atrophy might be *chronic systemic inflammation*: constant long-term inflammation throughout the body. Systemic inflammation is implicated in penis problems: deficiencies in blood flow and erectile dysfunction in Mr. (formerly) Happy.

Research does find that high levels of systemic inflammation are associated with vulvodynia and vestibulodynia—chronic pain in the vulva and in the vestibule, the foyer-like area by the vaginal opening, respectively. Vaginal atrophy was not studied. However, because chronic inflammation is implicated in so many degenerative disorders, it likely contributes to the rather rude ways our vaginal and other tissue tends to erode on us in menopause. This, too, suggests a role for progesterone, which you might recall has inflammation-curbing effects.

FIFTY SHADES OF GO AWAY
Are a third of women sexually broken or is there a problem with the standard?

There are women in relationships who feel unloved and ignored, who tend to be about as sexually approachable as a laundry basket of poisonous snakes.

No surprise, right?

However, these women are joined in their sexual unapproachability by another group of women: happy women in loving, satisfying relationships who once had satisfying sex lives. They don't find sex traumatic or painful, and their partner hasn't become physically offensive or otherwise a big no-go. They aren't opposed to sex; in fact, they want to want sex—they just have no desire to have it with their partner.

THE COMA SUTRA

In the 1990s, sexual medicine specialist Rosemary Basson, MD., read scientific surveys that suggested 30 to 35 percent of adult women experienced "low sexual desire." More than a third of the adult female population! That number took her aback. But "low" compared with what? Basson began to suspect the problem wasn't in women themselves but in the way the male sexual response was held up as the sexual norm, I reported in my syndicated advice column.

Basson explains that men have "spontaneous sexual hunger," meaning spontaneous lust: sudden, out-of-nowhere raging horniness, prompting a desire to get it on. Women, too, experience this spontaneous lust—in the early stages of a relationship or if they're away from their partner for a stretch of days or weeks. However, Basson finds that after a woman settles into a relationship, she tends to have a different cycle of sexual response. Her desire becomes "triggerable," meaning that she first needs to start fooling around with her partner, which is likely to lead to her experiencing arousal, and then to a desire to have sex.

Basson calls this the female "cycle of sexual desire." It tends to be a factor in any couple with at least one female partner. However, because most couples, whether straight, bisexual, or lesbian, don't know this, their sex lives (and often their relationships) go to pot while they wait around for the woman's (or women's) desire to spontaneously erupt—which is like waiting for a bus that never comes.

Starting in 2006, I wrote about Basson's finding in my syndicated advice column every few years because I heard from so many readers—especially those in heterosexual relationships—that their relationship was in peril because the woman no longer wanted sex. After each column ran, I'd get emails along the lines of "This saved our marriage!"

That's not all Basson's insight saves. She explains that women stop feeling "inferior" or broken simply because they had the *normal sexual response* of *women* in relationships.

Basson notes that there *are* some women who experience a physical disorder, called hypoactive sexual desire disorder (HSDD)—defined as low or absent sexual desire. Women diagnosed with HSDD are unable to experience "any responsive desire" *and* feel highly distressed because of it.

Gynecologist and sexologist Rossella E. Nappi, MD, notes that there's an idea that "HSDD is a made-up condition which serves only marketing purposes for lifestyle drugs." Pharma companies *have* come up with drugs to "treat" it—flibanserin (brand drug: Addyi) and bremelanotide (brand drug: Vyleesi). These drugs are only for use in perimenopausal women, have dangerous side effects, and barely work. There were major protests to the FDA that flibanserin was approved at all. In fact, both drugs are considered so seriously risky to take that they are restricted and only available through an FDA risk-monitoring and mitigation program called REMS.

Nappi and her colleagues cite research suggesting neurochemical and hormonal causes for low sexual desire and call for the development of "safe and effective hormonal and non-hormonal treatments of HSDD" for both menopausal and premenopausal women. The Nappi team points to research on lab animals and humans suggesting that amping up the activity of dopamine—the neurotransmitter driving seeking and wanting—and decreasing the activity of the sexual desire-inhibiting neurochemical serotonin, "may have a prosexual effect."

Ultimately, though some women may have biochemical issues affecting their desire, for many, what really needs curing is the assumption that women in long-term relationships are sexually dead. Additionally, not being into sex (and being good with that) or not wanting as much sex as one's partner—and especially one's male partner—should not be seen as the failings they are made out to be.

Men in general have much higher sex drives—which is probably why novelist Philip Roth wrote about a guy who molested a pound of liver in his mom's refrigerator, while decade after decade, I've never done so much as flirt with the pâté in mine.

THE LOST CITY OF CLITORIS

My fingers were my faithful sex providers throughout my life, and I am especially grateful for their excellent work during periods of sexual drought. Tragically, they were no match for the menopausal clitoris.

With loss of estrogen at menopause and the decreased blood flow to vaginal tissue, your clitoris doesn't just shrink. It becomes less sensitive, which means it takes longer to get to your happy ending, and by longer, I mean, think of that old movie with Lawrence of Arabia crossing the desert on a camel.

Hormone therapy is found to improve clitoral sensitivity. However, let's note that "improve" is not a synonym for "fully restore"—and you could lose a damn finger trying to make yourself come. Luckily, it's the 21st century. The answer? Automate! Retire your fingers and get your vagina a rechargeable friend! Yes—a vibrator!

For many of you, this is "Um, duh!-type advice, but there *are* women who are uncomfortable with it. If you are one of them, this section is mostly for you.

Here goes:

I bet you've worked hard and accomplished a thing or two. Well, don't you deserve to feel all the pleasure you can? Maybe you were raised to have (or just developed) sexual shame, but there's a way to see this vibrator thing that might help you cut the circuit powering it. Consider that, beyond the person part of us, *we're just meat*—bodies with meat that feels good when you rub it in some places. That's just a fact. And you harm not a person in the world by taking advantage of that fact.

So many of us in our 50s, and especially our 60s and beyond, have a hard time getting partners. That's tough, but if it's where you're at, look around your life. Is it satisfying and meaningful? Do you have some wonderful friends and family you love, whose presence in your life makes you feel happy and loved? Maybe instead of picking through the dregs on dating apps in hopes of having sex again before you die, you can cover the sex thing by opting for self-serve. In the words of one of my favorite, um, doctors, Dr. Seuss: "Oh, the places you'll go!"

As a vibrator newbie put it on Reddit:

A vibrator is changing my life.

This is absolutely so ridiculous, but I feel like it's true.

A few weeks ago in a moment of weakness I ordered a vibrator. I never had anything against them, or anyone who uses one, I had just always figured they weren't for me.

I like sex, it's fun and all, but I almost never come. I get it isn't always about the orgasm, but y'know sometimes, it is.

But anyway, the vibrator is awesome, and it makes me come like nothing else. I feel SO much less stressed, I look glowing, like physically I look nicer. I have no tension.

Anyway, I kinda just feel like telling every single person ever to buy a vibrator.

There are awesome inexpensive vibrators online, and you can choose one through reviews—or call a store like San Francisco's Good Vibrations and ask for advice from one of their "Sex Educator/Sales Associates," who spend their days matter-of-factly helping people choose the right vibrators, dildos, butt plugs, and the like. This store was founded in 1977 by sex educator Joani Blank, who, the GV site notes, "pioneered an alternative to conventional adult stores by focusing on sex education and women's pleasure."

Vibrator types of note include

- **Clitornados:** combo clit-sucker/vibrators that used to sell for around $200 when they first came out, but now can be had for $30 to $50.
- **Buzzzzzz bunny:** vibrators shaped like penises that rotate internally and have rabbit-ear (or sometimes anteater-nose) attachments to give your clitoris vibrating attention.
- **The vintage Cadillac of vibrators:** the famous Hitachi Magic Wand massager that sex educator Betty Dodson popularized as a female pleasure tool way back in the 1970s.

In January 2024, *The New York Times' Wirecutter* blog, reviewing "The Best Vibrators," deemed the Hitachi the absolute best friend you could give your clitoris. (And I would add: Especially if you are a menopausal woman.)

As sexual health educator Bianca Alba put it in her review: "No toy offers the level of power and intensity as the widely beloved Magic Wand. The intense stimulation it provides can be particularly helpful for people experiencing diminished libido or sensitivity."

If you're a first-time buyer, you might picture—with some horror—your postal carrier delivering the package with your vibrator all, "Look who's getting her freak on!" Look up the "discreet shipping" policy of an online sex toy retailer (which few could remain in business without). You're sure to see something like "All of our packages are shipped discreetly in plain packaging, with 'Barnaby LTD' as the name on the return address"—and not a word about what's inside: the best in vibrating power tools for your clitoris.

YOU JUST NEEDED TO BE SAVED BY PENIS MAN!*
(Spoiler: Um, no you didn't.)

Gynecologist Jen Gunter, MD, goes on this fabulous tear in *The Vagina Bible*, debunking the "use it or lose it!" woman-blamey myth "that a penis is the cure for everything." Supposedly, if you don't get some regular penis up in your vagina after menopause, your vaginal tissue will take this as a message to crap out on you, becoming thin, dry, and even scarred. The thinking behind this, writes Gunter, "is that the local trauma of sex keeps the tissues healthy, possibly due to increased blood flow (the body's response to injury is to send more blood to the injured site)."

She says this notion that "sexual activity with a penis preserves the vagina from GSM always sounded biologically preposterous and devoid of common sense" to her, "in addition to ignoring the experiences of women." Gunter adds that she went through menopause at 49, and "Sex did not protect my vagina."

She concedes that her personal experience does not count as scientific evidence. However, in a four-country European study called REVIVE, surveying 3,768 menopausal women (ages 45 to 75), a whole bunch who'd been riding the penis pony likewise did not find sex protective for them. (Or, in more scientific terms, 51 percent of the study participants experiencing "vulvar and vaginal atrophy" were sexually active.)

VAGINAL LUBRICANTS AND MOISTURIZERS
(If desert vagina is your only issue)

If your only problem is vaginal dryness, a little slippety-slide from lube or lotion—a vaginal lubricant or moisturizer—might be just the thing to grease your path back to pain-free enjoyable sex.

Dr. Gunter, a specialist in treating chronic vulvovaginal pain, explains in *The Menopause Manifesto* that lubricants and moisturizers are different. *Lubricants* are short-term dryness alleviators, used so you can stay wet during sex, while *vaginal moisturizers* provide vaginal lubrication over a period of days.

VAGINAL LUBRICANTS

There are three types of lubes: water-based, silicone-based, and oil-based. Which works for a woman is a personal preference thing, but Gunter observes that women with GSM "tend to do best with a silicone lubricant," making it "a good place to start."

***Silicone-based lubes* that Gunter says seem "well-tolerated":**
- Astroglide X—silicone only
- Astroglide X Silicone Gel—silicone and coconut oil
- überlube—silicone and vitamin E

***Water-based lubes* Gunter recommends:**
- Good Clean Love—pH 4.73 and 240 mOsm/kg
- AH! YES Water-Based Personal Lubricant—pH 4.08 and 154 mOsm/kg

Should you consider other brands, Gunter advises that water-based lubes should have a pH of 3.5 to 4.5, the premenopausal pH of the vagina. (Unfortunately, few products list the pH.)

Another important factor is "osmolality"—how concentrated the molecules of a product are. Osmolality should be less than 380 mOsm/kg, because vaginal secretions have an osmolality of 260 to 280 mOsm/kg, Gunter explains. Exceeding that can potentially *reverse-moisturize* your vaginal tissue—that is, drain it of moisture, leaving it drier than before you "moisturized."

Oil-based lubricants

Oil-based lubes can work, too, but Gunter cautions that they are incompatible with latex condoms. She didn't list any of these, but AH! YES sells one—AH! YES Natural Plant Oil Based Personal Lubricant—and that's a product line she has recommended (under the name YES outside of the US). Personally, I've grabbed olive oil in a pinch, and Gunter reports that some women also like coconut oil.

VAGINAL MOISTURIZERS

Vaginal moisturizers "rehydrate vaginal tissues and are formulated to be bioadhesive"—to adhere to human tissue—allowing them to stay on the vaginal tissue for several days, Gunter explains. "At times they perform as well as lower-dose estrogen" (prescription vaginally-applied estrogen).

"Vaginal moisturizers can be water-based," she adds. "Glycerine is a common ingredient" and "should be in a concentration of 8.3% or less." Moisturizers can also be silicone- or oil-based. Hyaluronic acid—a substance now in an increasing number of face creams—is a powerful option.

"Hyaluronic acid is a large molecule that is found in and around skin cells that lubricates and hydrates cells," writes Gunter. In a small randomized controlled study comparing hyaluronic acid vaginal tablets with vaginal estradiol tablets, urogynecologist Murat Ekin, MD, found that both "provided relief of vaginal symptoms," decreased vaginal tissue erosion, and improved vaginal tissue by increasing the percentage of cell layers in it. Ultimately, however, estradiol was "significantly" better (on average) and provided better symptom relief overall.

Vaginal estradiol—estradiol inserted into your vagina—has long been disgustingly pricey: vastly more than *systemic* patch or pill estradiol. Gynecologist Kirtly Parker Jones, MD, explains on the University of Utah's *The Scope* podcast in 2018 that she could get pill estradiol for hot flashes—a 90-day supply—for $10 at Walmart. "If I wanted to use the same hormone vaginally... and this isn't rocket-science drug technology, it will cost $520 depending on how the estradiol is delivered" to the body (like with an estrogen-dispensing ring). "$520 is the upper end; $300 is the lower end."

Since then, some less-expensive vaginal generics have been approved—generic Estrace cream (around $30 a month) and generic Vagifem tablets ($49 a month in twice-a-week doses after an initial daily dosing for a week). It helps to look for discount coupons or discount online pharmacies.

Hyaluronic acid vaginal moisturizers are probably $50 a month or less. They are available OTC; however, it's important to be mindful that the health supplements area (from vitamins to creams) is the unregulated Wild West.

ESTROGEN: GLOBAL VS. LOCAL
Differences in risk and effectiveness

A menopausal woman using estrogen may be prescribed systemic estrogen, vaginal estrogen, or both.

I'll start with a refresher on the two types because the comparison is important for understanding vaginal estrogen's more contained work space. Systemic estrogen is estrogen that's absorbed "globally": throughout the body (your "system"). Most vaginal estrogen remains "local." It's applied in one "locale"—up the old hoohoo, as I'm sure they say in ob-gyn training—which is where it goes to work. Its effects are said to be limited, meaning *contained to the area it's applied to*: the vagina and its neighbors, like the bladder and the urethra. However, you'll see below that there's a possibility of a bit of systemic estrogen "sneak-through"—mostly at first.

"Vaginal estrogen works by increasing glycogen in the vaginal tissues," explains Dr. Gunter in *The Vagina Bible*. Glycogen is a stored form of glucose—that is, sugar—and a glycogen-rich vaginal environment is a good thing. Vaginal bacteria called *lactobacilli* feed on and ferment glucose to produce lactic acid, which lowers the vaginal pH to a healthy level. "The net result, writes Gunter, "is an increase in lubrication, vaginal discharge, tissue elasticity, and resilience."

Gunter notes that estrogen "will take at least six weeks to work, but may take two to three months to get the full effect, so it's worth completing a three-month course and then re-evaluating." She adds that women may initially experience increased blood levels of estrogen and breast tenderness, but that "once the estrogen treats the vaginal inflammation, the levels drop" in blood serum (to levels considered normal for menopausal women).

In reading research on vaginal estrogen, I looked at study after study for serious adverse effects. A 2020 journal article, "Vaginal Estrogen—What a Urologist Should Know," sums up the findings: The scientific "literature supports the low risk of vaginal estrogen," reports gynecologist Christina Escobar, MD.

Systemic estrogen, in adequate doses, can also find its way to the vagina and manage vaginal symptoms. But for women whose vaginal symptoms aren't sufficiently alleviated, a supplemental prescription of vaginal estrogen can get the job done.

For women prescribed vaginal estrogen who need to avoid systemic estrogen exposure, the most important safety indicator is the estrogen levels found in the blood serum of women using vaginal estrogen, explains Escobar. (Serum levels would be significantly higher in women taking systemic rather than local estrogen.) In a research review by urogynecologist David Rahn, MD, vaginal estrogen in doses currently given did not elevate women's systemic levels beyond the normal range for a menopausal woman not using hormones.

Finally, Gunter explains that vaginal estrogen (unlike systemic oral or skin-patch estrogen) does not need to be paired with progesterone to be safe. She's correct, but we've seen that progesterone has vital roles beyond keeping estrogen from turning our endometrium into The Cancer Borg.

> **BONUS POINT**
>
> ### THE FDA GETS IT WRONG AGAIN
> *Their vaginal estrogen "fact sheet" is anything but factual*
>
> In the FDA-mandated "fact" sheet given out with a vaginal estrogen prescription, vaginal estrogen is falsely accused of having the side effects of *systemic* estrogen. This unfounded info sheet "frightens many women and their partners needlessly, as there is no evidence that low-dose vaginal estrogen is associated with cardiovascular disease, breast cancer, dementia, stroke, or blood clots," write gynecologist Andrew M. Kaunitz, MD, and his colleagues.

OTHER TREATMENTS FOR A PROBLEMATIC MENOPAUSAL "DOWN THERE"

DHEA

DHEA, dehydroepiandrosterone, is a hormone produced by the body that can be converted to male and female sex hormones (estrogens and androgens respectively). In 2016, the FDA approved it for vaginal use (as the vaginal suppository prasterone, brand name Intrarosa) to treat menopausal women who experience "moderate to severe pain" during sex due to menopausal atrophy of the vulva and vagina.

In a randomized controlled trial by endocrinologist Fernand Labrie, MD, women given a DHEA suppository experienced significant improvements in their symptoms of GSM, including reduced vaginal dryness, much less pain during sex, more robust vaginal tissue (in color, thickness, and quality), and improved vaginal pH. The Polish Menopause and Andropause Society, in a research review that included high-quality clinical studies, deemed DHEA "effective, safe and well tolerated long-term therapy for vulvovaginal atrophy."

DHEA appears to be converted to estradiol by vaginal tissue and is believed to act *locally*—just vaginally rather than systemically. It can have mild "androgenic" (male hormonal) side effects, but not on the level of *oral* DHEA, which can potentially cause acne, greasy skin, unwanted hair popping up in unwanted places, and stinky sweat.

Gunter notes that DHEA "has never been compared in studies against vaginal estrogen, so making statements about which product is better is not possible."

OSPEMIFENE

Ospemifene (brand name Osphena) is a pill, taken orally. It's often prescribed to menopausal women who've had breast cancer who cannot use vaginal estrogen therapy to treat "moderate to severe" painful intercourse and vaginal dryness.

Ospemifine was found to improve vaginal tissue and vaginal pH, reports a 2016 research review led by gynecologist Chiara Bondi, MD. It had neutral or minimal effects on the endometrial lining of the uterus and was not found to stimulate the growth of breast tissue, which suggests it does not elevate a woman's cancer risk.

Ospemifene is in the SERM family, meaning it's a selective estrogen receptor modulator. "It acts like an estrogen on some tissues and like an anti-estrogen on others," explains Gunter in *The Menopause Manifesto*. "On vaginal tissues it acts like an estrogen," though it is a "nonhormonal" medication. In other words, though it "plays" like a hormone, it is not a hormone, which is why oncologists may deem it safe for women with a history of breast cancer. Gunter reports that side effects from ospemifene include hot flashes and a "slightly increased risks of blood clots."

VAGINAL "REJUVENATION" BY LASER?

"Wanting to believe" isn't the same as "proven to work and safe"

I ran into a reporter friend I hadn't seen for a few years. I told her the subject of this book, and she told me she'd experienced "horrible" genital issues in menopause—basically destroying her vaginal tissue—and could no longer have sex. "You have to write about vaginal rejuvenation. This laser, the MonaLisa Touch, would've saved my vagina if I'd gotten treatment before it was too late."

I hugged her and promised to look into it.

"Vaginal rejuvenation" sounds like a medical miracle, but it's a marketing term. "MonaLisa Touch" creeps me out—calling to mind some handsy art gallery gropenfart—but it's actually a medical device: a probe inserted into the vagina that uses a heated laser to slightly "injure" vaginal tissues. The tissue trauma kicks off our body's repair process and is said to increase the density of fine blood vessels called capillaries in the area and to remodel and grow tissue.

The laser is approved by the Food and Drug Administration—*but only for reducing acne scars*. Gunter explains in *The Menopause Manifesto* that "some small studies indicate that" vaginal lasers "can restore glycogen in the tissues" (which you might recall leads to increased lubrication, tissue elasticity, and resilience). However, Gunter notes, "there is very little quality data about the safety of these devices and how well they perform when compared with estrogen" or DHEA or ospemifene "or even against a placebo."

Dermatologist Arisa E. Ortiz, MD, surveying the FDA database of patient injuries, reports that chronic injuries—continuing harms—from laser and energy-based vaginal rejuvenation devices include "long-term pain, numbness, burning, bladder disturbances, infections, scarring," disfigurement, and painful intercourse. In 2018, the FDA issued a safety alert, warning that these devices are *not* approved for "vaginal 'rejuvenation' and/or cosmetic vaginal procedures," for which their safety and effectiveness "has not been established."

Many women believe these devices are the answer. The anguish my friend and many other women feel at their destroyed vaginal tissue can, very understandably, shove *hoping* that these devices work into *believing* that they do. Disturbingly, Gunter writes in the *Journal of the American Medical Association* that "Websites, from small private practices to large academic health care systems, present bold claims, making it appear to an untrained eye as though vaginal laser therapy were well researched and the standard of care."

"There is an awful legacy of inadequately tested devices in obstetrics and gynecology," including the Dalkon Shield, the Majzlin spring, and vaginal mesh for pelvic organ prolapse, "with our patients suffering the consequences." Gunter adds, "To see that legacy continue with the ongoing promotion of inadequately studied lasers for GSM is tragic."

Tragic—and tragically likely to continue. Gunter writes:

> It is doubtful that the clinical practice of laser therapy for GSM will halt in the United States without FDA intervention, and many practitioners here and around the world will likely continue to use the offensive "vaginal rejuvenation" language to coax patients into paying thousands of dollars to treat GSM for what the most robust current evidence tells us is an ineffective procedure. There is simply too much money to be made.

IT'S ALL IN YOUR HEAD

*Menopause and Perimenopause:
Not as Bad as Brain-Eating Zombies*

— 15 —

CRAZY IS SOMETIMES A STATE OF OVARIES
Mental and cognitive health

I'M GENERALLY A happy, optimistic person—and not just classy-happy. In some ways, I've got the demeanor of a puppy—breathlessly excited about small things people tend to take for granted—though I lack my dog's bouncy enthusiasm for the opportunity to dash out and pee in the yard.

THEY SHOULD CALL IT MIDDLE RAGE

In my 40s, something changed. I began spending every day in the sort of zen state you see in TV shows where they attach car battery cables to some guy's nipples. But I wasn't just wired; I was a human hate fest: that person who eventually loses it, drags somebody out of Starbucks and crucifies them for their heinous behavior—such as texting with those keyboard clicking sounds enabled on their phone.

Given my extreme swerve from puppy-happy to homicidal uber-bitch, you'd think I would've worried about my mental health. In fact, I didn't realize anything about me had changed—probably because the change happened gradually.

If only I'd known to look for it. But because I knew nothing about perimenopause, I had no idea that my ever-aggro state might stem from a biochemical shift common to 40-something women: basically becoming possessed by that hormonal demonspawn, soaring perimenopausal estrogen, and the stress hormone surges that come with. When there's little or no progesterone for counterbalance, what goes missing is emotional composure: the ability to regulate your emotions—to stay calm and in control when you're under stress. Throw in perimenopausal sleeplessness and mood swings, plus bloating, weight gain, and insatiable hunger—and even the Dalai Lama could lose his trademark cool.

Piling on with all of this, a woman who has no idea that perimenopause could be the source of this tsunami of emotional suck is not only prone to go without treatment but often feels deeply ashamed. She has no idea where this new "her" came from—this person set off by the slightest irritation, screaming at three people in a single afternoon or rage-crying over a watermelon she bought that turned out to be rotten (as a 47-year-old woman on Reddit confessed to doing). She was terrified she'd blurt out something awful during one of her emotional "storms" and destroy her relationship with her husband and daughters.

Luckily, when a researcher friend of mine worried she was aging into a short-fused bitch, she confided in me. This kind, generous woman—the sort who makes you feel good just being around her—was bereft at how she'd been treating her husband, constantly snapping at him over nothing. The stupidest little things set her off.

She had no idea how to change back to her old self and felt sick about it. "I'm mean to him, and he doesn't deserve it," she lamented.

I practically yelled. "This isn't you! It's perimenopause, the stage before menopause. And it's temporary and fixable. Immediately fixable! I know because I went through this."

I explained that suddenly out-of-whack menstrual cycle hormones turn some women chemically nuts. Minor annoyances they would normally have ignored or shrugged off become detonators for the perimenopausal nervous system, jacked up by excess estrogen and progesterone gone AWOL into a state of DEFCON: WE'RE ABOUT TO BE NUKED BY NORTH KOREA.

"But remember—FIXABLE!" I told her. "This is not some 'new normal.' It's the 'shitty temporary'—fixable by filling in for the progesterone-gone-missing so you can be you again."

HER STORM MAY NOT BE YOUR STORM
But perhaps you could hold the umbrella

Not all women go ragey from the stormy hormones of perimenopause. Some suffer anxiety, depression, or precipitous mood swings and crushing stress in their wake—or a combo of these. Others take nary a ride on the mental-health crap carousel.

Whichever group you fall into, knowing that perimenopausal hormones can suddenly go all guerrilla warfare on midlife women allows you to step up for women like my friend if co-workers or others trash-talk them. Imagine if things were different—if we *all* knew enough to take a more charitable approach, both to our own symptoms and to others'.

Understanding the hormonal basis of the emotional turbulence allows us to see symptomatic menopausal and perimenopausal women the way we do people having a hard time with other medical conditions, like gastroenteritis or diabetes. We don't see them as morally suspect. We don't cut them off as friends or grumble about them as colleagues-turned-slackers. We get that parts of their body aren't working so well, so we sympathize with them and we might even offer to drive them to their colonoscopy.

HI, ANXIETY!

At first, I was surprised to see the low percentages of anxious women in menopause and perimenopause. Psychiatrist Andreea Seritan and her colleagues found that 11 percent of perimenopausal women and six percent of menopausal women reported feeling "more anxious" during their respective stage of the ladyhormone rodeo. However, these numbers don't tell the whole story; they only show how many women experienced anxiety alone. When Seritan and her team inquired about experiencing anxiety *and* depression, 50 percent of perimenopausal women reported suffering from both, as did 38 percent of the women in menopause.

I looked back on my own experience. Did *I* feel more anxious or both anxious and depressed in perimenopause or menopause? I don't think so—though it's possible I'm what the literary world calls an "unreliable narrator."

It turns out we can be anxious without recognizing it. Joseph LeDoux and other neuroscientists find that fear and anxiety can be triggered beneath our conscious awareness, with various parts of the brain and their neurochemical messengers kicking us into a heightened state of alertness. We experience this through the physical symptoms of anxiety—like a sweat-stache, gaspy breathing, and an unnerving restlessness (basically, "ants in your pants" but in your mind and all over your body). When we aren't able to trace these sensations to a particular cause, it can be psychologically toxic, leading to bewildering free-floating dread.

This dread that rises up in us seems like a bug—and it can be—but it's also a feature. Our threat-detection system evolved to err on the side of over-noticing threats, which psychiatrist and evolutionary medicine co-founder Randolph Nesse refers to as the "smoke detector principle." Nesse explains that we need to "ensure that the alarm sounds every single time there is a fire," so smoke detectors are calibrated to pick up on the slightest sign something's burning. Unfortunately, this can lead to some seriously annoying false positives, like a smoke alarm that goes off whenever the guy in the adjoining apartment uses his toaster.

DARK HOLE SWEET HOME

Perimenopause gave me a beatdown in about 35 different ways, but I didn't get depressed. Though the physical and emotional struggles were *depressing*, I didn't suffer symptoms pointing to *depression*, like persistent smothering hopelessness, constant crying, debilitating pessimism, and fatigue and sadness that just won't lift.

It's important to delineate the symptoms from the disorder. *Depression* is like being trapped under a giant invisible anvil with no idea of how you might get out. *Depressive symptoms* are different. They are physical and emotional manifestations *associated* with depression that come and go. They are disturbing and life interrupting but not so severe and persistent as to be immobilizing; for example, pessimism, low energy, irritability (a perimenopausal biggie!), intermittent sadness and hopelessness, and a lack of interest in engaging with people or doing activities you previously enjoyed.

A significant group of women in perimenopause experience *depressive symptoms*: about 18 percent in early perimenopause and about 38 percent in late perimenopause, according to SWAN (the Study of Women's Health Across the Nation). In menopause, an estimated 22 to 25 percent of women experience depressive symptoms, which tend to be worst in early menopause and then gradually decrease.

A key question is whether women's depressive symptoms and depression are *caused* by the shifting hormone levels and the related chemical chaos in menopause and perimenopause. Current evidence does not support this for depressive symptoms, and the same goes for depression itself. In general, the big risk factor for getting slammed by "a major depressive episode" in perimenopause or menopause is a previous history of major depression, reports experimental psychologist Pauline Maki.

However, in perimenopause, the emotional turbulence from those big sweeping high-to-low mood swings makes women prone to *feel* they are depressed. If a woman's mood gets elevated—especially if she experiences big happy highs—and then her mood dives, the accompanying low can feel much lower by comparison.

Factors triggering or contributing to depressive symptoms include social stressors, like ongoing conflict at work and at home—often driven by symptoms of perimenopause, like insomnia and irritability. Other contributing factors include recently diagnosed health problems and the physical effects of undiagnosed conditions, including vitamin and nutrient deficiencies, and bummer conditions associated with aging that cause chronic pain, such as osteoarthritis.

Abruptly cutting off estrogen through surgical menopause increases the risk of depressive symptoms, as do premature declines in estrogen—for example, from POI, primary ovarian insufficiency (aka premature ovarian insufficiency), a condition in which the ovaries stop producing or only intermittently produce estrogen and progesterone.

This gloomfest isn't without a bright spot. In perimenopause, if you do get dragged down by depressive symptoms and you don't have a history of major depression, your suffering is very likely temporary. The same goes for perimenopausal mood swings and other emotional mayhem. As neuropsychologist Eef Hogervorst and her colleagues put it: "For the majority of women going through the menopausal transition, psychological health symptoms are transient."

WHEN ESTROGEN BECOMES STRESSTROGEN

I spent *years* in a state of low-grade rage. But it turns out I wasn't just chronically angry; I was chronically stressed.

Looking for a definition of stress in science journals is, shall we say, *stressful*. Instead of definitions, there are a lot of sections with titles like "Difficulties Defining Stress."

Charming.

Because trying to get a grasp on things that are undefined is like trying to get a grasp on soup, I turned to the *Oxford English Dictionary*, which can be relied on to define words instead of making excuses about why it can't. It defines stress as I think many of us understand it: "A state of mental or emotional strain or tension resulting from adverse or demanding circumstances."

And sure, it is those things, but they forgot the brain and the body! The "mental or emotional strain" isn't just a floating idea or belief, like the words in a comic strip thought bubble. It has a physical home. It starts in the brain and manifests in chemical and physical changes in the brain and body.

Taking the *manifestations* of stress into account, I cobbled together a more complete definition: "Stress is the brain's perception of a threat or challenge to our well-being—real or perceived, internal or external—resulting in the brain and body's response: chemically driven physiological change within us and behavior to get threatening situations under control and protect our well-being."

This more comprehensive definition might seem like intellectual wank-off-ery. In fact, understanding the mechanics of how stress manifests in the brain and body is essential to both noticing pernicious levels of stress in ourselves and being motivated to resolve them—behaviorally and, if necessary, medically. The goal of each of these measures is positive chemical change: preventing or diminishing runaway stress hormones, along with the runaway inflammation that their release causes (and is also incited by).

The three most vital behavioral measures are making healthy sleep (and correcting unhealthy sleep) a top priority; modifying stressful areas of our lives, as much as that's possible—on our own or with the help of a cognitive behavioral therapist—and doable shifts in how we eat and exercise, targeted to keep us in our best metabolic health *(detailed in Chapter Twenty)*. Medical measures—various drugs used to reduce the chemical and thus physical manifestations of stress—are detailed starting a few sections below.

Though we spend a lot of time complaining about stress, having some emotional and physical adversity is good for us. It's like a gym for the self, making us stronger and more able to cope with hardship and discomfort. Of course, there are times we experience crushing stress—for a few hours, a day, or more.

If you occasionally get hammered by an all-day stress-a-thon—as probably most of us do—the result can be like overdoing it at the bar one night and waking up with what feels like the mother of all hangovers. You feel kind of chewed for a day or so, you do the stress-healing version of chugging Gatorade and vowing never to do shots again, and your system recovers.

However, chronic stress—like the unrelenting estrogen- and norepinephrine-driven stress I got battered with in perimenopause—means you're constantly in a chemically-infused state of tension. With elevated stress hormones undermining your physical and mental health daily, there's no time for recovery. You're living in a war zone, or rather, you *are* the war zone. Predictably, as endocrinologist Hans Selye discovered back in the 1930s, this chemical state of affairs is not exactly a wheatgrass-tini for peace of mind and bodily health.

Selye is sometimes called "the father of stress research." In 1936, Selye, studying rats, discovered that both emotional and physical threats led to the same ill effects in the body: most notably, enlarged adrenal glands, ulcers in the stomach and intestines, and lymph gland shrinkage.

His research led to our understanding that it isn't just yicky viruses and bacteria that make humans sick. As we saw in Chapter Ten, persistent stress is associated with serious health problems, including diminished immune function, bone erosion, an increased risk for heart attacks and strokes, and "other fun ways to get to the morgue ahead of schedule," as I put it in a column. The negative effects on health come from the cascade of chemical reactions stress kicks off in the brain and adrenal glands, resulting in "increased production" of stress hormones—"mainly cortisol in humans"—explains neuroendocrinologist Gareth Leng. They turn harmful when they're "continually activated" (that is, chronic).

Research suggests that chronically elevated stress hormones cause unwelcome long-term changes in the brain, eroding memory, emotional regulation, and other mental niceties. It's also starting to look like high cortisol levels may be associated with an increased risk for dementia—in particular, dementia due to Alzheimer's disease, according to a research review by psychiatrists Sami Ouanes, MD, and Julius Popp, MD.

In patients with Alzheimer's, increased cortisol in the years or decades prior to diagnosis "is associated with a poorer prognosis and a more rapid cognitive decline." Accordingly, taking steps to decrease elevated cortisol in midlife may prevent cognitive decline in later life. They add that "further studies are needed" to investigate potential cortisol-reducing interventions.

Very much in favor of that; however, those of us in perimenopause and menopause need to get on reducing elevated cortisol levels *now*. Lucky for us, a study investigating estrogen's effects on an unexpected audience points the way to potential treatments.

MEN WITH PMS DOING MATH

Estrogen spikes don't just do a stress hormone number on women. In a study that seems like some perimenopausal woman's revenge fantasy come true, German psychologist Clemens Kirschbaum and his colleagues administered estrogen to men and made them do math problems in front of an audience to see what it did to their stress levels.

The pressure of solving equations publicly would be stressful for most people, but the estrogen-dosed men's stress hormones shot up way higher than the guys dosed with the placebo. This effect is also seen in research on animals. Rodents that had their estrogen levels amped by researchers showed increased production of stress hormones. (Mercifully, I don't think the rats were asked to do equations in public.)

Reflecting on these findings, Dr. Prior observes that "elevated endogenous estradiol"—a perimenopausal woman's own estrogen going into flood mode, "amplifying the stress hormone response to life stresses"—can explain why women find themselves suddenly less able to cope with stress.

All of this trash-talking of estrogen in excess might give you the idea that estrogen is some kind of cognitive bad guy. In fact, you'll see in the next chapter that estrogen—in adequate rather than excess supply—does vital jobs in the brain.

WHY TAKING PROGESTERONE STOPS THE CRAZY

Dr. Prior describes progesterone as a "brain-stabilizing, calming hormone." While perimenopausal estrogen levels that soar and drop stimulate the stress neurotransmitter norepinephrine, progesterone suppresses it. Not surprisingly, Prior reports that the most severe mood symptoms "occur when ovulation is absent," no progesterone is made, "and estrogen is high."

Norepinephrine's ravages may even continue in menopause, despite the bottoming out of a woman's estrogen levels. Gynecologist Rong Chen, MD, the lead researcher in a 2020 paper with Prior and other co-authors, explains that as estrogen levels decrease in menopause, "serotonin levels also decrease by about 50%." The dropping serotonin has a seesawing effect, "causing an increase of norepinephrine" and the physical and emotional crapfests that come with, like the delightful experience of bolting awake in bed with your heart pounding for no reason whatsoever.

The fact that progesterone substantially improves sleep—increasing deep sleep and decreasing sleep interruptions and the depression and mood swings associated with insomnia—likely contributes to its anxiety-alleviating effects. In a couple of small clinical studies led by psychiatrist Lorraine Dennerstein, MD, 300 milligrams of nightly OMP was found to decrease anxiety, stress, and depression in premenopausal women (between 18 and 45 years of age), while one of the synthetic knockoffs, a progestin called dydrogesterone, had no effect.

You might recall that progesterone, through its conversion to the neurotransmitter Mr. GABA (gamma aminobutyric acid), helps inhibit excessive levels of the "excitatory" neurotransmitter, glutamate. Though glutamate is important and healthy in normal amounts, in excess, it's associated with increased anxiety (in addition to migraines). Chemical calm-downs instigated by Mr. GABA can help you counteract spiraling glutamate-driven intrusive thoughts—the emotional hamster wheel to hell.

An important consideration is whether progesterone might take the calming business too far, dragging you down into depressive symptoms or depression. Research finds otherwise. Dr. Prior, in 2018, notes that multiple randomized controlled trials "confirm that progesterone (300 mg daily at bedtime) does not cause depression."

Okay, so 300 milligrams doesn't, but different individuals metabolize a drug better or worse, so maybe we should look at bigger doses of progesterone. You know those rat studies where they dose them with some soft-drink sweetener—the amount you'd get if you drank 2,600 cans of Coke in a day—and then say the stuff causes cancer? That's the sort of be-on-the-safe-side test we'll turn to (though not to the excessive level of excess in those rat studies).

Our test lab is pregnancy. Progesterone rises to about 10 times higher than usual during pregnancy. Yet, gynecologist Inger Sundström-Poromaa,

MD, reports that "continuous exposure to high progesterone, such as during pregnancy, has not been associated with depressed mood." In fact, "evidence suggests that allopregnanolone—a steroid produced when progesterone is metabolized—may have protective and mood stabilizing effects during pregnancy and the postpartum period."

There are a few women who may have a heightened sensitivity to progesterone, such as women with a severe form of PMS called PMDD (premenstrual dysphoric disorder), covered at the end of this chapter. However, for most women in menopause and perimenopause, it seems likely that OMP will be a soothing, calming force that prevents the literally poisonous effects of chronic stress.

Progesterone may even protect the brain—in day-to-day functioning and when there's trauma. Day to day, it has neuroprotective and neuro-enhancing effects, such as improving the capacity of mitochondria, the energy furnaces of cells. Estrogen, also neuroprotective and neuro-enhancing, is a friend to mitochondria—while, as you'll see in the next section, MPA is quite the opposite.

DOCTORS AND RESEARCHERS CONFUSE MPA AND OMP, BUT YOUR BRAIN WON'T

Studies on animals and humans suggest that MPA is detrimental to mental health (our emotional well-being), cognitive functioning (like reasoning and memory), and the health of the brain itself.

However, because MPA was concocted to mimic some effects of progesterone, it isn't entirely without benefits. Again, like OMP, it stimulates breathing and has been helpful for women with obstructive sleep apnea because of it. In rats with brain injuries, reproductive endocrinologist Frank Stanczyk and his colleagues report that administering MPA reduced swelling, as progesterone does, but MPA didn't do that as well as progesterone and lacked progesterone's healing effects. For example, MPA, "unlike progesterone," did not improve the rats' ability to remember and navigate through an environment, like by finding their way back to the food stash.

In contrast, research led by neuroscientist Robin Roof found that male and female rats treated with progesterone in the wake of a serious brain injury showed "markedly" diminished damage compared with the untreated rats. Female rats with the highest levels of progesterone "were virtually spared from post-injury damage."

There's related research on people: patients with traumatic brain injuries. Such assaults on the brain are often deadly. Yet a 2007 study by a professor of emergency medicine, David Wright, MD, on 100 patients with severe brain injuries found that when progesterone was administered within 11 hours of injury, fewer patients died by the 30-day mark. While 30 percent of the group getting the placebo died, only 13 of those who got progesterone did. In patients who were only moderately injured, Wright likewise saw improved outcomes.

Later clinical trials on brain-injured patients didn't show the same effects. However, scientists are not in doubt about the benefits they've seen from progesterone in brain-injured animal populations. There are some important differences—and sorry animal lovers...just the messenger here! For example, the rats were all injured in uniform ways by the researchers to make the study methodology consistent, while the human subjects arrived at the emergency room with varied injuries—from car crashes, falls, and other disasters. Some had more injury to more areas of the brain and were injured in different areas than others. This mucks up the ability to understand the effects of progesterone and how much of a difference it might make.

MPA also leaves us open to neurochemical damage. Along with estrogen, only progesterone (whether produced by our body or as OMP) protects the brain from a toxic glutamate storm. Glutamate is an essential neurotransmitter in the brain, but excessive activation of it can cause it to flood the brain, killing brain cells and impairing normal brain function, leading to slurred speech and shaky movements.

MPA, in fact, *exacerbates* the toxic effects of excess glutamate (according to rat studies by neuroscientist Roberta Diaz Brinton and her colleagues). Their research also finds that MPA diminishes the neuroprotective effects of estrogen and damages mitochondria, those cellular power generators that both estrogen and progesterone help keep firing.

MPA may also contribute to the degradation of cognitive functioning as well as the progression of Alzheimer's. A 2020 study on rats by neuroscientist James Simpkins and his colleagues found that MPA suppresses the production of a vital enzyme, MMP-9, which plays regulatory roles promoting cell health and survival. By suppressing it, MPA compromises the clearance of beta-amyloid plaques that accumulate in Alzheimer's disease.

The Simpkins team adds that the MMP-9 enzyme is also "indispensable" for brain cell plasticity—the amazing ability of brain cells to remodel themselves and their actions in response to signals from our brain, body, and environment, enhancing learning and memory. In other words, beyond MPA's possible Alzheimer's-promoting effects, its suppression of this enzyme could suppress learning and memory.

CLUB PSYCH MED
Antidepressants for menopausal and perimenopausal women

For menopausal and perimenopausal women who are drowning emotionally and aren't helped by cognitive behavioral therapy, behavioral change, or hormone therapy, an antidepressant could be a life raft. It's likewise an important option for women who are advised not to use hormone therapy due to elevated cancer risk, current or pre-existing cancer, or other reasons.

In providing hot flash relief, the "chill pill" nickname for these drugs is apt. Recall from Chapter Ten that antidepressants alleviate hot flashes—doing so almost as well as OMP, though much less powerfully than the best hormonal weapon against them: estrogen.

Antidepressants are prescribed by primary care doctors, psychiatrists, and gynecologists. Unfortunately, psychiatrists and primary care doctors with a background in menopausal and perimenopausal mental health are about as common as chickens with buck teeth. (Sadly, the same applies to gynecologists—as you'll learn in Chapter Twenty-Three.) So, in prescribing an antidepressant, doctors are prone to default to a one-size-fits-all approach: giving a perimenopausal or menopausal woman the same drug they (or some colleague they hit up for advice) prescribed to the 20-something dude who came in just before her.

Certain antidepressants are better suited than others for menopausal and perimenopausal women. Reviewing research on depression, experimental psychologist Pauline Maki reports that bupropion (brand name Wellbutrin—a norepinephrine-dopamine reuptake inhibitor, aka NDRI) is sometimes prescribed to perimenopausal women, simply because "it does not lead to as much weight gain, sexual dysfunction, or sleepiness" as other antidepressants. However, Maki adds, these prescriptions for bupropion are based on clinical guesses alone; there are no randomized controlled trials validating its use in perimenopausal women, specifically.

The "other antidepressants" she's referring to are SSRIs—selective serotonin reuptake inhibitors such as Prozac and Zoloft—and SNRIs, serotonin-norepinephrine reuptake inhibitors. Two large randomized controlled trials examined the efficacy of the SNRI antidepressant desvenlafaxine (brand drugs Khedezla and Pristiq) for treating major depressive disorder in both perimenopausal and menopausal women. For both groups, treatment with 50-milligram and 100- to 200-milligram doses "led to significant improvement in depressive symptoms compared with placebo," reports Maki.

Menopausal women tend to have a "poorer response" to Prozac, Zoloft, and other SSRIs, meaning these drugs do less to alleviate their symptoms. However, the SNRI desvenlafaxine was found to work just as well in perimenopausal and menopausal women, meaning it could potentially be prescribed consistently across both stages.

That said, there could be a desvenlafaxine piper to pay: nausea experienced by 40 to 45 percent of the women taking it, depending on the dose. This may be decreased by doctors starting patients on a low dose (50 milligrams a day for at least three days, then 100 milligrams, and eventually 150 milligrams by the end of the week). Other common side effects include dry mouth, constipation, sleepiness, insomnia, anxiety, and sexual problems. ("Bye-bye, libido and orgasms!") These side effects were more likely to be experienced by women taking higher doses (150 to 200 milligrams).

There is a bit of potential pharma skulduggery to consider. At least one trial of desvenlafaxine—identified with the code name "Des 223"—has gone unpublished, reports psychiatrist and medical transparency researcher Erick Turner, MD, and his colleagues. This typically happens when the drug manufacturer needs to hide a negative finding: a finding that could harm their drug's marketability. What unsells drugs? Terrible side effects, a lack of effectiveness, and/or harm to patients—sometimes including death.

Turner and his team also spotlight two desvenlafaxine studies with negative results—that is, drug-unselling results—that were published in a way that obscured the findings. Instead of putting these trials out as stand-alone papers, as the drug company surely would have if the results had been rosier for their bottom line, they were mushed into a "pooled analysis" paper with multiple studies with positive results. That study was funded by Wyeth pharma, and two of the four authors were Wyeth employees—surprise, surprise.

MONTHLY TEMPORARY INSANITY
Caution regarding progesterone for still-menstruating women with PMDD

Premenstrual dysphoric disorder (PMDD) is a severe form of PMS (premenstrual syndrome). It slams women with a cluster of debilitating physical and psychological symptoms in the week or so before they get their period (and seems to linger a few days afterward). The core PMDD symptoms are similar to PMS symptoms—including irritability, anger, feelings of hopelessness or worthlessness, and anxiety, tension, and feeling wired—but they hit women with a merciless intensity. Simply put, PMS is like being jostled in a store; PMDD is being flattened by a speeding bus.

PMDD is estimated to affect between 3 and 9 percent of women during their reproductive years, with symptoms often worsening during perimenopause. According to the International Association for Premenstrual Disorders (IAPMD; iapmd.org), the cause of PMDD is not yet known. However, referencing research by behavioral endocrinologist Peter J. Schmidt, MD, they note that PMDD "is not a hormone imbalance," but "a severe negative reaction in the brain to the natural rise and fall of estrogen and progesterone."

Sound familiar? As we've seen with the dive in estrogen causing stress hormones to surge, it's the *fluctuations* in estrogen and progesterone that women with PMDD are sensitive to—but excruciatingly so. Because women with PMDD are highly sensitive to hormone shifts, the ups and downs of hormones in perimenopause can hit them especially hard, making their PMDD symptoms even worse.

OMP might help some women with PMDD, but for others, it's like using a barrel of gasoline as a fire extinguisher. Some studies found it ineffective. Though this is yet another under-researched area of women's health, PMDD's less brutal cousin, PMS, has gotten more attention—which isn't to say the findings are helpful. A 2012 Cochrane review of decades of studies concluded (rather inconclusively): "The trials did not show that progesterone is an effective treatment for PMS nor that it is not."

Recent European trials of a drug produced from a progesterone metabolite showed initial promise, and other drugs are being tested as well. The IAPMD website should have the most up-to-date information on treatments.

It's possible OMP might be problematic for PMDD sufferers *at first*—in the first month of taking it—and eventually be helpful. Doctor-researchers on the IAPMD site note that recent research—in 2017, by Schmidt and his colleagues—finds that for some women with PMDD, negative emotional reactions go away about one month after starting hormones. (They gave women a combo of 100 milligrams of skin-patch estradiol and 200 milligrams of twice-daily vaginal progesterone by suppository.)

So, contrary to Prior's advice that estrogen should be avoided in perimenopause, it may be necessary for a perimenopausal woman with PMDD to take estrogen as well as OMP to keep her hormone levels stable. However if you have PMDD, and taking OMP or OMP plus estrogen leads to all-day road rage or other scary symptoms, it's essential you call your doctor ASAP for advice on how to taper off. Though in women without PMDD, stopping progesterone isn't found to cause rebound effects, for PMDD sufferers, cutting it off abruptly could trigger even more horrible symptoms.

Drugs found to help women with PMDD include SSRIs, such as Prozac, Zoloft, Paxil, Celexa, Lexapro, and their generics, and the Yaz birth control pill (3 mg of drospirenone, a synthetic progestin, and 0.02 mg of ethinyl estradiol). All of these drugs have side effects and some of them are serious. Cognitive behavioral therapy helps women function better and Dialectical Behavior Therapy (DBT) has been found effective for preventing suicidal behaviors.

PMDD can be identified by tracking symptoms for at least two menstrual cycles (more on this at the IAPMD site) and by taking a symptom test posted there. If you think you might have PMDD, there's a doctor tracker on iapmd.org to help you find a specialist near you. The IAPMD site also has contacts for crisis support and links to peer forums where women with PMDD can get insight and emotional support from other women who have it (iapmd.org/peer-support). Reddit.com/r/PMDD/ is another source of peer support.

— 16 —

MENOPAUSE BRAIN

Untangling what estrogen does and doesn't do

DEMENTIA IS A savage thief of self.

My friend Stef Willen wrote movingly in her *McSweeney's* column about dementia's slow smash-n-grab on her strong, independent, woman-of-the-mountains grandmother. I quoted bits of it in my column: "I'd always thought she'd die of a swift heart attack, but death snuck in the back door and did a real hit-and-miss job," Stef wrote. "None of us even noticed until the essential parts of her began to go missing."

The neurologist told Stef that her grandma's neurons weren't communicating. Some were dead, and some weren't firing in the right pattern. As desperate as Stef was to have the solace of the scientific *why*, the mechanistic explanation for the looting of her grandma's once-sharp mind made it even uglier. As Stef put it: "Apparently, who we are is an electrochemical reaction, and my grandmother had blown her circuits."

As of 2022, about one in 10 Americans age 65 and older has dementia—one in 10 and counting, due to our living longer, along with improved diagnostic tools and standards.

Dementia is not a specific disease but a blanket term for a heartbreaking decline in cognitive ability, disrupting daily life. It ravages a person's memory and reasoning and leads to disorientation, anxiety, depression, agitation, and personality changes, among other symptoms. Alzheimer's disease, the most common cause of dementia, accounts for 60 to 80 percent of dementia cases, reports the Alzheimer's Association.

Like Stef, scores of us have gotten the worst front-row seat in the world. Even as late as the 1990s, cases of dementia were underreported due to less advanced screening tools and the symptoms often being mistaken for normal aging. The Borg-like ever-burgeoning prevalence of dementia makes it not some abstract idea—an occasional tragedy striking other people's families—but the reason so many of us in our 40s and beyond spend our days (and years) grieving the loss of someone who's still here.

Given this context, the headlines in 2003 hit like a nuclear blast. The Women's Health Initiative (WHI) trial's memory and cognition team accused estrogen-progestin therapy of wreaking serious destruction in the brain, announcing a shocking, nearly doubled rate of dementia in women 65 and older who'd received estrogen-progestin treatment: a rate "twice that of women in the placebo group." Their conclusion: "The risks of estrogen plus progestin outweigh the benefits."

Mirroring the 1995 birth control panic in the UK, garbage cans far and wide became home to American women's hormone-therapy pill packs. Premenopausal women not yet using hormone therapy were too terrified to consider it, and doctors began refusing to prescribe or continue prescribing hormone therapy for many patients—including those suffering life-wrecking hot flashes and other debilitating symptoms.

The reality?

Technically, the WHI researchers' "twice the risk" claim wasn't an *out-and-out lie*. However, it was disgustingly misleading. It was the sort of bamboozling with statistics briefly detailed in Chapter Two, with study results stated in a way that makes a small or even minuscule risk to an individual sound huge (and thus vastly scarier than it actually is).

THE HEADLINE-GRABBING STATISTICAL SCAMMERY
Absolute vs. relative risk

The WHI researchers conceded (buried in the weeds of their paper) that "the absolute risk is relatively small."

Recall from Chapter Two that *absolute risk* is the measure that's vital for us to know: the one that tells us our *actual personal risk*—allowing us to make fact-based medical decisions instead of going with the unwarranted panic-driven kind. Simply put, absolute risk is the likelihood of something bad happening to someone who fits within specific parameters: for example, a menopausal woman, age 65 or older, using estrogen-progestin therapy for a certain period of years.

Let's do a little forensic accounting on this "twice the risk" business from the WHI. The WHI researchers found a 1 percent rate of dementia in women who did *not* use hormone therapy and 1.8 percent rate in women who did. Yes, that's right: a whole honking eight tenths of a percent higher! (Not exactly what we picture when the headlines scream about a *nearly doubled* risk.)

The raw numbers of those diagnosed? 21 women out of 2,303 on the placebo (1 percent of these women); 40 out of 2,229 on estrogen-progestin (1.8 percent).

So, technically, sure, the risk *did* double—from one population *relative to another*. Helpfully, this is called "relative risk."

You are not a population. You are a person.

Relative risk numbers reflect not individual risk but population-to-population comparisons, *only* telling us how much the two groups differ from each other. For example: Kids from the north side of town had twice the home runs of kids from the south side. That number—100 percent more home runs—says nothing about how likely a kid from either side is to hit a home run (nor does it clue you in that one north-side kid scored all the northies' home runs, while all his teammates immediately struck out).

Likewise, the WHI's big, scary relative risk—that nearly doubled group-to-group risk *they* announced—tells you not a bent thing about your absolute risk: how much risk you, as a woman 65 or older, would incur from estrogen-progestin treatment.

To get to that, we use the raw numbers in their paper: the 40 women out of 2,229 in the estrogen-progestin group diagnosed with dementia, which we saw is 1.8 percent of the 2,229. The absolute risk from those numbers? A 1.8 percent risk, meaning that for every 100 women, 65 or older, getting estrogen-progestin treatment, 1.8 percent are predicted to develop dementia.

For the sake of example, let's assume you're a 65-year-old menopausal woman. Starting from the actual, absolute risk to *a woman* 65 or older, you and your doctor can home in on the actual risk to a specific 65-year-old woman—you!—by factoring in your individual health metrics, such as your genetics and any health conditions you have or could be prone to.

The more "data points" you factor in, the less uncertainty there is about the potential outcome from going with the treatment. It's a major informational leg up, allowing you to make the most reasoned decision about whether the level of risk makes sense for you to incur. *(Spoiler: Regarding the type of estrogen-progestin therapy used in the WHI,* conjugated equine estrogen [CEE] and MPA, *there are now safer forms.)*

A BIG FAT FLY IN THE RANDOMIZED CONTROLLED OINTMENT
(Estrogen, we hardly knew ye)

Though randomized controlled trials are referred to as the "gold standard" in research, the results are not always so golden. "Any study, whether randomized or observational, may have flaws in design or analysis," notes British medical statistician Stuart Pocock.

These flaws can be difficult to identify—or they can be flamingly obvious, especially to certain scientists: those who eat, sleep, and breathe the substance being studied. Bruce McEwen, for example, I picture languidly running a finger along the outline of the cortisol molecule the way other men trace the curves of their lover's body. Very often, scientists like this can immediately spot what should and should not be in a piece of research— "should" and "should not" per how bodies and substances have certain well-established properties and behave in well-established ways. (If a lab technician draws fluid from your vein, it will not be Green Goddess dressing. Nobody expects chickens to lay Tiffany bracelets or is irate that trees are not made of soup.)

In 2003, when WHI researchers announced that estrogen appeared to be *bad* for the brain—allegedly doubling a woman's risk of dementia—a number of scientists were shocked. They suspected there was something amiss with the WHI team's findings, and more pointedly, the methodology that led to them.

By the way, these doubters weren't junior researchers going contrarian to make a name for themselves, but all-in senior scientists like Bruce McEwen and neuroscientist James Simpkins, who are at the forefront of vital discoveries about estrogen and the brain.

Simpkins pointed out to *Science*'s Ingrid Wickelgren in 2003 that the findings from the memory and cognitive aging arms of the WHI fly in the face of *hundreds* of studies conducted over a decade—studies that suggest estrogen protects brain cells from damage and improves cognition in people and animals. Many more studies have been completed since, likewise finding protective, cognition-improving effects.

Sander Greenland's advice was helpful for making sense of the contradictory findings: "Look at how the data were generated"—meaning, for example, facts about the participants, the drugs or forms of drugs given, the length of the study (long enough to see an effect?), and compliance: whether the participants got lazy about taking their meds.

The WHI had methodological shortcomings in every single area of fact that I listed above, skewing the results, individually and in combination. We'll get to those issues in this chapter and in the next few. But because the various illegitimate, panic-inciting claims from the WHI still linger in public consciousness today, *still* deterring women and their doctors from considering hormone therapy, I want to spotlight one of the more egregious ways "the data were generated."

When, in one of the WHI's memory and cognition arms, the researchers failed to find evidence of harm from hormone therapy conforming with the results they'd previously announced, they found a way to "find" it, report oncologist Avrum Bluming, MD, and social psychologist Carol Tavris. Bluming and Tavris explain that in 2004, the WHI's memory and cognition research team discovered an inconvenient fact: their participants who were taking estrogen alone (sans progestin) did not show an increased risk of dementia.

Well, that wouldn't do! Instead of simply disclosing what would have been good news to menopausal women using estrogen therapy alone, the researchers engaged in a form of methodological cheating. They took the data from estrogen-only group with no increased risk and mushed it together with that of estrogen-progestin group, where they did find a slightly increased risk— which allowed them to report a slight increased risk of dementia for this combined population!

Though I have no crystal ball into their intentions, I can't help but notice that they went with the more headline-grabbing result, and whoopsy about all the menopausal women benefiting from using estrogen alone who'd be led to believe the *collective* reported risk, reflecting a drug they were not even taking, applied to them!

Sleazy-peasy.

The WHI's memory and cognition study (like the WHI as a whole) also includes outrageous failures in reasoning and errors in methodology. A particularly devastating methodological error by the researchers—a substantial factor driving the unwarranted panic about hormone therapy when they announced their findings in 2003—was their parameters for study participants.

Here they were, doing a study to look for dementia in the wake of estrogen-progestin treatment, yet before they dispensed the first pill, they'd already "found" indications of dementia in many of their participants: the signs of "mild cognitive impairment" that are often the beginnings of dementia: basically the foyer to dementia. (About 50 percent of cases of mild cognitive impairment "convert" into dementia, reports psychiatrist Gavril Cornutiu.)

Very obviously, this group should never have been mixed in with the women who were cognitively healthy when the study began—or included in the study at all.

Including already-cognitively-impaired participants was such a howler of an error that, in 2004, some of the WHI's memory and cognition team went back to their study data and ran a re-analysis—first removing the dataset of women with mild cognitive impairment. They crunched the remaining data from the cognitively all-there ladies (as women starting hormone therapy at menopause are likely to be!) and...whaddya know! Turns out the women who went into the study cognitively healthy *did not become cognitively impaired!*

Summing up, Bluming writes: Estrogen therapy and estrogen-progestin therapy were "indeed associated with cognitive impairments, *but only among women who were already cognitively impaired at the outset.*"

ESTROGEN IN THE PENTHOUSE
How estrogen benefits the brain

In the 1970s, it became clear—especially from research from neuroendocrinologist Bruce McEwen's Rockefeller University lab—that estrogen is not simply a reproductive hormone but is vital to the brain. As another pioneer in hormone research, gynecologist Frederick Naftolin, MD, put it: "There is not a cell in the brain that is not directly or indirectly sensitive to estrogen."

In short, estrogen seems to be brain food.

Some of estrogen's actions we're pretty sure about—"sure" in the scientific sense, meaning there's solid evidence to back them up—while others require further research.

For example, there's solid evidence—detailed in the sections below—that estrogen helps with memory, protects brain health, protects and enhances higher reasoning, and provides fuel (like glucose and oxygen). You'll see that estrogen also impacts mood, though the current findings are incomplete, often conflicting, and inconclusive.

MEMORY ENHANCEMENT

Memory comes in a number of different forms: short-term, long-term, verbal, spatial, and working memory are just a few. "Working memory" sounds like the opposite of "slacking-off memory" (which of course is a thing—not in official scientific terms). Working memory is like a mental whiteboard—a temporary workspace where we hold a few pieces of information we need to keep handy to work with in the moment, like a set of numbers we're adding together; say, 20 + 32 + 40.

In contrast, long-term memory is more of a storage facility. It's like the stacks in a university library: dusty shelves and file cabinets where you store stuff like your social security number and, in the thundering words of FDR, that "date which will live in infamy!" (March 8, 1979, when Jeremy, the cutest boy in elementary school, pulled down your pants *and underpants* while you were reciting your poem at the assembly.)

We'll get to some of the other forms of memory and how estrogen and the loss of it impacts them—after a brief visit with menopausal forgetfulness.

Many women in menopause feel their memory for words, names, and phrases isn't what it used to be. Of course, this could be due to the effects of aging and life stress rather than menopause—or simply perceiving that we have a harder time remembering things. In fact, that perception probably isn't off base. "Women show small but significant declines in verbal memory and processing speed as they transition through menopause," reports experimental psychologist Pauline Maki.

As for the geniuses who risk death by telling a perimenopausal woman with memory complaints, "It's all in your head," Maki notes that "Midlife women's complaints of forgetfulness are validated by studies showing that the severity" of their complaints "correlates with performance on tests of verbal memory."

Memory deficits are associated with declines in estrogen, which you'd think would be paired with a decline in estrogen receptors. In fact, less estrogen—lots more places for estrogen to dock! Brain imaging research led by neuroscientist Lisa Mosconi finds that the loss of estrogen at menopause leads to a progressively *higher* density of estrogen receptors in women up to their mid-60s (compared with that of premenopausal women).

More estrogen receptors sounds like a good thing, since estrogen needs to dock with them to get to work. However, in standard cognitive tests, a higher density of estrogen receptors is associated with *worse* memory performance and "self-reported mood and cognitive symptoms after menopause" (which isn't to say the increase in receptors *causes* the memory, mood, and cognitive processing issues). The researchers speculate that the receptor mania is a desperation move by the brain—an attempt to compensate for lowered estrogen levels with extra receptors so it can take up as much estrogen as possible.

Estrogen, when present in adequate supply, appears to play a major supporting role in the healthy functioning of memory. It boosts the concentration of an enzyme that's needed to synthesize the neurotransmitter, acetylcholine, which is essential for memory encoding (a computer-like process of converting information you take in into neural code that your brain can read and store). On the flip side—the process of remembering—acetylcholine helps facilitate memory retrieval, which isn't just a matter of grabbing a memory out of the file drawer and dispatching it to you. The stored neural code first needs to be converted—reconstructed into usable form; for example, into images and feelings from your first kiss and your thoughts about it.

Amazing, huh?!

Not surprisingly, the presence of estrogen is associated with improved verbal memory—the ability to recall a word or term instead of futilely racking your brain for it—along with "verbal fluency": the ability to express that word quickly and efficiently as speech. In menopausal women, research by Maki and others finds that estrogen therapy improves cognitive performance in both of these areas.

Research on both humans and animals finds that estrogen is associated with improved "spatial memory," which is also called "place memory": the ability to remember the location of objects or places. We use this for navigation—remembering the way to our friend's house out in the boonies, including the direction, the distance, and turning left at the erect penis dead tree. We also need spatial memory to recall items we've seen and where they're situated within a collection of other objects (a classic memory test from neuroscience research).

However, spatial memories and others we take in need to be saved in a stable and strong form to make them less prone to erosion. This is called memory "consolidation," and estrogen plays an important role in the process, while low estrogen levels appear to hamper it. For example, perimenopausal women with low estrogen levels are found to have "poor spatial reference memory consolidation" in research by neurobiologist Robert Astur.

Finally, there's some evidence suggesting estrogen improves "episodic memory": a form of long-term memory for "episodes," like the moment the entire elementary school got to see your vag.

BRAIN DAMAGE PREVENTION

Your cat wants to kill you and eat your face.

To an aspiring face-dining cat, humans have annoyingly long lifespans, so a popular strategy is using the cover of darkness to plant itself in your path to the bathroom and trip and kill you.

But good news! If, instead of becoming Ms. Meow Mix, you merely end up with a concussion, estrogen will be there for you. Numerous studies find that estrogen is "neuroprotective," shielding the brain from damage caused by physical trauma and toxic chemical assaults. Bruce McEwen's research found that estrogen prevents brain deterioration from damage and destruction to cells by Alzheimer's-associated beta-amyloid protein and by nasty, unstable atoms or molecules called "free radicals."

Another physical affront to the brain is the shrinkage of women's gray matter at menopause with the drop in estrogen levels. This is a serious problem, because gray matter is filled with brain cells essential to every aspect of our thinking and behavior—everything from reasoning, self-control, and movement control to seeing, hearing, and speaking to our memory, physical sensations, and emotions.

The loss of gray matter is particularly concerning for long-term brain health, as brain imaging research by psychiatric doctoral student Laurens van de Mortel and psychiatrist Guido van Wingen, MD, finds that going from "mild cognitive impairment to Alzheimer's dementia was associated with reduced grey matter volume in several brain regions." Encouragingly, other imaging research, led by Lisa Mosconi, suggests that greater lifetime exposure to estrogen is associated with less brain shrinkage.

Lifetime estrogen exposure is predicted through "reproductive history events" that signal increased estrogen exposure; for example, a longer span of years between puberty and menopause, having a higher number of children, and the use of hormonal contraceptives or hormone therapy. Mosconi found that greater lifetime estrogen exposure, as indicated by factors like these, was "associated with larger grey matter volume in women in midlife."

At menopause, inhibition of the loss of gray matter through estrogen therapy may decrease a woman's vulnerability to Alzheimer's disease, observe Mosconi and her colleagues. However, at the end of their paper, they include an important demographic note, explaining that their participant group was "healthy, well-educated...mostly white people of generally middle/high socioeconomic status," which limits the "generalizability" of their findings to women of other races and ethnicities. "Clinical evidence of higher frequency and severity of menopausal symptoms in Black and Hispanic women strongly argues for examination of outcomes across ethnic groups."

COGNITIVE MOJO

Estrogen helps out in our brain's Department of Higher Reasoning (the prefrontal cortex, or PFC, the area right behind the forehead). In both women and our hairy cousins—female monkeys—estrogen improves "executive functioning": mental skills like reasoning, planning, focusing, remembering, prioritizing, and resisting temptation.

Estrogen does its work by increasing the activity of neurotransmitters—serotonin, dopamine, and norepinephrine—which help protect and enhance executive function. McEwen explains that each of these neurotransmitters is central in its own whole *system*—serotonergic, dopaminergic, and so on. Collectively, these chemicals and their systems support the healthy functioning of everything from our emotions, memory, and navigational ability to our control of "motor activity": the movement of our body parts.

Connectivity is a must for dependable executive functioning. Like your cellphone, your brain needs a reliable network, and estrogen is part of that. McEwen explains that estrogen increases the density of small "dendritic spines" on neurons in the PFC (and larger ones in the hippocampus). These spines are basically tiny antennae that foster the development of synapses—junctions that pass signals from one brain cell to the next and are crucial for learning and memory. McEwen was referring to rat brains, but a review of research on estrogen's effects on the human PFC by psychiatrists Sheila Shanmugan, MD, and C. Neill Epperson, MD, suggests estrogen therapy may alleviate symptoms of "executive dysfunction" in menopausal women by selectively increasing the smaller dendritic spines in the PFC.

Executive *dysfunction* is the term for deficits in executive function skills, leading, for example, to difficulty with organization, time management, decision-making, and self-control—issues common to people with ADHD. Because norepinephrine and dopamine levels take a dive at menopause, these executive function issues tend to rise up or get worse in many menopausal women. Basically, it's like menopause ushers in ADHD, the functional (or rather, dysfunctional) result of lowered norepinephrine and dopamine levels. Research led by Epperson found that an ADHD med, Vyvanse, helped alleviate the executive function issues in both perimenopausal women and those in early menopause—none of whom had been diagnosed with ADHD.

Women in menopause who have ADHD and take meds for it may find, as I did, that the dose that worked fine for years, prior to menopause, no longer does the job. My psychiatrist (thankfully!) understands the neurochemical affronts of menopause and worked with me to adjust the meds I was taking. This allowed me to once again sit at the computer and write—instead of effectively being kidnapped by incessant ants in my pants, except throughout my entire brain and body.

BRAIN GRUB

Just as it's hard to think over the animalistic growling of your stomach, an underfueled brain is a poor source of cognitive mojo for memory or planning.

In addition to the memory-enhancing chemical effects triggered by estrogen, Maki and neuropsychologist Susan M. Resnick find that blood flow is increased in estrogen therapy users (compared with non-users) in the brain's primary memory organ, the hippocampus, and two other brain regions that form a memory circuit.

Blood acts as DoorDash for the brain, increasing the transport of glucose (aka sugar), the brain's main fuel, along with oxygen and other nutrients, across the blood-brain barrier. Neuroscientist Roberta Diaz Brinton and her team find that estrogen promotes enhanced utilization of glucose in the brain, which, in turn, boosts the capacity of mitochondria—the little energy furnaces in your cells—that help power you mentally and physically.

Keeping our mitochondria humming is looking more and more vital for hanging on to our marbles as we age. Brinton writes, "The role of mitochondria in health and disease has long been recognized, and the evidence for mitochondrial dysfunction as a key precipitating factor in age-associated neurodegenerative diseases such as Alzheimer's and Parkinson's continues to mount."

MOODUS OPERANDI

Estrogen has unclear but potentially beneficial effects on mood. Estrogen boosts the activity of the serotonergic, dopaminergic, and other systems of the brain in ways that positively affect mood. Women who experience the drastic cutoff of estrogen through surgical menopause tend to suffer depressive symptoms—symptoms that are found to be alleviated by estrogen therapy.

However, the *precise ways* estrogen affects mood remain undetermined—not because researchers forgot to run studies to investigate it, but because the research findings are collectively inadequate for making well-supported conclusions.

Take depression. Psychiatrist David R. Rubinow, MD, and his colleagues searched for methodologically sound randomized controlled trials to answer the question, "Does hormone therapy successfully treat depression during or after the menopausal transition?" (meaning in both perimenopause and menopause). Only five studies met the bare minimum methodological requirements. However, two of the five had a high risk of bias, and ultimately, the Rubinow team concluded that the evidence for hormone therapy's effect on depression is, "at best, 'C'"—as in "low quality evidence."

ESTROGEN THERAPY FOR MOOD AND COGNITIVE SYMPTOMS?
Current practice standards—and some counterpoints

Due to the conflicting, inconclusive, and insufficient findings on estrogen's effects on the brain, as of 2024, medical practice standards exclude estrogen as a treatment for cognitive and emotional symptoms or to protect the brain. As summed up by Maki in a 2022 paper on menopausal brain fog: "Based on current guidelines," estrogen is not prescribed "to treat cognitive issues at menopause or to prevent cognitive decline or dementia later in life." (The same goes for mood issues.)

However, it's important to understand that "Estrogen is not prescribed 'to treat'..." does not necessarily mean "Estrogen is not beneficial for..." Though there isn't sufficient evidence to conclude that estrogen should be given to menopausal women to improve cognitive and mood issues and overall brain health, as Maki puts it: "There's a biological plausibility that estrogen could enhance brain function."

In fact, that's something of an understatement.

"Biological plausibility" is a term used to reflect that evidence strongly suggests there's a cause-and-effect relationship between a treatment and an outcome. In this case, the *cause* is estrogen treatment and the *effect* from it appears to be improved cognition, mental health, and brain health. There is an important nuance to this, detailed in the next chapter: the timing of estrogen treatment—specifically, how soon after hitting menopause it should be initiated to have protective and beneficial effects.

Making a persuasive case for estrogen's benefits for cognition are studies on women who've had their ovarian estrogen supply abruptly cut off through surgical menopause or treatment with estrogen-blocking drugs. The elimination or blocking of these women's estrogen supply led to rapid declines in working memory and verbal learning, the ability to process and retain information we read or hear. However, when these patients were started on estrogen treatment shortly after their own estrogen was cut off or blocked, their cognitive declines were *rapidly reversed!*

More support for estrogen's benefits for cognition come from an observational study on a group of largely Mormon menopausal women, exploring the relationship between a woman's estrogen levels and cognitive decline. These women, all in Utah, were 91 percent Mormon, with an average age of 74—so primarily older women, 10 or more years past going into menopause.

The researchers, clinical neuropsychologist Joshua Matyi and his colleagues, were uniquely comprehensive, taking into account *lifetime estrogen exposure*: women's exposure to their own bodily estrogen from puberty through menopause. Like Mosconi, Matyi and his team estimated via "reproductive history events." However, they also factored in estrogen fluctuations: lowered levels in late pregnancy, prior to giving birth, and while breastfeeding, as well as increased levels of estrogen from any hormone therapy.

Their results, like Mosconi's, suggest that a longer duration of estrogen—a woman's own bodily estrogen being present for a greater stretch of time between puberty and menopause—helps decrease the cognitive decline associated with aging. Additionally, hormone therapy use at the onset of menopause was associated with further cognitive benefits, especially in the oldest women in their sample.

As for our takeaway from all of this, recall that epidemiologist and biostatistician Sander Greenland emphasizes the importance of seeing whether a finding appears consistently in a body of research to determine whether an effect might be real (as opposed to the result of fraud, bad math, or ludicrous methodology).

Well, as Simpkins and McEwen made clear, the benefits of estrogen on cognition are not some lone wolf finding in a single study. Again, there are hundreds of studies that find this—and more continue to be published.

PART 3

LONG-TERM HEALTH PROTECTION

*Estrogen, Progesterone, and
Hearts, Breasts, and Bones*

— 17 —

RETHINKING ESTROGEN

I GET WHERE feminist doctor-scientists like Prior and Susan Love are coming from in arguing that menopause should not be considered an "estrogen deficiency disease." In fact, I was right there with them in finding it denigrating to women. Until—eventually—I wasn't.

Sure, the notion that a natural state for women—the low estrogen level of menopause—is a sign of deficiency *can* seem offensive, suggesting, for one, that we women are just breed sows who lose all value once the piglet factory is closed.

However, three things led me to rethink the notion that "estrogen deficiency" is offensive—rather than *descriptive*. And not just *descriptive*, but *very helpfully descriptive*, with "estrogen deficiency" both identifying the problem and implying what we need to do to solve it.

First, I increasingly read research papers that found major benefits from estrogen in both female humans and lab animals and major detriments from a lack of estrogen (due to menopause, medical conditions, or estrogen-blocking drugs).

The fact that low estrogen levels at menopause are "natural" is no reason to slam the door on the benefits of prescription estrogen—succumbing to the "naturalistic fallacy": the erroneous "If it's natural, it's good!" belief that would've led me to have a funeral for my vagina.

Second, a few years into menopause, I had symptoms that OMP alone—the 300 milligrams of oral micronized progesterone I took nightly—no longer alleviated or alleviated enough, compared with its savior-like effects in perimenopause. These included intense hot flashes; sleep splintered into shards by bed-wetting night sweats and nocturia waking me up to pee; and, oh joy—vaginal dryness that no amount of shoving non-prescription lubricants up there managed to alleviate.

I'm miserable: Hot. Wet. Wetting. Sleep-starved. My vagina is about to be listed on Google Maps as desert wasteland. And yet, the Amy's Menopausal Shitshow Players decide to add a cast member.

About two years into menopause—out of nowhere—another symptom struck. I was ragingly hungry. *Monstrously* hungry—just like in perimenopause! And I started gaining weight. Suddenly—and *rapidly*. I stepped on the scale one day and—holy concrete block! I had somebody's jumbo-sized baby squatting somewhere inside my body.

THE MENOPAUSAL MIDDLE
Estrogen gone missing leads to weight gain and metabolic issues

We women tend to put on weight in menopause. If that weren't el sucko enough, there's a change in *where* we put it on: a redistribution of what I call "Jessica Rabbit fat"—curvy-lady hourglass-figure fat from our hips and thighs—to the beer gut area. (I don't believe in God, but if I did, I'd believe he hates women.)

Throughout my life, I'd been lucky, shape-wise. In my 20s, when I "medicated" with brownies and ice cream, the weight I gained made a beeline for my hips and butt. Even at my heaviest, my stomach somehow stayed flat and I had a small waist—well, at least relative to the double-wide caboose below.

A few years into menopause, I looked in the mirror and noticed something wild: My big, round junk-in-the-trunk babuttski had swapped itself out for a small butt! A small, rather flat butt. Hmm. The flat-ass-ening *was* dismaying, but, for about 10 seconds, I was into having a normal cute butt like some 20-something LA yoga hipster—until I looked again.

My butt fat had not gone away.

It had simply relocated to the belly area—becoming a buttfat gut! (Or, as I came to call it, "my butt gut.")

I've got plenty of company in this disturbing reapportionment. You see women on message boards bewailing this as "menopause belly" or "menobelly."

And that's only the beginning of the bad news.

This belly fat is the unhealthy "white fat" known as "visceral fat." Unlike muffin-top fat you can grab with your hands, visceral fat fattens you *from the inside out*, packing itself around abdominal organs like the liver, kidneys, and intestines.

In case you find that insufficiently disturbing, visceral fat isn't just an inert blob hanging around making your pants too tight. It's "metabolically active" fat: an evil fat-based factory pumping out nasty inflammatory proteins and other biochemical troublemakers—spiking your blood sugar, making you store dietary fat instead of burning it for fuel, and triggering chronic inflammation. So begins a vicious loop, with visceral fat jacking up inflammation and inflammation firing up more visceral fat, in an endless trashing of your metabolic health.

In your menstruating years, estrogen is basically the traffic director of healthy fat storage, working with other hormones and enzymes to guide fat to your butt, hips, and thighs. It also inhibits fat from taking up residence in your waist area (though it does a better job of this in some women than others).

However, when estrogen levels decline at menopause, so does the control it maintained over insulin and your blood sugar—and cortisol release. You can start wishing your wardrobe included a solid supply of Uncle Seymour–style elastic waistbands—just the attire for maximum comfort while getting medical tests for the elevated risk of type 2 diabetes, heart attacks, strokes, and cancer associated with visceral fat.

Though estrogen isn't a weight-loss drug, the Danish Osteoporosis Prevention Study (DOPS) found that women who take it early in menopause gain less weight. Other studies, including a Cochrane meta-analysis, echo these findings.

Pairing OMP (or MPA) with estrogen is not only an endometrium-protecting necessity for a menopausal woman who still has her uterus, but it also has metabolic benefits for *any* woman—more than estrogen alone. While progesterone itself does not cause weight loss, decades of research find that it is associated with "increased energy expenditure"—researcher-ese for *an increase in calories burned!*

We see this in a small study in menstruating women that investigated calorie expenditure in different stages of the menstrual cycle. Over the three months of the study, metabolic researcher Paul Webb, MD, found an 8 to 16 percent increase in calories burned during the progesterone-rich weeks following ovulation. In two out of the three months, one woman had a 14 percent increase in calorie expenditure—an increase that flatlined during the month she took an oral contraceptive, which works by *suppressing* ovulation.

In other words: No ovulation, no progesterone made, and calories don't budge.

The idea of boosting our estrogen level in menopause in hopes of inhibiting weight gain might be confusing, considering how elevated *perimenopausal* estrogen seems to leave some of us insatiably hungry and packing on the pounds.

It occurred to me that estrogen might not be a *cause* of perimenopausal weight gain—just a *participant* in it. Studies on stress, stress hormones, and weight gain in women by psychologist Elissa Epel and neuroendocrinologist Bruce McEwen suggest to me that it's not estrogen itself but estrogen's *acrobatics*—soaring and diving perimenopausal estrogen spiking cortisol—that turn us ravenously hungry and keep the scale inching upward.

Recall that the stress hormone cortisol has important roles in the body, like regulating our immune system, energy metabolism, and sleep patterns, as well as "helping us adapt to stressors," as McEwen puts it. However, *chronic stress* is associated with *chronically elevated, dysregulated cortisol*—which can lead to dysregulation of appetite-regulating leptin, insulin, and other hormones, triggering increased food intake and visceral fat accumulation.

But about that "increased food intake"—ravenous as we can get, we're picky-ravenous. We'll stress-eat Doritos, doughnuts, Double Stuf Oreos. But carrots? That crime against taste buds known as celery? That would be a big not gonna happen, no way, no how, N-O. And we aren't alone. Though "animal studies reveal that stress" mainly leads to "decreases in food intake," Epel notes that "when rats have a choice of highly palatable food, such as lard or sugar, stress increases intake of palatable food specifically."

CRUSHING IT AT THE ESTRO-GYM

Skeletal muscle is just hugely important to maintain—not just for bone health but because it helps determine our metabolic rate, supports healthy fat distribution, and helps us maintain a healthy weight. Accordingly, the loss of skeletal muscle leads to poor utilization of calories, meaning that calories that would've been burned for energy instead get socked away and turned into fat. This makes skeletal muscle loss "an important factor in the propensity to gain weight," endocrinologist Michelle P. Warren, MD, explains.

Remember mitochondria, those little energy furnaces in our cells? "Our overall skeletal muscle function and quality are largely determined by mitochondrial health," explains kinesiologist Rene Vandenboom. There's also a "goes both ways" effect: Exercise that generates skeletal muscle—especially endurance exercise and muscle-straining weightlifting—can stimulate the growth of new mitochondria, in turn leading to improved muscle health!

Estrogen is a major mitochondrial helper. As we saw from Roberta Diaz Brinton in the previous chapter, estrogen, throughout our brain and body, enhances mitochondrial function, increasing our cells' conversion of nutrients into energy and keeping our cells in healthy running order.

This reduces the wear on cells from "oxidative stress" (basically the biochemical rusting of cells), Vandenboom notes. However, "in estrogen-deficient states," such as menopause or when women are taking estrogen-blocking drugs, mitochondrial function is impaired.

"Impaired" mitochondrial function is a bit dry—or as I like to say, *beige*, which can leave us undermotivated to make changes. Picture hordes of wee, slack-faced cartoon furnaces inside your cells, all coughing and sputtering like chain smokers of yore. You and your body rely on these little fellas for energy provisioning, but it's just not there. Not surprisingly, this has some less-than-desirable effects—in fact, a chain of them.

For example, in menopause, there's a widespread tendency for women to engage in less physical activity—due in large part to lowered energy levels driven by estrogen decline and the accompanying mitochondrial dysfunction. Decreased physical activity leads to a loss of "fat-free mass," which refers to your entire body minus all the fat. It's a term for tissue—a large part of which is skeletal muscle, but also includes your organs, bones, water, and connective tissue like ligaments and tendons.

Estrogen therapy at menopause is muscle enhancing, helping improve muscle quality and metabolic health (through improving insulin sensitivity). It also helps decrease muscle erosion in menopausal women. However, as you'll see later in the chapter, timing matters. Vandenboom notes that estrogen therapy was most helpful for muscle health in women when it was initiated six or fewer years since menopause (meaning the day after that 12-month stretch without periods). In women 10 or more years past menopause, each of the benefits detailed above was reversed, leaving women with reduced insulin sensitivity (a factor in diabetes 2 and other metabolic diseases), along with increased muscle erosion and lower overall muscle quality.

If you're six years and 20 minutes past hitting menopause, please do not panic! This six-year figure does not mean estrogen won't be helpful, and the same could be true if you're eight years past. The six-year mark just happens to be the measure in these studies. And you'll see in sections to come in this chapter and others that our individual health plays a role—and may override the "numbers" to some degree: guidelines based on age and years from menopause, on average, from various studies.

Finally, in a bit of good news for menopausal women who cannot or will not take estrogen, Vandenboom reports that "exercise has been found to serve as a means of augmenting and/or mimicking the effects of estrogen on skeletal muscle function." He notes that exercise before menopause has a preventive effect, decreasing the "consequences" of lowered menopausal estrogen levels. It also "appears to lessen the significant losses in appendicular lean muscle."

Of the many forms of exercise, slow-speed, muscle-straining weightlifting *(see Chapter Twenty)* is the most effective at protecting and maintaining mitochondrial, muscle, and cardiometabolic health. Importantly, it does not require you to exercise for hours every day (or even every week) or move into the gym—or even *go* to a gym—making you less likely to slack off on it. (The left side of my living room floor looks like a weightlifting graveyard, with four dumbbells, a couple of kettlebells, a barbell, and a weight-loaded vest.)

GETTING WAISTED
The tape measure test for metabolic health

Waist size is important for more than fitting into your favorite pants. An excessively large waist circumference (aka waistline) is typically a sign of what can be "killer fat": excess visceral fat. Kinesiologist Robert Ross and his colleagues report that this organ-crowding abdominal fat is "strongly associated" with premature death—from "all-cause mortality" (death from any cause), as well as death from certain *specific* causes: heart attack, stroke, a bum aorta, or narrowed or blocked arteries.

To guesstimate how much visceral fat you have, find a measuring tape with a centimeter side, pull up your shirt, and wrap it around your waist. Annoyingly, nobody's standardized exactly where to measure or come up with any scientific rationale for the area they happen to recommend. Ross and his team suggest running the tape around the area between your lowest rib and the "iliac crest," the top of your hip bone—the largest part of your hips; the part you can feel if you jab your thumb in there when you put your hands on your hips.

According to the National Institutes of Health (from a paper by nutritional researcher Michael Lean, MD, and his colleagues), women with a waist circumference of 80 centimeters or less are considered to be a healthy weight. *(And by "women," they mean the usual suspects: white, middle-class women.)*

However, 80 centimeters marks the beginning of the danger zone, the "threshold above which health risks are increased." An 88-centimeter measurement is solidly *in* the danger zone: time to contact a doctor for tests to assess your cardiac health and other possible issues and to take steps to improve your metabolic health.

Granted, these are general guidelines, calculated from measurements from white women in the UK, who were around 5'3". (Globally, white women are 5'4" on average.) In other words, these measurements may not apply all that well if you are, say, five feet tall in shoes and golden brown like my Portuguese/black/native-Brazilian-descent friend, Liliane, or 6'1", like my pre-Raphaelite Scottish giantesse friend, Helen.

Helpfully, Ross and his colleagues lay out average measurements for women of various ethnicities and national origins (though it isn't a comprehensive global list). From their table, for Chinese women, 80 or more centimeters is problematic. For Korean women, 91 or more. Japanese: 90 or more. For Jordanian women, it's 96 or more. Iranian? 91 or more. Tunisian women: 85 centimeters or more.

BMI—body mass index, a number derived from your height and weight combined—was formerly the standard for determining healthy weight. It isn't as accurate as waist measurement; however, it may still be helpful in *combination* with waist measurement, especially for women who do not check the "average white woman" box. Calculating BMI involves a bit of a dance with math, but there are BMI calculators online to do it for you. Just enter your height and weight and click up your number.

"Normal weight" BMI, via Ross and his colleagues, is 18.5 to 24.9; "Overweight" is 25 to 29.9. "Obese I"—class 1 lower risk obesity—is 30 to 34.9; and "Obese II and III" is 35 and up—moderate risk and severe risk respectively.

BEYOND "E"
The T-zone: thyroid and testosterone

It's important that women experiencing weight gain in menopause get both their thyroid levels and their testosterone levels checked out—ideally, by a reproductive endocrinologist who is not just an infertility specialist but also specializes in treating hormone disorders.

Low thyroid levels (hypothyroidism) drive weight gain—though mildly low thyroid levels called "subclinical hypothyroidism" might not but should be watched (through periodic testing). Hyperthyroidism results from an excess of thyroid hormone and can have serious effects. Among its symptoms, it usually causes weight loss, but in about 10 percent of patients, it leads to weight gain.

On to the next "T," testosterone. PCOS—polycystic ovary syndrome—is a hormonal disorder in premenopausal women characterized by excessive levels of androgens (the category name for testosterone and other so-called "male" hormones). Women who had PCOS in their premenopausal years are more likely to have higher-than-normal "T" levels in menopause.

Both too little testosterone and too much can drive weight gain. Abnormal levels can also cause acne, hair loss, or hair growth (in the last places we'd want to lose it or grow it). Sure, we women *can* do anything men can do, and then some—or, in a remix of a Bob Thaves cartoon that former Texas Governor Ann Richards belted out in a speech: "Ginger Rogers did everything that Fred Astaire did...backwards and in high heels." (That said, thanks—but we'll take a pass on developing male pattern baldness or growing a goatee.)

MENOPAUSAL TESTOSTERONE THERAPY?

I suspect testosterone may eventually be seen as the third important hormone in menopause and perimenopause. However, there's a gigantic hole where decades of comprehensive research on testosterone treatment in women should be.

We know very little about when and how low testosterone levels in women should be treated (and whether they should be treated at all). Many doctors don't even test women's levels appropriately. Because women produce small amounts of testosterone compared with men, we should be given a high-sensitivity test capable of detecting the tiny and possibly important fluctuations in our comparatively very low levels.

If you're getting your "T" levels tested, it's wise to ask whether they're giving you a "high-sensitivity" (HS) test—because there's a good chance they won't, especially if they're general-purpose endocrinologists rather than specialists in women's endocrinology. These high-sensitivity tests have different names at different labs, but the testing method will have words and initials like "liquid chromatography" (LC) and "mass spectrometry" (MS).

By the way, I only knew to tell you about this after a female gynecologist I started seeing when my gyno got transferred ordered this for me, and I noticed it was higher sensitivity than the standard tests for males that an endocrinology bigwig gave me.

Hugely grateful.

I kept seeing her, and about a year later, I asked for some "T"-related lab tests: not expensive, but not the standard ones gynecologists order—especially if they aren't *intensely* menopause and perimenopause-focused.

When the results came back and I messaged her about an elevated level (really just to tell her my plans to fix it), she disclosed that she was "not an expert in interpreting" what the level should be.

I was blown away. And *not* because she (like probably most gynecologists) lacks expertise in this area. I didn't care *in the slightest* that she didn't know (nor did I need her to, because I *am* an expert—and know how to correct the elevated level without drugs).

The fact that she, unlike too many doctors, had *the integrity to be honest*—to volunteer that she didn't know instead of putting on a front of expertise—made me think even more of her than I already did from a year of seeing her.

Or, as I put it to a friend, "I love her!"

(More on this sort of ethical disclosure in Chapter Twenty-Three.)

And a final note on testosterone: Though I see recommendations on blogs and elsewhere for women to use testosterone, we lack sufficient evidence for its safety and effectiveness. Because of that, as of March 2024, there are no FDA-approved testosterone treatments for women.

REVERSING OLDLADYFACE
Estrogen's effects on skin

When I was 58, I was frightened by a prowler I spotted in the reflection of my darkened TV screen—this extremely drawn and tired-looking old lady burglar—and then, for the real scare, I realized it was me. Menopausal-faced me.

In menopause, with the decline in estrogen levels, many women experience "a swift commencement of skin aging," explains dermatology researcher M. Julie Thornton. There's an increase in dryness and wrinkling, skin becomes thinner, and there's a decrease in collagen and the skin elasticity it fosters. Collagen is a protein that's basically spandex for your skin, giving it resilience and stretch.

When your estrogen supply bottoms out in menopause, it's like your skinsuit has worn-out elastic. Though Thornton concedes that some of the effects on collagen and the level of moisture in your skin are due to aging, she notes that the deterioration correlates with the loss of estrogen more than with chronological age. For example, once estrogen declines in menopause, "skin thickness is reduced by 1.13% and collagen content by 2% per postmenopausal year." There's also a 30% reduction in collagen in early menopause (prior to the five-year mark).

However, Thornton adds, many of the negative effects on skin "can be reversed by estrogen replacement, which increases epidermal hydration, skin elasticity, and skin thickness as well as reducing skin wrinkles and augmenting" collagen levels and quality. She's talking about systemic estrogen therapy, which is also found to increase collagen content in bone, improving bone density.

Though research finds both estrogen and progesterone *creams* to be wrinkle-reducing, there's a problem: As I noted previously, OTC and compounding pharmacy progesterone skin creams, unlike FDA-approved drugs, are unregulated. This means the one you get has not been validated for safety and effectiveness, and there's no watchdog over the purity of their ingredients or the safety of the manufacturing process.

Again, you could be getting huge amounts of a hormone—and not necessarily the one listed on the label.

THE TIMING HYPOTHESIS
The critical window for estrogen to be helpful instead of harmful

The neuroscientists were right. The findings from the WHI that made it look like estrogen harms the brain just didn't make sense.

What wasn't clear at the time was why. Where could this increase in dementia be coming from?

"Look at how the data were generated."

That was key.

We've seen what Simpkins, McEwen, and the other neuroscientists saw: substantial evidence, down to the mechanics of estrogen—the processes and chemical reactions it triggers—that estrogen protects our cognitive function and the long-term health of our brain. This isn't wrong. However, what had yet to be recognized was the confounding study methodology: the absolutely dunderheaded inclusion of women who should never have been given estrogen.

It turns out that probably most of the women in the 2003 WHI memory and cognition study—maybe even 70 percent—*never had a chance* for estrogen to protect them. Three things stood in the way: their advanced age (70-plus), their extended distance from menopause (15 or more years), and the poor health associated with both.

This made these WHI participants very different from the younger, healthy, recently menopausal women who'd normally be prescribed estrogen. Most women who start hormone therapy do so between age 51 and 55, initiating it upon hitting menopause or just a few years afterward to alleviate disturbing menopausal symptoms. As a result, the lion's share of prescriptions for hormone therapy go to women between the ages of 40 and 60, reports gynecologist and reproductive endocrinologist Wulf Utian, MD.

Gynecologists, reproductive endocrinologists, and other menopause researchers know this. However, the WHI trial was designed by the National Heart, Lung, and Blood Institute of the National Institutes of Health (NIH), "largely by cardiologists and epidemiologists, initially without accurate input from reproductive endocrinologists or menopause experts," reports Utian. Sure, cardiologists and epidemiologists conduct research, too, but having them design a study on menopausal endocrinology is a bit like hiring a mailman to bring your baby into the world because he's a "delivery specialist."

Their lack of knowledge and expertise in the menopause arena led to big blunders in the initial design of the trial that spilled into the various arms of the study. For example, the 2003 cognitive aging arm of the WHI included *only* women age 65 and older, in hopes of increasing the odds of finding a link with dementia. A whole 54% percent of the participants were over age 70, and 18% were over 75.

In the initial mass-panic-inducing WHI trial, published in 2002, the results from the many participants in their 60s through age 79 in deteriorating health do not generalize to the population of much younger and generally healthier women who tend to start on hormone therapy at, say, age 51 or so, to alleviate their menopausal symptoms.

Not surprisingly, with the inclusion of so many elderly and infirm women, 35% of the so-called "healthy" participants (per the WHI announcement) were overweight; 34% were obese; 35% were being treated for high blood pressure; 39% had been smokers and 10% still were; 4% were being treated for diabetes and 12% for high cholesterol. And that's just a selection—not a comprehensive list. Their advanced age and multiple serious health issues were reflected in the WHI findings—"increases in breast cancer, coronary heart disease, stroke, and pulmonary embolism in study participants on estrogen plus progestin compared to women taking placebo pills"—put out to the media by the NIH in 2002.

The risks from hormone therapy in older women are likely due to how estrogen—in multiple areas of the body, from the heart and blood vessels to the brain—has a positive effect when women are healthy but often causes harm or just doesn't help when disease starts taking hold. In the brain, for example, estrogen preserves healthy brain cells, but it does not repair already-"broken" ones.

In lab tests of estrogen's effects on brain cells, neuroscientist Roberta Diaz Brinton finds that the health or unhealth of these cells determines whether estrogen will be helpful and protective or harmful and destructive. Timing is everything. As Brinton explains her findings, if brain cells "are healthy at the time of estrogen exposure, their response to estrogen is beneficial for both neurological function and survival," with estrogen "inducing a proactive defense state." Conversely, if harm to brain cells is already present—"if neurological health is compromised"—"estrogen exposure over time exacerbates neurological demise."

This is the basis of the hypothesis Brinton calls the "healthy cell bias of estrogen action." In the simplest terms, get the estrogen in there while you're healthy and it'll keep you healthy. Wait till you're unhealthy, and estrogen will be your cellular enemy, running with the destruction that's present and making it worse. In other words, a woman's own health is the "critical variable" in whether estrogen will be health-protecting or health-eroding.

Supporting her "healthy cell" hypothesis, Brinton notes that the results from her lab tests "are remarkably consistent" with data showing that women who initiate estrogen therapy right at menopause enter into "a prevention mode well before age-associated degeneration is rampant." These women "have a lower risk of developing Alzheimer's disease" compared with women who have never used estrogen therapy or hormone therapy.

Age and proximity to menopause tend to be stand-ins for good health. In line with Brinton's theory, between 2004 and 2007, when the WHI researchers reanalyzed their data by age, setting aside the datasets with elderly, unhealthy participants, there was a "crucial turnabout" in their previous doom-and-gloom conclusions, reports gynecological endocrinologist Andrea Genazzani, MD. In younger, recently menopausal women—those who'd initiated hormone therapy between age 50 and 59 or within 10 years of menopause—"the data pointed toward a reduced risk of heart disease, a lower risk of death from any cause, and no apparent increased risk of stroke," as well as a reduced risk of dementia.

This finding has plenty of company: both from observational studies and randomized controlled trials. In the cognition area, for example, that observational study on Mormon women by Joshua Matyi and his colleagues found that "Women who initiated hormone therapy earlier"—closer to when they went into menopause—"showed higher cognitive test scores than those who initiated it later."

Collectively, these results are part of a growing body of research supporting the "timing hypothesis" or "critical window theory." This suggests that once a woman hits menopause, there's a limited window of time for her to initiate estrogen in order for it to have protective effects (as opposed to having no effect or causing harm).

The most generous version of this—the greatest span of years from menopause—calls for a woman to begin hormone therapy between the ages of 50 and 59 or within 10 years of hitting menopause (which starts 12 months from a woman's last period).

However, you'll see evidence in the chapters on cardiovascular health for a narrower window for initiating estrogen: six years or less from menopause. Ultimately, it's important for women to start hormone therapy as soon as possible upon reaching menopause, especially because cardiovascular health slides fast with the disappearance of estrogen.

Because a woman's health drives whether estrogen will be a friend or foe, for some women, *to some degree*, age could be "just a number" (as could their years from menopause). Current health could be determined through results from cognitive tests (which include questionnaires, neuropsychological exams, and/or MRIs) and tests to assess the condition of other areas of the body, such as cardiovascular and metabolic health.

Pauline Maki, reflecting on Brinton's finding in the cognitive health arena, explains the potential for leeway on age and distance from menopause: "The healthy cell bias predicts that older women who are 'healthy'—who perform at or above expected levels on cognitive tests—would benefit from [hormone therapy] even if they are outside the window." "Similarly," Maki adds, "the healthy cell bias predicts that women whose cognitive performance is poor, regardless of age, would experience the most adverse cognitive effects" from hormone therapy.

ESTROGEN FOREVER?

After the 2002 WHI trial falsely accused estrogen of being the hormonal Grim Reaper, the FDA stuck a "black box warning" on estrogen and the estrogen-MPA combo, calling for them to be used at the "lowest effective dose" and for the "shortest duration" that's needed to control menopausal symptoms.

Absurdly, nobody knows what either of these measures happen to be. Take the "lowest effective dose." The WHI tested only *one* of the available doses of CEE (0.625 mg conjugated equine estrogen), so whether lower (0.3 mg) or higher doses are generally more effective is anyone's guess!

In 2012, The North American Menopause Society (NAMS) publicly acknowledged that the scientific flaw factory known as the WHI trials "had several characteristics that limit generalizing the findings to all postmenopausal women"—the understatement of understatements. Despite that, the WHI team's 2013 call to limit treatment to five years or less became the standard for medical practice—five years for estrogen-only therapy and four to five years for estrogen-progestin.

Limiting the years of treatment means limiting estrogen's benefits. In recent years, research has increasingly shown that estrogen does not just alleviate symptoms but provides decades-long protective effects—not only in the brain but in our muscles and bone, the cardiovascular system, and the bladder and vagina and thereabouts. Cut off the estrogen and you cut off those protections.

A big question for women who opt for hormone therapy in menopause is exactly how long they can keep taking it. Though many doctors still cling to their WHI-driven belief that hormone therapy use should be limited to five years or less, this stance does not align with current evidence on the substantial benefits from long-term use.

For example, a 2024 study led by biostatistician Seo H. Baik investigated the use of menopausal hormone therapy in women 65 or older, using the medical and prescription records from 2007 to 2020 of 10 million senior female Medicare patients. They examined the effects of hormone therapy on health according to the type of estrogen and progestogen, the delivery system (oral, transdermal, etc.), and the dose.

They found that the use of "estrogen monotherapy" (estrogen alone) at age 65 and beyond was associated with "significant reductions" in mortality, breast cancer, lung cancer, colorectal cancer, heart failure, blood clots, atrial fibrillation (irregular heart rhythm), heart attacks, and dementia. "Progesterone monotherapy was associated with a 22% reduced mortality risk," while "progestin monotherapy was associated [with] an 11% increased risk" of mortality. Additionally, "Progesterone, when used alone, was associated with a 10% reduction in breast cancer risk," while progestins "increased the risk by 21%."

Baik and his colleagues note that there appear to be greater reductions in risk with low rather than medium or high doses of estrogen; with vaginal or transdermal estrogen rather than oral estrogen; and with estradiol (same as our body makes) rather than the CEE given to WHI participants—either with or without MPA.

The Baik team's finding joins previous findings of benefit that, as Baik puts it, suggest "the possibility of important health benefits with use of menopausal [hormone therapy] beyond age 65." In light of these findings, there is now "no general rule for stopping hormone therapy based on age alone," reports The Menopause Society in April of 2024, in line with their 2022 position (before they changed their name from The North American Menopause Society).

The NAMS 2022 position statement deemed extended use of hormone therapy "a reasonable option with appropriate counseling, regular assessment of risks and benefits, and shared decision-making" (between a woman and her doctor, considering medical options through the lens of her values and preferences). Whether you, personally, can or should use hormone therapy—and for what duration—requires you and your doctor to factor in your age, overall health and individual risk of breast cancer, heart disease, gallbladder disease, and other conditions that might make this treatment a no-go.

Referring to "shared decision-making," Genazzani adds that "tailoring treatment also means considering a woman's needs, such as her right to have a satisfying sex life or her obligation to preserve body image, her work, or her athletic performance. These are all critical factors to consider in choosing the right treatment option."

Finally, it's important to note that even if you've enlisted a statistical and medical genius for risk prediction, you may experience harm from estrogen (or another drug or treatment) that they can't foresee. What they're doing is making their best guess. You can supplement that best guess by getting other opinions and seeing whether the "best guesses" are in alignment.

My own best guess—based on my individual health stats—is that I have a very low likelihood of gallbladder disease, heart attacks, or stroke. I also don't have liver disease or a history of blood clots and other conditions that would make estrogen prohibitive. I, of course, worry about breast cancer, but I get regular mammograms. I also get regular Pap smears and pelvic exams.

In my risk-benefit analysis, opting for all the benefits of estradiol and OMP—especially for long-term cardiovascular protection—while continuing to get regular cancer look-sees in my boobs, vagina, and nearby territory seemed the wisest course of action. I asked my doctor to prescribe transdermal estrogen—the FDA-approved bioidentical estradiol patch—at the low dose of 0.0375 milligrams. I went up to 0.050 and, eventually, to 0.075—the level at which my hot flashes become *not flashes* or, at least, *not very hot, long, or often flashes*.

— 18 —
DROP DEAD, GORGEOUS
There's a heart-eating serial killer on the loose

IF THERE WERE a crazed killer slaying 1 in every 5 American women, we'd know, right? The news media and talk shows would cover little else. We'd all be seriously freaked and take major steps to protect ourselves.

Well, that ruthless perp *is* out there right now: the worst mass killer of women in human history. Statisticians predict that the death toll will eventually be 1 in 3 women—their deaths often preceded by years of debilitating suffering.

The killer is heart disease—causing death from blocked arteries, heart attacks, strokes. That's how it ends, anyway. But on the way, heart disease (technically "cardiovascular disease") doesn't work alone. It's got a goon squad of accomplices vandalizing our health: runaway inflammation, a broken insulin response, and high blood sugar. The destruction they wreak opens the door to a continuing pile-on of ruinous conditions: most notably, obesity and high blood pressure—which fuel further inflammation and jack up the risk of heart disease and diabetes.

Diabetes *doubles* the risk of heart disease and can damage the heart and blood vessels—while torturing women: chaining them to dialysis machines and even stealing their toes and feet through tissue death and amputation. However, heart disease manages to show up diabetes in the ugliest way—as the number one killer of new moms. It accounts for *over a third* of maternal deaths, with black women experiencing some of the highest maternal mortality rates, according to the American Heart Association.

With heart disease and its vile co-conspirators killing so many women in such horrific ways, and with a vast number of these deaths preventable, there should be huge crowds of us marching the streets, protesting and raising awareness: "Take back the arteries! Cardiology is a feminist issue!"

I'm not kidding.

We can't stop what we aren't aware of, and only 56 percent of women are aware that heart disease is *the leading cause of death in women!* Tragically, few of the women who are in the know will get serious about prevention or get serious in time—but understandably so. To be human is to put off what we should do today till the second Tuesday in never—especially when we're unclear on what exactly should or could be done (and how quickly dire the consequences of doing nothing can be).

Say you're 45 and your ticker is still ticking okay. If you think about your arteries at all, you figure you've got time before you need to worry about the state they're in—which you actually don't. Once arterial damage sets in, it's too late to stave off the impending disaster. At best, you might chip away at the severity of the destruction as it marches on, triggering escalating harm throughout your tissues and organs.

BLOCKED ARTERIES RUIN EVERYTHING

"During a heart attack, a clot in one of the arteries of the heart suddenly blocks the flow of blood to the heart, and within minutes, heart muscle begins to die," explains cardiologist Joseph Ornato, MD. "The more time that passes without treatment, the greater the damage." Fixing the damage is not an option. "The part of the heart that dies during a heart attack cannot grow back or be repaired."

Heart disease is the meanest monster of a mugger, robbing you of your health in every possible way—but not *just* your health. A heart attack that doesn't kill you right away can be death to your quality of life, leaving you frail and weak, gasping to breathe, and unable to walk even short distances. (Getting down the driveway to your mailbox and back seems like the Bataan Death March.)

Of course, even *seeing* the mailbox could be a problem in the wake of a heart attack, stroke, or other manifestations of heart disease. Reduced blood supply to your eyes starves them of oxygen, stealing your vision. Impaired blood flow from your heart to your kidneys can damage your kidney function. Damaged kidneys put strain on your heart, forcing it to go into overdrive trying to pump your weakened kidneys the blood they need to do their vital job: clearing waste products from your system. Eventually, dangerous levels of waste can build up—your blood basically turns into a poisonous swamp—and you can entirely trash your kidneys in a matter of days.

HOW TO PREVENT A BROKEN HEART

At menopause, there's this fork in the cardiovascular road nobody tells us about: One path is suffering and death and the loss of everything that makes you you (like when just breathing is a struggle). The other path is maintaining your health and living as the healthy old lady you.

Assuming you don't already have existing heart disease (or other risk factors that make estrogen prohibitive), you give yourself the best shot at the healthy old you path by initiating estrogen therapy (and its cardiovascular protections) right when you hit menopause. That timing means starting estrogen therapy *before* the rapid onset and progression of arterial damage—taking off when your body's estrogen bottoms out in menopause—can make it too late to save you from cardiovascular decline or even destruction. Things won't be that dire for every menopausal woman, but most probably experience at least some decline in arterial health and overall cardiovascular health with the loss of estrogen's cardio-protective effects.

This doesn't necessarily mean you're doomed if you *don't* take estrogen. For those of you who don't, it's especially important to be disciplined about eating and exercising in the targeted ways that are most powerful for protecting and enhancing menopausal and perimenopausal health. *(Chapters Twenty and Twenty-Two.)*

At the end of Chapter Twenty, I list lab tests and other measures for determining your level of cardiovascular health, and through that, your risk of disease. My results showed me my risk is low. Could I have gone without estrogen therapy at menopause, at least for cardiovascular health, and been okay? Possibly. However, research on menopausal women suggests that hormone therapy (estrogen, paired with progesterone) is such a powerful force for maintaining our cardiovascular health that I saw a strong argument for using it protectively, *preventively*. (Even by women who have no bothersome menopausal symptoms.)

Regarding the duration of treatment, we saw the scientific support in the previous chapter for age alone no longer being a reason to stop hormone therapy. Depending on your individual health, you might be able to maintain the cardio-protective (and otherwise protective) effects of hormone therapy throughout your lifetime.

HEART IS WHERE THE HORMONES ARE

Our "ovarian hormones," estrogen and progesterone, get around. They do some of their best work in our cardiovascular system.

Estrogen decreases significant risk factors for cardiovascular damage. Among its cardiovascular benefits, it maintains the stretchiness and flexibility of our blood vessels and their smooth, undamaged surface, and it helps prevent high blood pressure by keeping them relaxed and open. This, in turn, helps prevent the sludgy, artery-narrowing buildup of plaque that eventually ends very badly—causing a stroke that deletes a chunk of our cognitive ability or a heart attack that destroys part of the heart, leaving us in a weakened and progressively weakening state.

Dr. Prior's and others' research shows progesterone is likewise protective—relaxing the blood vessels, preventing arterial stiffening (particularly during perimenopause), and helping balance the sympathetic nervous system, which regulates blood pressure and our heart rate. It also decreases inflammation, a key factor in the progression of cardiovascular disease. However, in perimenopause, when anovulatory or weakly ovulatory menstrual cycles leave us short on progesterone, we lose the protections it normally provides—unless we make up for the shortage with a prescription for OMP.

In menopause, when our estrogen levels join progesterone in bottoming out, we can experience a rather rapid decline in our cardiovascular health—a *pointless decline* if we are among those who can replace estrogen and its protections with a prescription.

For those who can't or won't use hormone therapy, sticking to two out of the three options below is a way to keep yourself in the best possible health.

THE POWER OF THREE
Hormone therapy + targeted eating + targeted exercise

As essential as estrogen and progesterone are for maintaining healthy "pipes," they alone are not enough.

While availing yourself of the benefits of hormone therapy, if you live like a potato—spend your days (or even one day!) largely sedentary—you chip away at your cardiovascular health. Sitting or lying down daily for extended periods of time is ruinous. It can lead to "poor circulation," meaning slowed-down blood flow. This can mess up your ability to regulate your blood pressure—a serious issue since high blood pressure basically opens the floodgates to heart disease through the injuries it causes to the lining of your arteries. Being sedentary can also raise your blood sugar and diminish your body's ability to metabolize and use lipids (fats in your blood). Fats that don't get used get stockpiled!

The blood sugar-spiking standard American diet joins being sedentary in trying to kill us, negatively affecting blood pressure, blood sugar, and lipid metabolism. You're basically munching your way to a broken insulin response—the inability to control your blood sugar called insulin resistance—as well as chronic inflammation. Chronic inflammation, in turn, ignites and amplifies both the harms of being sedentary and eating a diet that keeps your blood sugar doing the high jump.

As I briefly noted in the "Symptoms, Symptoms" intro to Part 2, to prevent these harms, menopausal hormone therapy must be paired with two other vital measures—guidelines for exactly how to eat and "move" (aka exercise). Like hormone therapy, each of these is independently protective and health-sustaining. But in line with the ole saying "the whole is greater than the sum of its parts," this trifecta—these three measures, working together to prevent inflammation, insulin resistance, and heart disease—give you *the* most powerful and effective cardiovascular protection. And by doing that, they send you off into oldladyhood in the best possible health.

Yes, I get that you, like me, probably have crush injuries from all the dietary advice constantly dumped on all of us—with every other breathless headline claiming to reveal THE "heart-healthy" diet. These articles do have one thing in common: the obligatory credibility booster, "Science finds..." or "Recent research finds..."—which, by the way, it probably hasn't and can't.

Most dietary "science" cited in articles and other advice to the public is dietary fiction—fatally flawed and beyond worthless—because it relies on research participants "self-reporting" what they ate over weeks or months. Hello? Have these researchers never met any people? We forget. We estimate badly. We *lie*—especially when we're embarrassed by the Krispy Kreme-littered truth.

Likewise, in many articles about menopause and perimenopause, the hormone therapy station wagon typically has the obligatory exercise advice trailer hitched to it—complete with a bullet-pointed list of eight or so types of workouts we could or should be doing.

Seeing a variety pack of exercise options like that is typically a sign—that the author moved over like 26 seconds ago from covering celebrities to the health beat and that there isn't the slightest bit of scientific anything behind it. This isn't to say it gets better when there's a scientific veneer. Doctors and medical plans likewise hawk scientifically unfounded exercise advice—that is, exercise measures they *assume* are beneficial but, in fact, have little effect on the health problem they're intended to prevent or solve.

In other words, this exercise advice tends not to be validated in any scientific way for having any major (or even meaningful) effects for protecting and maintaining our health in the ways we need. What doesn't get asked is the essential question we need answered to tell us the ideal way to exercise—for example: "Why and how would this exercise improve a woman's health in menopause or perimenopause?" And then there's an essential follow-up question: "Is this the best possible exercise to achieve that?"—meaning, "Does this give us the most health bang for our time-and-effort buck?"

Take the absolutely ludicrous advice I still see in articles telling women to swim to improve their bone health! It isn't that swimming is a waste of time in and of itself. It's nice to be in water; you're moving instead of being sedentary; and you are working your muscles, heart, and lungs. But because you're suspended in water, you aren't putting weight on your bones. That's how you "tell" them they're needed (a "Grow, grow!" or "Yo, stick around!" message they get in chemical form), which helps maintain the bone you have in menopause or, if you're in perimenopause, possibly builds bone.

In other words, your time is wasted for your goal of improving bone, because you're spending maybe a half hour or more in the pool, plus time to get to the pool (unless it's in your backyard or your penthouse), yet the most weight you put on your bones in this splashy endeavor is in walking from the locker room to the water's edge.

The advice in these pages is different. It respects your time and advocates for the life you could have if you know the absolute best ways to eat and exercise—to live strong now and to go off into old age at your healthiest. And by "absolute best," I mean according to strong scientific evidence.

I looked at the various ways our bodies go in the crapper: what bad stuff goes on in our cells and tissues and which chemicals or behaviors cause it. From there, I reverse engineered: figuring out exactly what we need to do—chemically, physically, behaviorally—to provide ourselves with the most powerfully effective protections for our health.

Ultimately, with the collective power of this hormone-diet-exercise trifecta, our daily and long-term health becomes something we continually foster rather than chase hopelessly after, like we would a purse-snatcher.

— 19 —

SISTER SLUDGE

*Estrogen and progesterone prevent
blocked arteries and an early exit*

ATHEROSCLEROSIS IS DEATH by sludge.

Imagine some rotten neighbor kid shooting wet cement into your garden hose—not entirely blocking it, but making the inside so narrow that only a trickle of water comes out the other end. That's atherosclerosis—only the hose is your arteries and the "cement" is plaque, and it isn't thirsty posies that are endangered but the continuing existence of your heart and brain.

Atherosclerosis is the underlying cause of about half the deaths in Western society. It wrecks the arteries, health, and lives of a huge number of Americans over age 45. A huge number of *unwitting* Americans. "About half of Americans between ages 45 and 84 have atherosclerosis and don't know it," reports the National Institutes of Health. Making it particularly sinister, there are often no symptoms until you have what the NIH tactfully refers to as a "medical emergency." (Becoming incapacitated by a heart attack or stroke while speeding down the freeway would qualify.)

THE MOST IMPORTANT PART OF YOUR BODY
YOU'VE NEVER HEARD OF

The health of your endothelium drives the overall health or ruin of you

The lining of your arteries. It's everything.

I'm talking about the endothelium, a smooth layer of cells just one cell thick that is crucial for maintaining what's rather blandly referred to as our "cardiovascular health." You know, little things...like keeping our heart pumping, our lungs fully functioning, and our blood traveling smoothly and unfailingly through our arteries—delivering the oxygen and nutrients our organs and tissues require to survive. The red blood cells that do the delivery then act as garbagemen, removing carbon dioxide waste (keeping your body from turning into New York City after a weeklong garbage strike). Blood is also the transpo system for hormones. If they can't get to the organ or tissue they're being dispatched to act in, they can't have the necessary effects.

The endothelium is actually an organ—*the largest organ in the body*, due to its length (an estimated 60,000 miles, if you lay your blood vessels out in a line), which makes it larger than the skin. (The skin, laid out, covers about two square meters, while the vascular endothelium spreads out over 3,000 to 6,000 square meters.)

Because endothelial health is essential to the healthy functioning of *all* of your organs, tissues, and bodily processes, it determines your overall health and well-being: whether you wake up as the energized (if wrinkled!) full-of-life you—or weak and sick, dreading your daily painful trudge to the toilet, and hoping to make it through another day without being zipped into a bag.

What, specifically, does the endothelium do? Actually, better question: What *doesn't* it do?

Its job description is really its *jobs* description.

To give you a few examples: It's the doorman—a selectively permeable barrier between the bloodstream and the tissues, regulating what gets in and out. It's the "Clot or not?" manager, producing substances that facilitate clot formation—and anticoagulants to keep it from getting out of hand. It's the foreman of the dam, regulating blood flow: either constricting blood vessels to reduce blood flow or opening them up (through the release of nitric oxide it produces) to increase it. And it's the fire marshal, seeing that inflammation does just enough to heal us when we need an immune response, but doesn't go chronic and turn into that fire that burned down Chicago.

CAN'T TAKE A CHOKE

Recall from the previous chapter how healthy arteries are flexible and stretchy? They're relaxed and open and the endothelium is smooth and free of buildup—like arterial Teflon for frictionless blood flow.

In contrast, in the clogged arteries of atherosclerosis—with the endothelium narrowed with piled-up plaque—blood flow is reduced along with the delivery of oxygen carried in blood. This leaves your heart, brain, arms, legs, pelvis, and various organs oxygen-starved. Your heart pumps harder and faster to try to compensate and your blood pressure rises.

Chronic high blood pressure—blood continually shooting through narrowed arteries with abnormally high force—damages your endothelium or accelerates existing damage, causing plaque (or more plaque) to build up within injured areas. As atherosclerosis progresses, your arteries not only become more obstructed by plaque but increasingly injured and unhealthy. Over time, as your heart struggles to pump blood, the constant stress on it leaves it progressively weaker.

Plaques can become unstable and rupture, triggering a clotting response: a maladaptive hijacking of our immune response that keeps us from bleeding to death from a cut. If a clot forms in a coronary artery, one of the arteries that supply blood to your heart, it can cause a heart attack: the reduction or blockage of the oxygenated blood flow to your heart, inflicting damage or destruction to the heart muscle. Cutting off the blood flow causes the oxygen-starved part of your heart muscle to start dying. After as little as 30 minutes of blockage, irreversible damage can set in.

THE ENDOTHELIAL DEATH SQUAD

Plaque narrowing our arteries is just *a* contributor to jacked-up blood pressure. Anything that forces the heart to consistently work harder to pump the necessary amount of blood through the body can lead to an increase in blood pressure. In addition to plaque buildup, there's a lack of physical activity (which can weaken the heart and impair its pumping efficiency) and chronic stress (which releases artery-constricting hormones). Other BP elevators include smoking (damages and narrows the arteries and makes the heart beat harder and faster) and being overweight or obese (which can lead to sodium and fluid retention and increased demand on the heart and is associated with health issues like diabetes that raise blood pressure).

High blood pressure likewise has company in injuring and weakening the endothelium. Other damage-inciters are hyperlipidemia (dangerously high LDL cholesterol and triglycerides), the above-mentioned smoking and obesity, high blood sugar, type 1 and type 2 diabetes, and premature menopause (either surgical menopause or menopause before age 40)—all of which are associated with increased inflammation.

This is one of the areas where risk varies greatly by racial and ethnic group, with black women the hardest hit. Cardiovascular disease strikes a staggering 1 in every 2 black women. Black women are *two times as likely* to have a stroke as white women and around 58% have high blood pressure, compared with 43% of white women, 38% of Asian women, and 35% of Hispanic women, according to the American Heart Association.

Black women are more likely to die of heart disease, and at a younger age, compared with white women and women of other races. Per 2021 Centers for Disease Control data *(the latest available as of October 2024)*, cardiovascular disease kills 22.6% of black women, compared with 18% of white women, 18.6% of Asian women, 11.9% of Hispanic women, 15.5% of American Indian and Alaska Native women (combined), and 18.3% of Native Hawaiian or other Pacific Islander women (combined).

Heartbreakingly, even web pages targeted to black women often fail them—like a January 30, 2024, Scripps Women's Heart Center web page, "Heart Disease and Black Women: Risk Factors, Prevention Strategies." It includes links to health metrics, such as the triglyceride levels indicating heart disease risk in white women and other groups, but never mentions the disparities in how triglycerides present in black women! *(See Chapter Twenty for details on black people's naturally lower triglyceride levels that can mislead doctors unschooled in the differences into believing their black patients' heart disease risk is nonexistent or less significant than it actually is.)*

It's amazing how much damage to our health we can incur via the one-cell-thick lining of our blood vessels. To understand that, it helps to think of the endothelium as a jacket lining with superpowers. It won't provide any "Up, up, and away!" action, but it's metabolically active, with a set of vital protective jobs to do: preventing inflammation, chemical and physical damage, plaque buildup, and blood clots.

These protective effects are impaired by smoking, diabetes, artery-choking chronic stress, and the rest of the above gang of endothelium-attacking nasties. They get right on elevating endothelial inflammation and the chemicals and processes that fuel and promote it. This makes the endothelium leaky and primed for harm and produces "adhesion molecules" that make it sticky, causing janitor cells—cleanup-crew white blood cells called "macrophages"—to get stuck to damaged areas.

These cells are normally helpful. However, when they're basically glued into the endothelium, they turn on us—gobbling up whole LDL cholesterol molecules and transforming into foam cells. These contribute to plaque formation—along with cholesterol, a bunch of cellular garbage that collects, plus calcium (in a place it shouldn't be), and fibrin, a blood-clotting protein.

And, yes, yet again, it's vicious circle time: Plaque contributes to high blood pressure and high blood pressure contributes to further plaque formation and buildup. Gunk and repeat!

OVARIAN HORMONES ARE ENDOTHELIAL HORMONES
A healthy endothelium is an estrogen- and progesterone-rich endothelium

Estrogen—produced by the body or prescribed—is crucial for keeping the endothelium healthy and protective. It's basically the endothelial Mini-Me, doing much of what the endothelium itself does to maintain healthy cardiovascular function, in addition to protecting it from damage.

For example, estrogen is not just an ovarian hormone but a cardiovascular gas station—a nitric oxide gas station. Like the endothelium (and also exercise), estrogen ramps up the production of nitric oxide gas, which relaxes the smooth muscle cells in the walls of your blood vessels, "dilating" them—opening them up—so your heart doesn't require the PSI of a pressure washer to move blood around. Maintaining normal blood pressure keeps our organs supplied with the oxygen and nutrients they need and helps prevent plaque formation and ruptures in the arterial wall.

Persistently high blood pressure can lead to weakened bulging areas in the arterial walls called aneurysms—basically IEDs in the arterial "road" that are prone to explode and take you out. Not all are deadly, but ruptured aneurysms in the brain and the aorta, the heart's primary artery for delivering blood to the body, tend not to leave "happily ever after" (or "alive five minutes from now") in their wake.

Should endothelial tissue somehow *get* injured, estrogen promotes repair—preventing the injured tissue from repurposing itself as a clot farm. As a backup plan, estrogen, just like the endothelium, hikes production of anti-clotting proteins called "anticoagulants" and increases the levels of a clot-busting enzyme so any clots that have the audacity to form can't get big and pluggy.

Estrogen improves blood delivery by growing more vessels to deliver it: off-shoots of existing blood vessels like branches on a tree. These collectively boost blood flow to your heart and other important locations, such as your vaginal tissue, where extra blood flow can help diminish desert vagina and its unfun friends.

And finally, estrogen produces molecules called "antioxidants" that curb or neutralize biological deathlords called "free radicals" (a type known as "reactive oxygen species"): vicious inflammatory molecules that engage in chemical warfare, weaponizing our own body against us in numerous ways. These toxic buggers both incite and turbocharge endothelial damage and atherosclerosis (and contribute to chronic inflammation and insulin resistance).

For example, free radicals induce oxidative stress (basically biochemical rust) that damages our cells—down to the DNA—prematurely aging them and turning them inflammatory. They degrade LDL cholesterol into its most toxic, endothelium-destroying form and give our energy-producing endothelial mitochondria a beatdown, weakening their ability to support our blood vessels' health and functionality. And adding what would best be called *injury to injury*, the pernicious chronic inflammation that free radicals generate rewards them by generating *more free radicals* to help them kill us more quickly and efficiently.

Progesterone is likewise a vital protector of our endothelium and cardiovascular health. As we saw in the previous chapter, it offers a number of the important protections estrogen does; for example, helping keep our arteries open so our blood pressure can remain normal and maintaining their flexibility and stretch. Regarding the latter, in healthy, regularly-menstruating young women around age 30, on average, reproductive endocrinologist Robert

Spaczyński found that blood vessels had the lowest amount of unhealthy stiffness when progesterone levels were highest. Because high levels of progesterone require robustly ovulatory cycles, this suggests healthy ovulatory cycles have a role in maintaining healthily elastic veins and arteries.

In Dr. Prior's words, "Basic and clinical studies" show that progesterone is involved in maintaining healthy blood pressure and control of our blood flow. It protects our "cardiovascular electrical system," the electrical signals controlling the steady pumping of our heart, and helps prevent coronary artery disease.

SECRETE ME RIGHT
Atherosclerosis prevention starts in perimenopause with adequate progesterone

Because the symptoms of atherosclerosis tend to show up in menopause, that's when doctors start treating it: when it's largely irreversible. However, research suggests its insidious effects could be prevented (or at least substantially decreased) if only researchers and doctors understood the need to take preventive steps in perimenopause: ensuring that women are producing adequate progesterone and having doctors prescribe OMP if they are not.

Progesterone deprivation due to anovulatory cycles during perimenopause is associated with "significantly more" acute myocardial infarctions (AMIs)—heart attacks from a blocked coronary artery—once a woman hits menopause, explains cardiovascular researcher Wim Gorgels, MD. In his study, a whopping 29 percent of the menopausal women who suffered an AMI had a high frequency of anovulatory cycles.

Research on our hairy tree-swinging relatives echoes this finding. In a study on female monkeys, those with anovulatory cycles were hit with the high levels of artery disease seen in male monkeys. In contrast, female monkeys that ovulated regularly—regularly producing progesterone—developed little or no arterial plaque.

Progesterone is not just important in perimenopause. It keeps protecting us in menopause. In a 1985 randomized controlled trial led by kidney disease researcher PB Rylance, MD, treatment with OMP led to a substantial decrease in blood pressure in menopausal women and in men, especially in those in the study given the highest dose: a 300-milligram dose twice daily.

(The 200-milligram twice-daily dose also decreased blood pressure—just not as much.)

The study had an inadequate number of participants—only a handful—but other studies with far more participants find OMP to have a blood pressure-lowering effect, in line with the Rylance team's conclusion: "We suggest that progesterone is a 'protective' female hormone."

MPA, on the other hand—the drug my multistate healthcare provider, Kaiser Permanente, made the standard on their formulary—seems to be quite the opposite: potentially destructive. In 2017, the American Association of Clinical Endocrinology and its educational arm, the American College of Endocrinology, put out a position statement deeming OMP safer than MPA and other progestins: "In general, MPA use seems to have greater risk with regard to multiple outcomes, including cardiovascular effects, blood pressure, VTE" (aka blood clots), and "probably stroke and breast cancer."

HOW ESTROGEN IS LIKE CINDERELLA
Start it too late in menopause and it'll turn on you

The estrogen molecules that protect our endothelium need landing pads to do their work: estrogen receptors they "dock" with in the endothelium and the layer of smooth muscle beneath it.

Uh-oh—because estrogen receptors in the endothelium and the muscle below "begin disappearing soon after menopause when circulating estrogen levels drop," report cardiologist Howard Hodis, MD, and epidemiologist Wendy Mack. With every one that disappears, we lose a work station for estrogen, meaning we lose the protective work estrogen could otherwise have done for us.

We preserve the estrogen receptor population by starting estrogen *as soon as possible upon hitting menopause*—ideally, like 20 seconds after the clock strikes 12 months with no periods. Starting estrogen right away is critical, because the more of these docking slots we hang on to, the more powerful estrogen therapy can be in maintaining and protecting the health and functionality of our endothelium. Conversely, with every receptor that disappears, we lose a work station for estrogen, meaning we lose the protective effects estrogen could otherwise have provided.

Cardiovascular studies on humans and animals from the 1980s on "clearly show that the anti-atherosclerosis action of estrogen is dependent on a healthy intact endothelium," write Hodis and Mack. This led to their "healthy endothelium hypothesis"—echoing neuroscientist Roberta Diaz Brinton's "healthy cell bias of estrogen action" in the brain, reflected in findings such as the lower risk of Alzheimer's disease in women who start estrogen therapy right at menopause. In short, estrogen is two-faced: In a healthy endothelium, estrogen gets right in there with "early beneficial effects," but in an unhealthy endothelium, it can cause harm.

Supporting their healthy endothelium hypothesis, Hodis and Mack, in their randomized controlled trial, EPAT (Estrogen in the Prevention of Atherosclerosis), found that initiation of estrogen therapy in healthy menopausal women without pre-existing cardiovascular disease "maintains vascular health, and reduces vascular aging and [the] progression of atherosclerosis." In contrast, in a damaged endothelium, estrogen has "adverse effects on established plaques," increasing inflammation and making these plaques more prone to rupture, lead to clotting, and cause blockages.

The body of science in this area suggests that by age 60, deterioration and plaque buildup in the endothelium prevent estrogen from doing its important work to inhibit atherosclerosis. Translating this into practical terms, it seems that estrogen initiated by a woman at 60 won't have the same protective effect it does in younger, just-menopausal women—and if the 60-year-old woman has enough arterial plaque in progress, it could cause harm.

However, chronological age is just a rough gauge for when endothelial health falls off into unhealth. Remember how atherosclerosis often shows no symptoms—only revealing itself in the form of a medical emergency? The term for this is "subclinical atherosclerosis," meaning atherosclerosis without significant signs or symptoms detectable by a "clinician" (that is, a doctor). This is not some rare medical phenomenon. Danish researchers led by cardiologist Klaus Fuglsang Kofoed, MD, found it in 30 percent of women age 40 and older.

This suggests we have to just meander along cluelessly, crossing our fingers we aren't playing host to the slow-speed devastation of atherosclerosis. In fact, that's not the case. With the set of lab tests in Chapter Twenty that detect cardiovascular risk factors like chronic inflammation and insulin resistance, there's a low-radiation imaging test called a coronary artery calcium (CAC) scan that shows how much calcified plaque is hanging around in Coronary Arteryville.

However, because normal aging amplifies atherosclerosis, Hodis, Mack, and other researchers advise that estrogen *initiated* after age 65 is probably harmful. In practical terms, if you are cresting 60, you should be mindful that you might be putting yourself at risk by starting estrogen—but also that one woman's 60 might be another woman's biological 55 and a half. As Pauline Maki pointed out about age and estrogen timing relative to cognitive health: "The healthy cell bias predicts that older women who are 'healthy'—who perform at or above expected levels on cognitive tests—would benefit from [hormone therapy] even if they are outside the window."

HICKORY DICKORY HEART ATTACK
Seeking a more precise heart-protection cutoff point

Hodis and Mack were determined to drill down to a more exact cutoff point for initiating estrogen. In 2016, they published the first randomized controlled trial investigating how the timing of hormone therapy affects atherosclerosis prevention in menopausal women, the ELITE study (Early *versus* Late Intervention Trial *with* Estradiol).

Healthy menopausal women showing no evidence of cardiovascular disease were randomized into two groups—"early" and "late," reflecting the length of time since they'd hit menopause—and given estrogen (with vaginal progesterone for women with a uterus):

- **The "earlies" group**: women *six years or less since menopause*, with a median (average) age of 55.4, who had gone into menopause 3.5 years before (on average).
- **The "lates" group**: women *10 or more years since menopause*, with a median age of 65.4, who had gone into menopause 14.3 years prior (on average).

In the earlies group, within six years of menopause, the women given estrogen had a *significantly lower rate of plaque progression* than the women given the placebo. However, in the "lates" group, 10 or more years past menopause, both the estrogen group and the placebo group had a *similar progression of plaque,* meaning the estrogen was no longer able to do the job to protect these women.

Of course, it could have been worse, because as disease progresses, estrogen can become harmful. For example, Hodis and Mack note that estrogen therapy in the first year of treatment in women with some already-present atherosclerosis—especially older, long-menopausal women—is found to jack up enzymes and processes that "destabilize" atherosclerotic plaques; that is, cause bits to break off and lead to clotting that can cause heart attacks or strokes.

TIME BALM
The six-year, be-on-the-safe-side window for initiating estrogen

Hodis and Mack's research suggests the general timing hypothesis for women in menopause—within 10 years of hitting menopause—is likely too broad a stretch to protect our endothelium. They call for initiating hormone therapy within six years of hitting menopause.

That six-year window is an average they came up with, and some women might be able to initiate estrogen at, say, eight and a half years, and be okay. As the daddy of the timing hypothesis, veterinarian and animal/human "comparative medicine" specialist Thomas Clarkson points out, it isn't the years themselves that are significant but the likelihood a woman has existing heart disease—like arterial plaque—that is advanced enough for estrogen to either be useless or cause harm. Again, however, because endothelial decline takes off immediately in menopause, the earlier in menopause a woman initiates hormone therapy, the more protective it is likely to be.

Hodis and Mack's research has had some mixed results—for example, one study had participants that were thought to be too young and healthy to find a difference between the treatment group and the placebo group and were probably studied for too short a time. We need more studies investigating the six-year cutoff (along with seven-, eight-, and nine-year cutoffs, for example). However, we won't put ourselves at increased risk by initiating hormone therapy within the six-year window, which is simply narrower than the one suggested by the general timing hypothesis. It's just a more conservative timetable—one that echoes decades of findings of estrogen's beneficial effects in research on humans and animals that applied a broader timetable: the 10-year cutoff of the general timing hypothesis.

In 2012, cardiologist Louise Lind Schierbeck, MD, led a large randomized controlled trial on menopausal women in Denmark that gave the participants hormone therapy over a 10-year period—oral estradiol and the progestin norethisterone acetate for women with a uterus. Women who'd started treatment "early after menopause had a significantly reduced risk of mortality, heart failure," or heart attack, "without any apparent increase in risk of cancer, venous thromboembolism [blood clots], or stroke."

In a 2006 meta-analysis of 23 randomized controlled trials in women younger than 60 initiating hormone therapy, geriatrician Shelley Salpeter, MD, found a *32 percent decreased incidence of coronary heart disease "events"*—including heart attacks, strokes, heart failure, and death.

The harms to elderly women initiating estrogen might lead you to believe that *staying* on hormone therapy as you get older could *get* harmful—as if there's a certain point it goes evil on you. In fact, it seems there's a "foot-in-the-door" effect in initiating hormone therapy.

Hodis and Mack cite 40 observational studies, some with decades of follow-up that consistently show long-term benefits—a reduction in heart disease risk and premature death—lasting for up to 10 to 40 years in women who initiated hormone therapy at or right around menopause. For example, a "longer duration of hormone therapy"—nine to 10 years, compared with shorter stints—is associated with "significantly less" plaque-driven coronary artery gunkage, with maximum benefits from hormone therapy "after 23 years of use." And though stroke risk goes up with age, Schierbeck and her team in Denmark followed up with their subjects at the 16-year point and found no increased stroke risk.

Basically, it seems that by initiating estrogen in time for it to be protective and then continuing to take it, you set yourself up for *continued protection*. This doesn't mean you won't experience *any* cardiovascular decline, since aging itself chews on our arteries and the rest of us. However, you're likely to experience far less and maybe even a minimal amount (depending on your individual health, lifestyle, and genetics) compared with what you'd get socked with if you didn't use hormone therapy or started it just before the critical window slammed shut.

Finally, I should mention that even healthy people—like the healthy menopausal women *without* vascular disease in Hodis and Mack's EPAT study—tend to have *some* deposits in their arteries. Vascular disease—aka atherosclerosis—gets diagnosed when the level of pipe blockage gets foreboding, as seen in imaging tests or when the movie you appear to be starring in is *Defibrillators on a Plane*.

ESTROGEN PILLS VERSUS ESTROGEN "STICKERS"

Whether estrogen acts as a protector or a destroyer may also be influenced by the form of delivery: oral versus transdermal "patch" estrogen.

German gynecologist and pharmacology nerd (my admiring term for him) Herbert Kuhl, MD, reports that older, long-menopausal women with pre-existing atherosclerosis *who take oral estrogen*—but *not* those using transdermal estradiol—increase the risk that unstable, renegade plaque bits will break off and lead to clotting and blockages.

He explains in a research review that oral estrogen destabilized plaque by amping up the level of an enzyme that drives collagen degradation—both eating away at the collagen scaffolding that holds arterial plaque together and *decreasing* the concentration of the chemical police force that would inhibit this munchdown. Transdermal estradiol, on the other hand, behaved itself—refraining from boosting the collagen-vandalizing enzyme, but pumping up the chemical police force that holds them at bay.

However, there was an interesting difference—right in line with the healthy endothelium hypothesis. The oral estrogen only got destructive in older, unhealthy women with plaque to derail from its moorings. In younger women without any meaningful plaque buildup, there was no similar first-year harm.

Transdermal estradiol is increasingly recommended as *the* form of estrogen to take by researchers and medical societies, as it has more helpful effects than oral estrogen and lacks its risks and harms.

Transdermal "E" comes in a stick-on, disposable abdominal patch form as FDA-approved transdermal estradiol. It also comes in gels, creams, and sprays, but these haven't been well-tested and might sometimes provide an inconsistent dose (if the dose rubs off onto your clothes or some inadvertently gets washed off).

Oral estrogen is pill estrogen. It comes, most commonly, either as CEE (conjugated equine estrogen) or estradiol (the FDA-approved bioidentical form of estrogen).

Systemic vaginal estradiol acts throughout the body, unlike most vaginal estrogens, which remain "local." Systemic vaginal estradiol *might* act like other estrogens on the cardiovascular system and elsewhere, but it's understudied and is rarely, if ever, tested in comparison with oral and transdermal estrogen.

Below, I lay out the differing cardiovascular effects of transdermal estradiol and oral estrogen (both estradiol and CEE)—followed by the "why" for these differences: how the estrogen is delivered to our system by each.

BLOOD PRESSURE

Transdermal estrogen keeps our blood pressure low and healthy. However, women taking oral estrogen showed a 14 percent greater risk of developing high blood pressure (compared with women using transdermal). That risk increase shoots up to 19 percent compared with women using vaginal estrogen.

GOOD CHOLESTEROL, BAD CHOLESTEROL

Oral estrogen alone causes unhealthy spikes in cholesterol-test blood lipids called "triglycerides." (Low triglycerides are referred to as "heart healthy." High triglycerides are cause for cardiovascular alarm.) Oral estrogen does elevate "good cholesterol" (aka HDL), while transdermal does not. However, that benefit alone does not outweigh oral estrogen's risks and harms.

BLOOD CLOT RISK

Oral estrogen, but not transdermal, is associated with elevated blood clot risk (compared with the risks in non-users). How elevated? In healthy women who initiate treatment with oral estrogen or estrogen plus MPA right around hitting menopause, there are 8 additional cases per 10,000 women, according to a Cochrane Collaboration research review. There are also 4 additional cases of pulmonary embolism—the clot-driven blockage of the blood flow to the lungs—per 10,000 women (compared with women who are *not* using estrogen or women using estrogen with MPA).

Though transdermal estrogen is not associated with increased blood clot risk, this finding may not apply to all women. For example, being overweight or obese can increase blood clot risk even in women using transdermal estrogen, reports cardiovascular epidemiologist Clare Oliver-Williams.

STROKE RISK

The risk of stroke is found to be very *slightly* increased by *oral* estrogen, prescribed by itself or with a progestin, according to the Cochrane review.

How increased? A healthy 50-year-old woman, *not* taking oral estrogen, has a clot risk of 6 out of 10,000, while a healthy 50-year-old woman using oral estrogen increases her risk to 12 out of 10,000.

That's *6 more strokes per 10,000 women* in women who use oral estrogen.

This is a seriously small risk. Tiny, even. Of course, a "tiny" increased risk, if you are one of the additional 6 out of 10,000 women who has a stroke, is not tiny at all!

For practical application of the finding, you need to figure out how likely you are to be one of the unfortunate 6, which you do by sitting down with your doctor and taking a methodical look at the facts: the findings from research and your individual risk factors for stroke.

As for transdermal estradiol, "Limited evidence indicates no increased risk of stroke" in low-dose amounts (lower than 50 micrograms a day), observes Oliver-Williams. This evidence is from observational studies as opposed to clinical trials, so it's considered "low-quality evidence" per the GRADE system for assessing research. This means the effect may or may not be real.

SLEEP

Insomnia is a major risk factor for cardiovascular disease. Any kind of systemic estrogen or estradiol is likely to alleviate menopausal insomnia at least somewhat—indirectly, by diminishing the occurrence of night sweats.

SNUBBING THE LIVER

It might seem odd that there are such differences in risks and benefits between oral and transdermal estrogen—until you look at how they get into your system. (We saw this as a potential explanation for the conflicting findings on prescription estrogen's relationship to migraines in menopause.) Because oral estrogen, after being swallowed and dissolved in the stomach or intestines, has to go through the liver, where much of it gets metabolized away, a higher dose is needed—"ten to twenty times higher," compared with other routes of delivery, like transdermal estradiol, explains pharmacist Jeannie Collins Beaudin.

Transdermal estrogens first go through your skin and into your circulation and only reach the liver to be processed after they've had a chance to act on your system. This means not as much is needed to have an effect. So, for example, "a common transdermal dose" of estradiol, "in the form of a patch, is 50 micrograms," while "an average dose of oral estradiol is 1 mg (1000 micrograms)," 20 times greater, notes Beaudin.

She adds that the "dramatically" lower doses of transdermal estrogen mean the liver has less work to do, leading, for example, to a decreased risk of gallbladder disease compared with oral estrogens. And because there's higher clot risk associated with a higher dose of estrogen, it makes sense that oral estrogen is associated with elevated clot risk, while moderate- and low-dose transdermal estradiol is not. The higher oral dose also leads to a risk of side effects such as elevated breast density from hormone metabolites—byproducts of metabolism, the mostly liver-centered process of breaking down, transforming, and eliminating nutrients and drugs we take in.

TRANSDERMALLY EVER AFTER

On a number of subjects, if you get 10 researchers together, you're likely to end up with 12 conclusions. However, the evidence supporting the use of transdermal over oral estrogen is so strong that both The North American Menopause Society and the American Association of Clinical Endocrinology, in their 2017 position statements, deemed transdermal estradiol safer than oral estrogen.

EFFECTIVELY NOWHERE
The estrogen dose that does the job

There are two questions we need answered on estrogen dosage: How much is safe and how much is effective.

Short answer: Nobody knows. (Including doctors who prescribe it for us!)

Research is *sorely lacking* on what dose of transdermal "E" is *effective* for cardiovascular protection and bone protection, and also alleviates menopausal symptoms, and at the same time, is not likely to be a welcome mat for breast cancer.

It isn't that nobody's *done* studies on the effects of this dose or that. They exist. But in the studies there are, the conclusions are all over the place because there's so little uniformity in the methodology from one to the next—including the dose tested, the delivery form, and even how they define cardiovascular disease. (For example, in one study, you can't just experience the heart pain of angina; you have to be *hospitalized* for it.)

Participants are also wildly un-uniform. One study tests older women with this health problem or that and another tests just-menopausal women who have small ears, small dogs, and live in Cleveland. (Okay, exaggerating—but not all that much!) The forms and amounts of estrogen given and the drugs they're paired with (including progesterone, MPA, other progestins, and cholesterol-lowering drugs) are likewise all over the map.

So one study could have a result, and you look for other studies with similar findings, but nobody tested *precisely* the same combination of factors—which means every conclusion is an unconfirmed floating island among unconfirmed floating islands!

Plucking out one study taking on the safety question, data from the UK's General Practice Research Database (from 400 general medical practices), low-dose transdermal estradiol therapy—0.050 milligrams or less—was not associated with an increased risk of blood clots or stroke. Doses greater than 0.050 milligrams, however, like the 0.075 milligrams I take, were associated with increased risk: 8 additional cases per 10,000 women per year.

This is a single observational study and it's seriously in need of company: more research comparing the safety of various doses of transdermal estradiol, and especially randomized controlled trials.

Where does this leave us? Guessing our asses off.

Now, looking only at these results, it might seem wise to assume that the itsy-bitsiest dose of estrogen is the safest to take. There's a problem with that: the "dose-response" relationship. A dose-response relationship is the amount of a drug needed to effect change in your body. A dose that's too low to incite change is the chemical version of somebody giving you a super-important message about what you absolutely, simply *must* do—but whispering it so softly that it's too quiet to make out.

Taking a high-enough dose is particularly important for cardiovascular health, because as Dr. Hodis and his colleagues on KEEPS (the Kronos Early Estrogen Prevention Study) note: "the arterial wall is dose-responsive to estrogen." In other words, without much of a dose, there may not be much of an effect.

Various pharmacology papers report that the *minimum effective dose* of oral conjugated equine estrogen (CEE) for most women—*for CEE to be powerful enough*—is 0.625 milligrams daily, 62.5 percent of a milligram. That's the dose that was used in clinical practice at the time of the WHI and given to WHI participants. The transdermal dose of 0.050—the 50 microgram patch—is *said* to be equivalent (on estrogen type and dose comparison charts used by pharmacists).

It shouldn't be.

There are big inconsistencies in how powerfully or unpowerfully the same transdermal dose manifests in individual women, reports pharmacology nerd Kuhl. Take the 0.050 milligram patch. On average, the women given the 0.050 dose of transdermal estradiol in the KEEPS study had *very low levels*—just over the bare minimum, 44 pg/mL—"which is considered minimally above menopausal levels," Kuhl noted. (This may have something to do with the researchers using a participant group too young and healthy to have arterial damage and the study going for too short a time.) But because individual women metabolize hormones differently, some KEEPS participants in the transdermal group—those with moderate-to-severe hot flashes—had *severely* low "E" levels—of just 9 to 11 pg/mL. That's an estradiol level of menopausal women taking no estrogen at all.

Basically, nailing down a transdermal dosage number we can go by—which, believe me, I am desperate to have!—is a scientific fool's goal. I'll give you a personal example.

The generic "dot" stick-on estradiol I decided to take comes in five strengths in the US:

0.025 milligrams
0.0375 milligrams
0.050 milligrams
0.075 milligrams
0.1 milligram

Using everything the science had to tell me, which was not one good, clear damn thing, I took a wild guess and went with the second dose from the top: 0.0375 milligrams of estradiol—which I paired with 300 milligrams nightly of oral micronized progesterone. Estrogen can take about three months to fully do its thing in your system, meaning show its effects. I waited not the slightest bit patiently for that three-month mark.

As you might remember from Chapter Seventeen, because my hot flashes remained hot and flashy, I talked with my gynecologist and went up to 0.050 and then 0.075—which did dial down the heat, frequency, and intensity a good bit.

I'd like to tell you I eventually estro-stickered the heatmonsters away—as many women do—but the sad fact remains: Save for a tiny shrug I pull out of my purse when the AC's set on "Tundra," I haven't been able to wear sleeves since 2017.

— 20 —

THE ESTROGEN, DIET, AND EXERCISE TRIFECTA

Kill inflammation overload and insulin resistance so they can't kill you

CARDIOLOGIST PETER LIBBY, MD, has spent his career investigating the pernicious effects on the endothelium from chronic inflammation—constant unhealthy low-grade inflammation.

In a 2006 PBS TV interview, Libby graphically describes atherosclerotic plaques as "hotbeds of an inflammatory process that can be prone to break open like a boil ruptures, or a pimple pops, and spew very potent blood clotting substances into the artery, [which] causes a sudden blood clot to form."

This—and the general focus on preventing plaque buildup—can make it seem like plaques are to blame for atherosclerosis. However, Libby emphasizes that chronic inflammation is a driving force behind it from start to finish—from the initial injury to the endothelium to what he calls "the clinical complications of the disease": blood clots, strokes, heart attacks, and death.

Chronic inflammation also underpins "inflammaging," which I explained back in Chapter Eleven is the low-grade, ruinous chronic inflammation throughout the body that tends to develop in middle age and increase with aging—significantly raising the risk of disease, suffering, and premature death in elderly people.

Inflammaging results from the chronic overstimulation of our immune system, which can become damaged, explains immunologist Claudio Franceschi, MD. The damaged cells of "older individuals" fall into a state of constant production of low levels of toxic inflammatory substances—like those nasty free radical/reactive oxygen species—despite there being no injury, bug, or disease to fight. However, "Inflammation is a highly demanding process," Franceschi writes, and when there *is* a problem—when immune cells get called on for a repair job or fighting off some disease or infection—they're out of gas. They become "paralyzed" and "non-functional": unable to come up with an adequate chemical response.

This ugly state of immuno-affairs occurs after we hit some inflammatory limit: cross some lifetime threshold of physiological stressors (the chemical expression of psychological and bodily stress within us) and overload our immune system. Other contributors to inflammaging include aging itself, mitochondrial dysfunction leading to "oxidative stress" (harmful molecules damaging your cells), changes in gut microbiota, and inflammation-elevating diseases such as obesity, note Franceschi and his colleagues.

As a way to understand the overload and how we get to that point, remember Bruce McEwen protesting that the stress hormone cortisol is misunderstood? That it does all sorts of good and important things to keep us alive—like revving up our immunity when it's there short term—and that only when it's chronically elevated do we have a problem?

Franceschi and his colleagues explain that "'Good' minimal stress trains the system, while 'bad' toxic stressors kill and paralyze the system." What this means is that stress, when it's not in overload quantities, can be adaptive—good for us—and lead to better management of diseases and longevity.

As we saw in Chapter Eleven, how we think is an important factor in keeping the effects of stress at an adaptive level. To paraphrase the Stoic philosopher Epictetus, *It is not events that disturb us but the view we take of them.*

In other words, perception actually *is* reality; that is, we can use it to create our *biological* reality—for example, by fostering resilience: the ability to cope with adversity and experience positive emotions in its wake. This reduces the release of stress-related hormones and pro-inflammatory cytokines within us. These chemicals are critical for fighting off infections, but when they're in excessive supply or chronically elevated, they can contribute to the development and progression of depression, autoimmune disorders, cardiovascular disease, and cancer.

Genetics and environment—the level of stress in our environment over time—play a role in the set point of our overload "threshold," or as Franceschi calls it, our "pro-inflammatory point of non-return." As he explains it, this is the point at which "there is no more possibility" to contain the pro-inflammatory toxins constantly raging in us, resulting in aging "characterized by uncontrolled diseases and frailty, which leads to early functional decline and death."

"Uh, thanks. We'll pass."

STOP THE SLOW-SPEED ARSON
We're being burned alive from within

In short, minimizing inflammation—keeping the level of inflammation in our bodies as low as possible throughout our lives—is probably the single most important thing we can do: both to hang on to our health and to live every day at our strongest, healthiest, emotionally healthiest best.

Understanding this makes for a very simple health directive: choosing how we eat and exercise by asking the question, "Will that help me decrease or avoid inflammation?"

An essential guideline for answering that is how a food or behavior affects our insulin response, a major player in triggering and exacerbating chronic dysregulated inflammation. (It's a two-way street, as inflammation can also trigger and exacerbate insulin resistance.)

Insulin is a hormone made by our pancreas. Its primary job is regulating our blood sugar levels, maintaining them within a normal range.

Our blood sugar rises when we eat. It's insulin's job to lower blood sugar levels back to normal by facilitating the transport of sugar from our blood into our muscle, fat, and liver cells. There, it is either stored as glycogen (a sugar reserve) or burned to supply us with energy. Excess glucose gets converted into fat (triglycerides) for storage in fat cells. As my investigative science journalist friend Gary Taubes puts it: "Raise insulin levels and we accumulate more fat in our fat cells. Lower insulin and fat is released from the fat cells and our lean tissue can burn it for fuel."

Insulin doesn't do all of this alone. "Insulin signaling" is the process of triggering reactions in other cells (to get them to do the necessary work). When blood sugar levels rise, the pancreas releases insulin. Insulin then helps glucose move from the bloodstream into cells for energy or storage. If there's more glucose than cells can immediately use for energy or store as glycogen (in the liver), insulin promotes the conversion of that excess glucose into fat for storage in fat cells.

When your insulin response is functioning well—called "insulin sensitivity"—insulin receptors in your muscles, fat, liver, and brain are responsive to insulin; that is, *sensitive* to it. This means insulin is used efficiently, in normal amounts, to maintain your normal blood sugar level.

Eating a diet high in sugary and starchy carbohydrates disrupts this response, spiking your blood sugar and requiring your body to produce much more insulin to do its blood-sugar-lowering job. This is basically a meal-by-meal blood sugar crisis. Eventually, your body's insulin signaling capability grows increasingly deadened, leading to a diminished ability to move glucose from your bloodstream into your tissues: a broken insulin response called "insulin resistance."

Your cells, deprived of their sugar ration, go into a panic, sending an SOS to your pancreas. Your pancreas responds in panic mode—putting out a *flood* of insulin—which works about as well as trying to persuade somebody by cranking your conversational volume to a yell. Of course, yelling merely increases the conflict level—possibly to the point where somebody loses teeth.

The loss of estrogen at menopause increases women's risk of developing insulin resistance and metabolic diseases. However, a research review led by Tiziana Ciarambino reports that estrogen treatment in menopausal women improves insulin sensitivity overall, as well as in fat cells and the liver. In the heart, it helps prevent insulin resistance-mediated cardiomyopathy—the thickening, stiffening, or enlargement of the heart that impairs its pumping ability. And we've seen in previous chapters that it has important protective effects for our muscles, some of which are due to how it improves insulin-stimulated glucose absorption. Other scientists report that it's found to delay the onset of diabetes, though more research must be done to conclude that it helps *prevent* diabetes.

Endocrinologist Gerald Reaven, MD, who originated the concept of insulin resistance, showed that insulin's impaired ability to clear blood glucose is linked with a cluster of disorders known as "metabolic syndrome" (also called "insulin resistance syndrome").

These five conditions are called "cardiometabolic diseases" because they affect both the cardiovascular system and metabolism (the breakdown and use of food for energy). Each of these substantially raises a person's risk of heart disease, diabetes, stroke, and cancer (including liver cancer, endometrial and breast cancer, and colorectal cancer).

THE FIVE UNHEALTHIES OF METABOLIC SYNDROME

- **High glucose:** Fasting glucose (a lab measurement) of more than 100 mg/dL.
- **High blood pressure:** Blood pressure greater than 130/85.
- **Too-high triglycerides (measured in a lipid test):** Triglycerides of more than 150 mg/dL.
- **Too-low HDL ("good cholesterol"):** HDL of less than 50 mg/dL (in women).
- **Excess body fat around the middle:** Waist circumference of greater than 35 inches (in women)—except for Asian women (greater than 32 inches). *(How-to: Chapter Seventeen, "Getting Waisted.")*

These cardiometabolic conditions tend to co-occur, and guidelines from the National Institutes of Health and the American Heart Association (AHA) call for diagnosing metabolic syndrome when a person has at least *3 out of these 5 risk factors* (all lab-based measurements except for waist measurement).

However, for black women, having just *2 out of the 5 risk factors* raises heart disease risk, according to an AHA study. If they do have two or more, also being obese or overweight *almost doubles* their heart disease risk. Complicating matters, black patients tend to have higher levels of HDL and lower triglycerides compared with whites, so these two measures may not be very accurate for determining heart disease risk in black women.

THE FIRE WITHIN SHOULDN'T BE FROM WHAT YOU EAT
Eating to prevent insulin resistance and chronic inflammation

Eating a carb-heavy diet (like the USDA Food Pyramid diet, which encourages carb consumption equivalent to about two cups of sugar a day), leads to a regular output of high levels of insulin to handle all the glucose coming in, explain nutritional medicine specialists Michael Eades, MD, and Mary Dan Eades, MD.

Because you now understand the mechanics of our insulin response, and how devastating insulin resistance can be, the benefits of reducing or substantially cutting carbs become clear. The healthy way to do this is through what dietary researchers Jeff Volek and Stephen Phinney, MD, two of the world's top experts in carbohydrate-restricted diets, call a "well-formulated" low-carbohydrate diet—containing adequate (saturated) fat and protein (1.2 grams of protein per kilogram of body weight).

This advice clashes with a lot of the dietary mythology pushed on us for years. For example, from Chapter Two, there's the unscientific health-harming advice to avoid saturated fat—which I noted the American College of Cardiology did an "Oops, sorry—our bad!" on in 2020 (noting that the evidence just doesn't support the claims that it's harmful). Again, research clearly shows that it is sweet and starchy carbohydrates—in bread, desserts, pasta, vegetables like potatoes, and even juice—that cause excess insulin secretion and put on fat.

Avoiding these sugary and starchy carbohydrates and replacing them with saturated fat lowers insulin levels, which helps reverse unhealthy sodium retention by the kidneys and promotes sodium excretion. This typically makes blood pressure levels drop, explains Gary Taubes, in *The Case for Keto*.

About that word, "keto," a low-carb diet is "ketogenic," referring to "ketosis," a state in which our body burns fat for energy instead of glucose (blood sugar). Sustaining this state requires consuming a "general range of 30 to 60 grams per day of carbohydrate (closer to 30 grams for those who are more insulin resistant)," explain Volek and Phinney.

"Using various blood tests that monitor various inflammatory signals, nutritional ketosis has been shown to reduce these signals to a degree comparable to the most powerful drugs currently available," they add. "Importantly, it appears to do so without the serious side effects that characterize most pharmaceuticals."

Consistently eating this way leads to "reduced inflammation and improved insulin sensitivity—in addition to a reduction in hunger and cravings," they note. These benefits "predictably lead to improved metabolic health and major weight loss" in those who are overweight.

I have to emphasize the importance of two words: "well-formulated." Volek and Phinney note that many people—those assuming that this diet simply requires cutting back on carbs—consume "poorly formulated ketogenic diets that put them at risk for unpleasant side effects and potential adverse events."

Phinney warns that people on medications for high blood pressure or type 2 diabetes should seek medical advice in order to safely go on a keto diet. Others who have or might have other medical conditions would be wise to do this, too. But even as a relatively healthy person, it's wise to find a doctor who knows the science and can partner with you to help you safely and effectively begin and maintain a low-carb/keto diet.

To find a doctor, Taubes suggests googling "low-carb, keto, or LCHF (low-carb/high-fat) doctors near me." Another possibility, he adds, is to use a program like that offered by Virta Health, Volek and Phinney's company, so you'll "at least have an informed physician handy on the other end of a telephone."

HOW TO KEEP THE CUPCAKES AWAY
(And pry yourself off the couch)

If you start a ketogenic diet, a big initial issue will be maintaining it. Some powerful helpmates for this include positive reframing of cutting out carbs, pre-powering willpower, building eating keto into your environment, and joining a supportive community. Last on the list—and extremely helpful for adhering to exercising (the subject of the next section)—there's ignoring the hell out of your feelings and doing what needs to be done.

Reframing: Consider how resilience involves reframing crappy situations through the lens of positive thinking, like realizing that the adversity you went through led to valuable shifts in your thinking you wouldn't have gotten to otherwise.

Reframe cutting out carbs similarly—as both Gary Taubes and I do. In his words, "If you think of keto as maximum carb restriction, you aren't denying yourself certain foods; you're abstaining from the foods that harm you."

Pre-powering willpower: Human "willpower" would rightly be called human "will weak and will give in to everything." Understanding that, when I started out eating this way in 2009, I knew to prepare in advance for challenging situations, like a friend's plate of delicious golden French fries trying to lead me down the devil's path.

I came up with a "list" in my mind, pictures of a bunch of sweet and carby foods, telling myself: "We don't eat these things"—basically, because they're poison. I know this probably sounds completely inane, but because it takes advantage of how human memory and learning work, it really helps. (Or, really helped me, anyway.) It's a sort of inoculation: reflex training for your psychological immune system like the way your physiological one is trained to recognize and quickly repel dangerous intruders.

Make your environment keto-supportive: I learned from psychologist Art Markman about how important it is when initiating a habit to build it into your environment. I both build and *unbuild* sticking to low carb into my environment with the foods I do and don't keep around. In case I get hungry while I'm out, I've always got food in my purse or bag: a Ziploc of some slices of bacon, some mini dried sausages (keto, sans sugar), or a tin of smoked herring with a fork and napkin rubber-banded to it. And at home, there's what I *don't* build into my environment: ice cream or anything else with sugar in it. If it's not there, I can't stick my snout in it and scarf it down.

It takes a keto village: It helps to have a community to support what you're doing. There are keto and low-carb communities on Reddit and Facebook (including a group of vegan low-carbers that Taubes says has over 50,000 members). You can also check for local meetup groups at Meetup.com.

Ignore your feelings: To be disciplined about exercising, I apply thinking from my book *Unf*ckology*: "Your feelings are not the boss of you." Basically, the fact that you have a feeling—"I don't wannnnaaa!"—is no reason to give in to it. Assuming nobody's cast a spell on you, freezing you in place, the fact that you don't "wannnnaaa!" is completely immaterial. Force yourself to pick up each foot and then put it down and start running or force your arms to hoist that barbell on the floor and get lifting!

You should also prep for doing this: Tell yourself you're going to force yourself to move and then do that in the moment. The more you do, the more it'll just be what you do—until *doing* rather than *not doing* becomes your habit.

EXERCISE AS MEDICINE

Simply getting exercise *of some kind* isn't enough. "I moved my body!" Well, okay, you weren't sedentary, but the question is: "To what end?"

Exercise as medicine means exercise that's chosen because it is most powerful for preventing the ways our bodies break down and, through that, is most powerful for protecting, enhancing, and maintaining our health. As I briefly mentioned in Chapters Ten and Seventeen, the exercise that does that better than any other is the kind that puts serious stress on our muscles: weightlifting—specifically, slow-speed, muscle-straining lifting with weights heavy enough that you can do only eight to 10 reps before your muscles give out. This is called "high-intensity training" or "HIT"—not to be confused with the cardio called "high-intensity *interval* training" or "HIIT." *(See the HIT how-to below this section.)*

Skeletal muscle plays a major role in preventing insulin resistance and inflammatory overload. For example, after we eat, our muscles are responsible for 80 percent of the uptake of glucose from our bloodstream so it can be turned into energy. If you think back to a day your energy level was between meh and half-dead, you get how vital this glucose uptake business is to whether you feel take-big-bites-outta-life energized or like you're dragging an anvil around.

Skeletal muscle is not just tissue; it is now recognized as a "major immune regulatory organ," inflammaging researcher Niharika Duggal explains. Maintaining healthy skeletal muscle is vital to the maintenance of a healthy immune system as we age, she adds. In contrast, physical *inactivity* and the resulting muscle frailty "limit the immune regulatory function of muscle in old age" and are linked with "age-related immune decline and the chronic diseases of old age."

Healthy muscles—muscles put to work *(hard)* every single day—keep both inflammation and insulin resistance at bay. In contrast, "The less we move our body, the more insulin resistant it becomes," writes metabolic researcher Benjamin Bikman in *Why We Get Sick*. His advice, in brief: "Use it or lose it."

Bikman explains that as healthy muscles contract, "they are able to take in glucose from the blood *without* using insulin." When we don't use our muscles, they become less sensitive to insulin. He gives the example of one leg that's in a cast. That immobilized leg "becomes half as insulin sensitive as the mobile leg within just days."

Even moderate-intensity walking counts for keeping inflammation and insulin levels lower, reports Bikman. In one study, people with insulin resistance who did this for three months lost 2 percent of body fat, on average, most of which came from unhealthy abdominal fat—the visceral fat that's associated with inflammation and inflammaging. "A 2% change isn't much," writes Bikman, "yet it was still enough to improve participants' insulin sensitivity." Another study—with a three-month exercise intervention—reduced markers for inflammation even in the absence of weight loss.

Walking is better than sitting, but its effects don't reach the level of exercise as medicine that we need for long-term prevention of insulin resistance and inflammatory overload.

Duggal reports that the strongest evidence for vigorous exercise as an immune booster comes from vaccination studies in older adults. Exercising regularly and habitually in old age and even single bouts of exercise before vaccination amped up immune responses to the flu and pneumococcal vaccines. However, it seems the intensity of exercise matters. Both aerobic exercise and lifting weights heavy enough to build muscle (through tiny tears made in muscle) increased the immune responses to the vaccine. More moderate exercise, such as 45 minutes of brisk walking, did not.

Finally, high-intensity weight training—weight work done *to a muscle-straining level of intensity*—improves not only the health of your muscle and bones but also significantly improves your cardiovascular health, *on a level comparable to that of aerobic exercise!* That sounds unbelievable, but once again, we need to look to the effects in the body to make sense of this claim.

Exercise scientists James Fisher and James Steele did a comprehensive research review looking for three essential "variables of cardiovascular fitness" in research participants doing high-intensity, muscle-straining weightlifting—seeking to determine whether this exercise produced the fitness-enhancing "physiological adaptations" in the body seen with intense cardiovascular exercise.

The essential fitness variables include "maximum oxygen uptake" (called "VO_2max"—with "V" for "volume"), the highest amount of oxygen your body can transport to your muscles and use during intense exercise—leading to more powerful athletic performance and better cardiovascular and overall health. Also vital is "economy of movement," the efficiency of your body's use of oxygen and energy (calories, etc.) during exercise, allowing you keep going longer with less fatigue.

Finally, there's "lactate threshold" (Tlac), the point at which lactate, a chemical byproduct of exercise, accumulates in the blood faster than the body can clear it. The better your lactate clearance (your body's ability to remove lactate or recycle it into energy), the longer you can exercise at a high intensity before your muscles start to crap out.

Fisher and Steele found strong evidence that resistance training performed to muscle failure induces these effects at levels comparable to those achieved through aerobic endurance training. (Their finding is joined by subsequent research reviews with similar results.)

What *doesn't* prevent insulin resistance and inflammatory overload? Chugging Gatorade (or other sugary "sports" drinks). There's this belief that we need carbs for energy for exercise. In fact, Dr. Phinney, an endurance cyclist riding 200 miles in a day, found that fat supplies almost all the energy used by high-caliber cyclists—once a period of "keto-adaptation" takes place. Keto-adaptation is a shift from burning carbs to burning fat for fuel, "both at rest and during exercise," write Volek and Phinney in *The Art and Science of Low Carbohydrate Living*. This doesn't happen instantly; it appears to take between four and 12 weeks to change over. They report that "biomarkers of inflammation in the body, such as C-reactive protein...are uniformly and strikingly reduced during the keto-adaptation process."

HIGH-INTENSITY TRAINING (HIT) HOW-TO

The absolute best source of exercise advice I've found is Drew Baye, a highly respected trainer whose thinking is based on rigorous scientific evidence. I will give you a brief how-to below, but please turn to his site, Baye.com, to get the expert advice that will serve you best. (If you're elderly, look up exercise for seniors. He's got that covered, too!)

Baye is very safety-focused, emphasizing developing good form with lighter weights before going to heavier ones. He suggests erring on the side of supervised training for anyone who is frail or otherwise prone to injury.

Baye describes "High Intensity Training" (HIT) as "a method of strength training performed with a high level of effort and relatively brief and infrequent workouts." He explains that the philosophy, summed up by Nautilus inventor Arthur Jones, who helped define and popularize HIT in the 1970s, is "Train harder, but train briefer" or "Train harder, but train less often."

Baye writes that "Exercise, to be productive, must be *brief* and *infrequent*." He explains that "Exercise does not directly *produce* any improvements in one's overall physical condition. It merely acts as a *stimulus* which causes the body to produce the improvements." For example, straining your muscle with heavy weights creates tiny tears in it. The process of repair that goes on is how new muscle is created. In contrast, if you don't lift heavy-enough weight, you don't challenge muscle enough to make those tears, which means all you've done is raise and lower items a bunch of times with nothing to show for it.

Other factors in building muscle are mechanical tension and metabolic stress. Mechanical tension, the force exerted on muscles when you contract them, stimulates muscle fibers to adapt to the load you're putting on them, leading to muscle strengthening and growth. Metabolic stress results from the buildup of exercise byproducts like lactate while you're lifting, chemically inciting muscle growth.

Baye notes that "The most fundamental principle of exercise is *overload*"—placing "greater demand on your muscles than they are accustomed to." In an HIT workout, "exercises are usually performed to momentary muscle failure, the point at which it is impossible to continue positive movement with good form." Going to that point "ensures you have recruited all the fibers in the muscles targeted and stimulated them to grow bigger and stronger." He notes that "The harder an exercise is, the closer it is performed to the point of momentary muscular failure, the greater the degree of overload and stimulus for improvement."

HIT can be done with machines or free weights. It must be done extremely slowly. Like, crazy-slowly. (No fast or jerky movements.) For example, I began to lift for 10 whole seconds up and 10 seconds down, copying what I saw Drew doing in videos. I keep doing reps until I can't do another with "good form"—meaning I stop before I contort myself into some injury that leaves me in pain for a month. The 10 seconds each way will seem freakishly slow at first. I had to use a clock, and some people use metronomes.

However, it turns out you don't have to do 10! Drew advises "taking at least 5 but not more than 15 seconds to perform each lifting and lowering phase."

After he told me this, I began doing just 5, which required slightly heavier weights.

This "to the point of muscle failure" thing is harsh—as in, your muscles are screaming and you want to join in. (Exercise scientist Brad Schoenfeld's research suggests you can come *close* to muscle failure and still do the job improving your muscles, and it's possible he's right.)

Because I'm a weenie and can take just one harshing a day, I do just one set six days a week—in what I described as the barbell and dumbbell "graveyard" in my living room. I do two sets on Sunday, for a total of eight sets a week—about sixteen minutes total.

I am, at age 60 as I write this, strong and fit and in the best health of my life.

TESTING, TESTING
*Get your cardiovascular report card
before you initiate estrogen (and even if you won't)*

Even if you're a perimenopausal age 49 and plan to ask for estrogen milliseconds after the clock strikes 12 months without a period, you shouldn't just assume your arteries are healthy enough for estrogen to be helpful in menopause. Cardiologist Frederick Naftolin, MD, advises that women considering initiating estrogen in menopause get a cardiovascular workup to ensure they don't have disease that's already taken off. Tests for inflammation and insulin resistance are a major part of determining this.

Of course, not all women have a medical care plan—or an affordable one. Thankfully, there's an awesome researcher who gets el cheapo prices for all the lab tests he orders in bulk, and he gives the public access to the discounts he gets.

BONUS POINT

LAB TESTS WITHOUT THE HUGE PROFIT MARGINS

For those who don't have a medical plan, ownyourlabs.com is a nonprofit service that allows people in the US to get heavily discounted lab tests through normal, legit labs near them. It was started by Dave Feldman, an engineer and citizen scientist doing important research on cardiovascular disease with a team of cardiologists, after his research participants asked him to connect them to the labs they were using so they could order tests for themselves.

The prices are just beautiful—and I use the "B" word because they are low enough that many people will be able to order important tests they can't get affordably from their doctor or can't get because they have no health plan.

For a general idea of how their rates compare, website talktomira.com sampled prices from three labs for an HbA1c (blood glucose) test. Least expensive? CVS MinuteClinic in New York City: $32. Second highest was in Chicago: $146. And the princess price? Here in LA, at Cedars-Sinai: $245.

HbA1c at ownyourlabs.com? $7.70! (As of December 2023.)

Whether or not you plan on using estrogen, it's important to monitor your cardiovascular health—including inflammation and insulin resistance—and way earlier than menopause or perimenopause, should you happen to be 22 and reading this. The earlier you identify and fix any issues, the healthier and more protected you'll be at menopause and beyond.

Monitoring involves observation and investigation across multiple areas:

- Lab tests
- Blood pressure
- Quantitative Basal Temperature (QBT), the daily first morning temperature-taking for ovulatory status *(Chapter Twenty-Four)*
- The waist circumference measurement that's more effective than BMI stats *(Chapter Seventeen)*
- Logging any daily issues you're having, such as sleep problems

The log gives you powerful "data" to present to your doctor, like, "I'm only sleeping about four hours a night" or "On most days, I have about 10 hot flashes." Getting specific like that is more powerful and helpful for guiding treatment than the more general, "I'm not sleeping well, and I'm having hot flashes."

With the waist measurement and lab tests, you're looking for signs of chronic inflammation, insulin resistance, and "subclinical" atherosclerosis: the beginnings of the inflamed, plaque-narrowing destruction of your endothelium.

Indicators your body is headed in a grim direction include the metabolic syndrome five: high blood pressure, high blood sugar, an accumulation of unhealthy belly fat, high triglycerides, and low HDL cholesterol (high-density lipoprotein). (The lab report will tell you whether you exceeded or are within normal ranges.) Remember, too, that chronic sleeplessness and hot flashes are associated with elevated cardiovascular risk.

The following is a list of the lab tests that appear to be the most important to get. If you have a primary care doctor, they'll likely test some or all of these (and add in thyroid, vitamin D, and other general health tests)—but they'll likely have some myth- rather than science-based conclusions about cholesterol (lipid tests) that I detail below.

The single most important lab test to get:

C-reactive protein (CRP): C-reactive protein is a protein in your blood plasma made by the liver that rises in concentration in response to inflammation (in response to injury and disease within you). Elevated CRP tends to be a reliable indicator of cardiovascular problems. The CRP test detects inflammation. It won't tell you what's inflamed or where. It only tells you *how much inflammation* is present. This tells you there's a problem to deal with; the next step is figuring out what it is and taking steps to treat or manage it. *(This test is $23.10 at ownyourlabs.com as of December 2023.)*

There's also a more sensitive CRP test:

High-sensitivity C-reactive protein (hs-CRP): This is a finer measure than straight-up CRP that detects lower levels of inflammation. This is the one to get if you have meaningful risk of heart disease—like a 10 to 20 percent chance of having a heart attack in the next 10 years.

Other tests to get:

Glucose: Tests to get are long-term glucose, measured by hemoglobin A1c (HbA1c), and short-term glucose, measured by fasting glucose or an oral glucose tolerance test. "Long-term" and "short-term" are my descriptions, not official medical terms. HbA1c (long-term) measures glucose levels over the previous two or three months. However, it may indicate falsely higher or lower levels, leading to overdiagnosis or underdiagnosis of diabetes, according to research by endocrinologist Mary Rhee, MD, and her colleagues.

Rhee and her colleagues recommend *both* HbA1c and either a fasting glucose test or an oral glucose test (where you drink a glucose drink), which measures the body's current glucose levels (short-term glucose).

Fasting insulin: The hormone involved in regulation of glucose—blood sugar. Eating spikes our blood sugar; it's insulin's job to yank our level down by driving the sugar into our cells, where it gets burned or stored to supply us with energy. Mary Dan Eades told me an "insulin challenge test" is better, because "it actually measures insulin sensitivity in action," but she says it's very non-standard for doctors to order.

Here's the one that gets misinterpreted by doctors:

> **A lipid panel, measuring fats (lipids) in your blood:** Those measured are total cholesterol, HDL (high-density lipoprotein), TG (triglycerides), and LDL (low-density lipoprotein).

Contrary to current medical practice standards, research strongly suggests there are just two measures to care about in a lipid panel: triglycerides and HDL. In women, a healthy triglyceride level is low—under 150 mg/dL. Healthy HDL is high—over 50. *(However, if you're a black woman, see "Black Women's Unique Lipid Profile" below.)*

An elevated triglyceride level "puts you at the highest risk of all for having a heart attack," explain the Eades. They call for keeping triglyceride levels below 100 mg/dL—and usually find "dietary changes alone" (shifting to eating low-carb) "will accomplish that goal."

To predict heart attack risk, they look to the ratio of triglycerides to HDL, which you get simply by dividing your triglyceride number by your HDL. As for the result: "A number over 5 warns of increased risk; a number below 5 is a good sign, and the further below the better."

Depressingly, there's a high likelihood your doctor is unaware of any of this, as is my primary care doctor—who (absurdly!) believes I'm in serious danger of a heart attack.

My triglycerides? 50. My HDL? 102.

Again, a healthy ratio: "A number below 5."

My TG/HDL ratio?

0.49!

Diagnosis: I'm as likely die of a heart attack as I am to be kicked in the knee by a unicorn!

Doctors also tend to have unwarranted freakouts about high total cholesterol (which is found to be protective in women over 50!). This can lead them to treat a lab value—one that does not actually indicate a problem—and harm you in the process; typically by giving you statins, drugs with horrible adverse effects.

These drugs have no benefit for preventing "all-cause mortality" in women, which means they don't do a thing to stop you from dying prematurely, no matter what you end up dying of. Statins are also linked with an increased risk of developing type 2 diabetes—especially in women—as well as cognitive issues, sometimes horrible muscle and joint pain, and fatigue. Also, because statins have mostly been studied in men, there may be undiscovered adverse effects that hit women who take them.

These two ratios, via MedicalNewsToday.com, are helpful for understanding whether you have real or medical myth-driven risk:

Total cholesterol to HDL ratio: The higher the ratio, the higher the risk. Most healthcare providers want the ratio to be below 5:1 (meaning 5 to 1). A ratio below 3.5:1 (3.5 to 1) is considered very good.

Triglycerides to HDL ratio: Echoing the Eades, health experts grade triglyceride/HDL ratios from low (and ideal) all the way up to "Uh-oh." Ideal: 2.0 or less. Good: 4.0 to 6.0. Bad: over 6.0 or above.

Contrary to what most doctors believe, the incidence of heart attacks is not worse in people with very high total cholesterol levels—even in the 400 to 600 mg/dL range, note the Eades. This makes it "questionable to worry about total cholesterol or LDL."

Unfortunately, most doctors are stuck in cardiovascular antiquity and believe keeping LDL low "is the be-all and end-all of heart health," explains Gary Taubes—despite substantial evidence that *low* levels of LDL are associated with an elevated risk of death.

In fact, it is not the mere LDL number that matters but its makeup. The harmful form is oxidized LDL, LDL turned noxious via the inflammatory effects of smoking, high-carb foods, and sedentary behavior. These oxidized LDL particles (unhealthy "Pattern B" LDL) are small and dense and associated with greater risk of cardiovascular disease—possibly because they are the right size to sneak through the "cracks" in an injured endothelium and promote plaque buildup. In contrast, healthy LDL particles ("Pattern A") are large and fluffy, bouncing around your blood vessels instead of settling into the walls. *(Note that having Pattern A does not rule out cardiovascular risk, as you may have other risk factors.)*

Determining whether you have the healthy Pattern A or unhealthy Pattern B LDL takes an expensive "particle size test": called LDL-P. (If you're getting one, ask for HDL-P, too, which is looking like an important measure of actual heart disease risk—though there's a good chance this information has yet to trickle down to your doctor.)

I learned a great frugalista stand-in for the LDL-P test from Mike Eades: your triglycerides level. *(Price for triglycerides test in a "lipid panel" at own yourlabs.com: $10!)* If you've got low triglycerides (under 100), it's a reliable sign of Pattern A: large, fluffy LDL. If you're Pattern B or untested but have high triglycerides, eating a low-carb diet is found to have a beneficial effect on LDL-P: turning dangerously small and dense particles into the larger, fluffy Pattern A—in addition to decreasing insulin levels.

The panic to lower LDL and total cholesterol basically involves treating lab numbers in ways that do nothing to fix the actual problem: the elevated insulin and inflammation in our system destroying our endothelium and us in the process.

BONUS POINT

BLACK WOMEN'S UNIQUE LIPID PROFILE

In a study led by pediatric endocrinologist Stephanie Chung, MD, premenopausal black women had fasting triglyceride levels approximately 21.74% lower, on average, than white women in that group, while menopausal black women had levels 17.57% lower.

Because black women (and men), on average, tend to have higher levels of HDL and lower triglycerides compared with whites, these lipid measures may not be very accurate for determining heart disease risk in black women. For example, black women with insulin resistance, which is typically associated with high triglycerides, often have lower triglyceride levels than would be expected.

When I searched for more predict-worthy tests for black women, I found sparse and conflicting information, along with the annoying, "Well, we researchers had better get on figuring something out!"

There was one exception: a test for coronary heart disease risk called the "PLAC Test for Lp-PLA2" that measures an enzyme in the blood indicating inflammation. In black women with Lp-PLA2 levels over 225, there was an elevated risk of coronary heart disease "events."

The price for this test seems to range from $119 to around $199. However, I had a hunch and checked ownyourlabs.com: $53.46! *(As of December 2023. Listed as "Lp-PLA2.")*

Your body is a whole system—an interplay of factors—and it's important to look at your risk factors collectively to get a complete picture of your inflammation level and overall metabolic health.

Great blood pressure? Really low numbers on CRP tests? Healthy levels of glucose and insulin? These are signs of metabolic health. However, there is one test—an imaging test—that will give you a highly reliable idea of what's going on in your arteries. I suggest this last because doctors will not take this as a first step—or give you this test at all, unless there's reason to suspect you might have dangerously mucked-up arteries:

Coronary artery calcium (CAC) test: This is a "calcium scoring test"—a scan of your heart with pretty minimal radiation (about the same as a mammogram) that tells you the extent of calcium buildup in the arteries to your heart. You get a calcium score afterward, on a scale that goes from zero to about 400 (or higher). A score of zero is ideal. Australian cardiologist Alexander Chua and his colleagues note that calcium scoring "has been shown to convincingly predict future cardiovascular risk...across a wide range of ethnicities, ages, and sexes."

Finally, some supplemental tests the Eades suggest:

Apolipoprotein B (ApoB): ApoB is a protein attached to each LDL particle—one ApoB molecule per particle—so the concentration of ApoB in the blood reflects the number of LDL particles in your blood. LDL particles can contribute to plaque buildup, and high ApoB reflects a greater number of these particles, so doctors tend to assume high ApoB means high cardiovascular risk. However, this may or may not be the case according to recent research.

ApoB is highly influenced by genetics and diet. For example, in people like me who eat keto, ApoB can be elevated without it necessarily reflecting increased cardiovascular risk.

Learning that, I asked for a test of the protein ApoA1, the main component of HDL, along with my ApoB test. In fact, I told my new primary care doctor I would *only* take an ApoB test if he would test ApoA1, too.

An ApoB result alone can be misleading. It's only half the story. The ApoB-to-ApoA1 ratio matters because it shows the balance between LDL and HDL. A high ApoA1-to-ApoB ratio is good because ApoA1 basically works as a janitor, clearing excess cholesterol from your tissues and transporting it to the liver for excretion, reducing cardiovascular risk.

Lipoprotein(a) [Lp(a)]: Lp(a) is a type of LDL cholesterol with the protein apolipoprotein(a) attached. It's an inflammation-promoting lipoprotein—a package of fat and protein—produced by the liver. Lp(a) can stick to your arterial walls, promoting plaque buildup and clot formation, while also impairing your body's ability to break down clots. High levels of Lp(a) (above about 30 mg/dL) are associated with a significantly increased risk of heart disease.

What drives Lp(a) up? Lp(a) levels *increase* with menopause, kidney disease, and hypothyroidism (too little thyroid). Diet matters, too. Replacing dietary saturated fat with the so-called "heart-healthy" diet of carbohydrates, protein, and unsaturated fat (like in vegetable oils) *increases* Lp(a) levels by 10 to 15 percent, reports cardiovascular researcher Enkhmaa Byambaa, MD.

What *reduces* Lp(a) levels? Byambaa and her colleague report that Lp(a) levels *decrease* with a diet high in saturated fats and low in carbohydrates. Hormone therapy likewise reduces Lp(a).

Black people tend to have higher levels of Lp(a) than white, Hispanic, or Asian people. In black research participants, reducing saturated fat intake—replacing it primarily with carbohydrates—resulted in a 24 percent increase in Lp(a) levels. However, most Lp(a) studies have been conducted on white people—and primarily men. So whether elevated Lp(a) translates to more deaths from heart disease is not conclusively known. The African American Heart Study, an observational study announced in 2023, will investigate whether Lp(a) is associated with more atherosclerotic "events"— that is, those caused by arterial plaque buildup.

Lp(a) is 70 to 90 percent genetically determined and remains largely unchanged after the age of five, so it can usually be tested just once.

— 21 —

THE TROPIC OF BREAST CANCER

JUST AS *TAKING* a drug comes with risks, so can *not taking it.*

Being diagnosed with breast cancer is the greatest medical fear of many of us and the biggest deterrent from using hormone therapy in menopause—which makes it the biggest deterrent from protecting our cardiovascular system and the rest of us.

Of course, not every woman will want to use hormone therapy, and some will have pre-existing conditions that prohibit it. However, decisions about whether to use or avoid it should not be driven by that Socrates of emotions, panic.

I say that like I'm able to manage my own risk in some coolly detached "Keep calm and science-on" way.

I am not.

Breast cancer terrifies me. Due to family history, I was tested for the cancer-risk-increasing BRCA gene mutations (thankfully negative!), and I get called in for annual mammograms. These come with a special bonus: intermittent howling fear in my head for days after they take the pics while I wait to hear whether I (yet again!) will get called back in for an ultrasound, biopsy, and/or an MRI.

Even an "all clear" isn't much comfort. My boobs are so dense, I basically get back a remark from whichever radiologist reads them along the lines of "Can't really see shit in there, but we did our best, and you don't seem to be slated for chemo or a steel drawer at the morgue."

On top of all of this, probably like many of you, I'm not just terrified for myself. Just months ago, yet another dear friend called me crying with the results of her biopsy. I think we've all gotten a number of those calls. Absolutely heartbreaking.

BOOBS BEFORE BLOOD PRESSURE?

Our boobs get all the attention—and not just from benevolently minded individuals who share their perceptive insights from the windows of passing cars.

Our breasts are a major part of our self-image. They're a front-and-center sign of femininity—welcome or, for some, uncomfortably unwelcome. In our teens, they announce to the world that we've shoved off from the dock of childhood. We spend piles of money pushing them up, squeezing them down, and hiring plastic surgeons to remodel them. For many women, they're a 24/7 diner for babies, and for probably most of us, they're an essential part of our erotic life. All of this makes the prospect of being diagnosed with breast cancer and needing a mastectomy loom terrifyingly large.

Our heart? We can't *see* our heart. We never check whether we're showing too much aorta through our tank top. Nobody yells from cars, "Whoa...pump on!" or "Hey, baby! I wanna lick your vena cava!" Then there's how only about half the population has heard that heart disease is the leading cause of death of women—and how little of a dent that makes in anyone's behavior. As vital as our cardiovascular system is to our survival, it's just yet another part of the internal factory of us, and unless it's on the fritz, we tend not to think of it at all.

Because of this, we prioritize avoiding breast cancer—which *is* horrible but usually curable today and can often be caught on a mammogram in the early stages—at the expense of suffering heart disease, which is horrible, irreversible, and deadly.

DYING TO SAVE OURSELVES
Our fears make poor statisticians

Remember the heart disease risk stats? Again, 1 out of every 5 women now dies of it, and 1 in 3 is projected to die of it in coming years, making heart disease the leading cause of death for women in the US—including women with breast cancer!

That 1-in-5 figure is more than *seven times the current rate of women dying of breast cancer*: 1 in 39 women (per the American Cancer Society, 2022).

But let's have a second look at that 1-in-39 number. Like my friend Roxanne Brown, who died in 2018, these are women who were diagnosed with breast cancer sometimes decades ago—before the amazing advances by breast cancer researchers that now allow more and more women to (so beautifully!) call themselves "breast cancer survivors."

Oncologist Avrum Bluming, MD, makes a vital point: "Given that the cure rate for newly diagnosed breast cancer is currently approximately 90%, breast cancer survivors are at far greater risk of dying of heart disease than of breast cancer, a difference that grows as they age."

Ironically, protecting your cardiovascular system (and cardiometabolic health) by taking estrogen in menopause may have a side benefit: protection against breast cancer through its beneficial effects on insulin.

Unhealthy high levels of fasting insulin—driving the insulin resistance we see in pre-diabetics—are associated with a greater risk of breast cancer. Estrogen helps you maintain insulin sensitivity, keeping your insulin receptors responsive to insulin so it can do its job regulating your blood sugar.

In women who are diagnosed with breast cancer, elevated insulin is associated with much poorer outcomes. "The average breast cancer tumor has over six times more insulin receptors than noncancerous breast tissue," explains metabolic researcher Benjamin Bikman in *Why We Get Sick*. "Six times more! That means this malignant tissue is six times more responsive to insulin and its growth signals than normal tissues."

The well-documented connection between insulin resistance and breast cancer led researchers to begin treating breast cancer patients with insulin-sensitizing medications, leading to reductions in the disease, reports Bikman. "Essentially, the researchers found that controlling insulin resistance helped control the breast cancer."

ELEVATED RISK OF BREAST CANCER OR ELEVATED SLOPPY ERROR?

Of course women panicked when the WHI researchers announced that hormone therapy led to "increased risks of invasive breast cancer." (That's pretty much all we need to hear to hop on the "Estrogen Is Evil" train.)

To be fair, an increased risk of "invasive breast cancer" *is* what the WHI researchers found: 1 additional case per 1,000 women per year, after 5.6 years of therapy. However, this result was not from estrogen therapy alone (which did not lead to an increased risk of breast cancer) but from estrogen paired with MPA. MPA, we saw in Chapter Seven, has a chemical makeup that increases women's breast cancer risk (in contrast with OMP's protective effects).

However, it turns out there was something amiss with this finding. Cardiovascular researcher Howard Hodis, MD, reports in a 2018 paper that the elevated risk of breast cancer reported in the CEE estrogen plus MPA arm of the WHI trial was wrong: based on a methodological screwup by the researchers!

Women who'd used hormone therapy in the past were sloppily included in the placebo group—a control group that was supposed to be women who'd *never* used hormones. Hodis and his colleague, gynecologist Philip M. Sarrel, MD, spotted the error because they'd noticed something weird about that control group: There was a *way* lower incidence of breast cancer than would've been expected in "never users."

The unusually low incidence of breast cancer stemmed from the fact that women who'd used hormone therapy in the past *had a lower rate of breast cancer.* And yes, you read that right—*hormone therapy users had a lower rate of breast cancer!*

Wrongly including these prior hormone therapy users in the "never users" control group caused the breast cancer rate in that group to be inaccurately low—making the WHI's hormone-treated group of women seem to have higher breast cancer rates by comparison.

Hodis and Sarrel pointed the error out to the WHI researchers. Once the dataset of previous hormone users was removed from the "never users" group, the previously announced elevated risk of breast cancer in the hormone-treated group *disappeared.*

Remember that saying, "Science is self-correcting"?

You'd think we, the public, would have heard about this error—maybe even gotten a public apology from the WHI researchers for all the menopausal women they (oops!) panicked into ditching their hormone therapy, and with it, its protective effects.

If only!

In the wake of Hodis and Sarrel's discovery, oncologist Avrum Bluming took the WHI researchers to task in a 2021 medical journal commentary: "The senior authors, aware of this criticism, have continued to publish updates without commenting on nor correcting this critical misinterpretation."

Nice.

My take? Reputation before responsibility to women.

We see you.

BLAMING ESTROGEN AND PROGESTERONE FOR MEDROXYPROGESTERONE ACETATE'S CRIMES

Estrogen itself, long accused of causing cancer, may actually *prevent* it—in healthy menopausal women, with no existing breast cancer, who initiate it when they're just-menopausal (or within the bounds of the "timing hypothesis"). For example, after excluding the elderly, unhealthy women from the WHI dataset, a 20-year follow-up study found a 37 percent *decreased* risk of breast cancer from CEE estrogen-alone therapy.

Though researchers I respect argue that the methodological issues in the WHI should knock it down from its randomized controlled trial status to something more on the level of observational research, it helps that five smaller RCTs echo this finding.

The women in this WHI follow-up group had hysterectomies and thus had no uterus to protect with MPA. However, for women who need combination therapy, OMP is the clear choice over MPA. We saw in Chapter Seven that progesterone is like a police force for your boobs and uterus, protecting them against runaway cell overgrowth that can lead to cancer.

MPA, on the other hand, accelerates the proliferation (rapid multiplication) of breast cells as well as breast cancer cells. For example, in a study on macaques, a kind of monkey, "estradiol+MPA resulted in significantly greater proliferation" in breast tissue compared with placebo, "while estradiol+micronized progesterone did not," reports epidemiologist Agnès Fournier.

Unfortunately, there are no randomized controlled trials on OMP and women's breast cancer risk, and other research is scarce. However, referring to a body of European research—large observational studies in France and Finland—plus a controlled trial on monkeys investigating the effects of OMP as well as MPA and other progestins, UK-based cancer researcher Jason Carroll concludes: "Collectively, these findings provide evidence to indicate that the increase in breast cancer risk is restricted to formulations containing certain progestins, such as [medroxyprogesterone acetate]."

In fact, in observational studies, OMP plus either transdermal or oral estrogen has been associated with a *protective* effect—decreased breast cancer risk—as has the progesterone our bodies produce during our menstruating years. The 2005 EPIC study, which took blood samples from menstruating women in 10 European countries, found an association between high levels of progesterone and a decreased risk of breast cancer.

Conversely, it's possible that anovulatory, progesterone-starved menstrual cycles play a role in breast cancer development. A few older studies (from the early 1980s) find an association between chronic anovulatory cycles and an increased risk of breast cancer. For example, anovulatory cycles were associated with a higher risk of breast cancer after age 55—three to four times greater—compared with regular cycles, according to research by the late reproductive immunologist Carolyn Coulam.

Epidemiologist Linda Cowan found that infertile women with anovulatory cycles had a breast cancer risk prior to menopause 5.4 times greater than those whose infertility was *not* hormonally driven (meaning it was caused by something other than anovulation).

Ideally, we'd have more recent research investigating this, applying advances in methodology. Instead, we're left to guess. That said, in light of the evidence we do have suggesting progesterone offers protection against breast cancer, it seems wise to test for anovulatory cycles (using QBT, Quantitative Basal Temperature [©CEMCOR], detailed in Chapter Twenty-Four).

ESTROGEN AND OMP, SITTIN' IN A TREE

There is recent reinforcement for the safety of OMP over MPA (along with various forms of estrogen)—from a 2022 observational study of 43,000 cases of breast cancer in women age 50 or older in a UK healthcare database. Gynecologist Haim Abenhaim, MD, and his colleagues explored which formulations of hormone therapy were associated with an increased incidence of breast cancer.

They looked at two forms of estrogen—bioidentical estradiol and "animal-derived estrogens" (that horse-pee CEE). They also looked at micronized bioidentical progesterone compared with "synthetic progestin": "predominantly" medroxyprogesterone acetate, MPA.

Estrogen on its own—whether bioidentical or "animal-derived" (as CEE)—was not associated with increased breast cancer risk, nor was OMP. That said, we've seen that transdermal estradiol is the safest form. Both oral CEE and oral estradiol increase inflammatory markers due to their being metabolized by the liver, while skin-delivered transdermal estradiol does not. Transdermal estradiol also does not lead to the small increase in stroke risk that oral estrogens do.

The Abenhaim team found that the various synthetic progestins women took—most of which were MPA—were associated with increased breast cancer risk, identical to that found in the long-term follow-up of WHI participants who were dosed with CEE plus MPA. As the Abenhaim team put it, "Synthetic progestin" (mostly MPA) "appears to be the single agent independently associated with an increase in breast cancer risk."

Summarizing their results, they explained, "Although menopausal hormone therapy use appears to be associated with an overall increased risk of breast cancer, this risk appears predominantly mediated"—that is, brought about—"through formulations containing synthetic progestins."

Science might not be self-correcting, but some scientists with integrity are. Noting the Abenhaim team's 2022 finding on the safety of progesterone over MPA, one of the investigators on the WHI study, ob-gyn Andrew Kaunitz, MD, publicly announced—in a 2022 video on Medscape.com, "The Safest Option for Menopausal Hormone Therapy"—that he would be shifting his prescribing standards. "Going forward," he said he would counsel women considering hormone therapy "that from the perspective of breast cancer risk, the safest progestogen appears to be micronized progesterone."

Recall those childhood obesity researchers in the Gary Taubes talk who refused to even *consider* they might be harming their patients—which would involve admitting they'd been wrong or, at least, might've been? Kaunitz is the other kind of researcher—the sort of scientist and doctor who puts evidence-based science and the welfare of his patients first.

More Dr. Kaunitzes, please.

BONUS POINT

THE BREAST CANCER RISK CALCULATOR

I got a sense of my percentage of breast cancer risk by using an amazing online risk-calculating tool—the Breast Cancer Risk Assessment Tool—via the US National Cancer Institute. It was created for doctors to use with their patients, but it's completely easy for any of us to use on ourselves and only asks a handful of questions.

It estimates a woman's risk of developing breast cancer within five years and in her lifetime—spitting out both percentages—plus the average risk for women in the US by race and age group. Through the questions you click to answer, it factors in your medical and reproductive history and asks for your family history of breast cancer (among close relatives: mom, sisters, daughters).

For perspective on your results, the NCI website advises: "Although a woman's risk may be accurately estimated, these predictions do not allow one to say precisely which woman will develop breast cancer. In fact, some women who do not develop breast cancer have higher risk estimates than some women who do develop breast cancer."

And if you're using the tool as a patient, they also suggest, "You are encouraged to print these results and discuss them with your provider." Current URL: **bcrisktool.cancer.gov** (then click "calculate patient risk"), but if this URL goes away, just google "breast cancer risk tool" and the US National Cancer Institute and you should find it.

HAZARDOUS CURVES
Breast cancer risk factors

From the Memorial Sloan Kettering Cancer Center (except where noted), general risk factors for breast cancer that increase your individual risk include:

Age—as in getting older:
- Women in their 30s have a 1 in 227 chance of developing breast cancer (0.44%).
- Women in their 60s have a 1 in 28 risk (3.6%).
- Women in their 90s and beyond have a 1 in 8 risk (12.4%).

Early menstruation and late menopause:
"Early menstruation" means starting before age 12 and "late menopause" is menopause after age 50. There's speculation that increased lifetime exposure to estrogen plays a role—and a lack of evidence to make that anything more than speculation.

Never being pregnant or being pregnant after 30:
These are associated with slightly higher risk factor. "This may be due to the protective changes in breast tissue that occur with full-term pregnancies," according to Sloan-Kettering.

A prior history or family history of breast cancer:
Only 5 to 12 percent of all breast cancer cases are hereditary. However, if a "first-degree relative" (mother, sister, or daughter) has had breast cancer, you may be two to three times more likely to develop it.

Genetic mutations BRCA1, BRCA2, and PALB2, due to abnormal genes inherited from either parent:
BRCA mutations are common in Ashkenazi Jews but they are also found in other groups. For example, a study led by epidemiologist Esther M. John found, in women under 65 diagnosed with breast cancer, 8.3% were Ashkenazi Jews; 3.5% were Hispanic; 2.2% were "non-Hispanic whites"; 1.3% were African-American; and 0.5% were Asian-American.

Having a BRCA mutation does not mean you WILL get breast cancer; it just points to an increased risk of breast cancer—an estimated 45 to 65% increased risk by the age of 70, reports clinical epidemiologist Heidi Nelson.

BRCA testing is expensive and is recommended only for women who have meaningful risk factors, reports Nelson. Such risk factors include close female relatives with breast cancer, "breast cancer in male relatives, multiple cases of breast cancer in the family, both breast and ovarian cancer in the family, family members with two primary breast cancers, and Ashkenazi Jewish ancestry."

PALB2 testing can be added to BRCA testing, because having a family history of breast cancer is a risk factor for it. PALB2 is a protein-coding gene, and mutations in the PALB2 gene likewise increase breast cancer risk, though generally not as much as BRCA mutations. By age 80, a woman has a 53% increased risk of breast cancer if she has this gene, according to a 21-country, 524-family study led by statistical geneticist Xin Yang.

If you have risk factors and don't have health insurance, you might be able to get free or low-cost testing from an organization near you. In that case, Google may be your boobs' best friend—and calling local breast cancer charities for information may also be helpful.

High breast density:
This is a term from mammography—basically the radiologist's-eye-view of breasts. It describes the amount of hard-to-see-through fibrous and glandular breast tissue versus fatty tissue (the kind that shows up more transparently on an X-ray). Dense breasts are associated with a higher risk of breast cancer and can obscure small tumors on a mammogram.

Per the CDC, there are four categories of breast density. The top two are the ones you want to be in: the "low-density" or "fatty" breast categories. The bummer categories are the bottom two: the "dense" or "high-density" breasts.

- Breasts that are almost entirely fatty (about 10% of women, meaning one in 10 women)
- Breasts with a few scattered areas of dense tissue (about 40% of women—four in 10)
- Breasts that are evenly dense throughout (about 40% of women—four in 10).
- Breasts that are extremely dense (about 10% of women—one in 10).

COMPARING APPLES AND ~~ORANGES~~ ZEBRAS
The scientific big nowhere on hormone therapy and breast cancer

Very reasonably, we all want the big question answered—not what estrogen tends to do in this population or that, but "Will *I* get breast cancer if I use hormone therapy?" And then there are companion questions, like, "What duration is safe for me?"

In other areas of research for this book, I'd start out with a big scientific muddle, then read and read and dig into the biology on a cellular level. Eventually, the evidence would turn into an arrow pointing in one direction or another: probably safe for most women or some women or probably harmful for some or most, and you could see which group you fit or generally fit into and have at least a starting idea of what might be a wise option for you.

However, the results on hormone therapy and breast cancer risk remain a giant sinkhole of whirling inconclusiveness: numerous conflicting findings with conflicting variables that make many studies islands unto themselves. They test varying hormone preparations, in varying doses, for varying lengths of time—some not long enough to actually see an effect—on women of varied ages, with varied conditions... (I could go on till next Tuesday or till sanity and I part company, whichever comes first).

In short, we're left with numerous conflicting findings saying much and collectively telling us nearly nothing. For example, there's a troubling amount of missing information on the long-term effects on breast cancer risk from using hormones. The conflicting findings we do have swing from showing no increased risk from 22 years of use of CEE plus MPA (according to a 1992 randomized controlled trial by reproductive endocrinologist Lila Nachtigall, MD) to recent studies suggesting just five years of use may increase the risk of breast cancer.

More recently, there's the 20-year follow-up WHI re-analysis and those five other RCTs that find estrogen either doesn't cause cancer or decreases cancer risk substantially. (Though MPA tends to get bad marks, longitudinal studies on estrogen and OMP and breast cancer risk are sorely lacking.)

And take how breast cancer risk goes up with age. Research by epidemiologist Katie M. O'Brien and her colleagues found that use of hormone therapy in women younger than 50 was not associated with an increased risk of breast cancer. The WHI re-analysis likewise found that women ages 50 to 59 had no increased risk of breast cancer. However, *a later age at menopause*—going into menopause after age 55—was found to increase risk in the Nurses' Health Study.

Questions fly to mind: Could it be that ages 50 to 59 are the sweet spot for starting hormone therapy—but only if you hit menopause before 55? Should researchers control for the age menopause begins? And in studies that find an increased risk of breast cancer, is it due to aging or the hormone therapy or a bit of both?

Without these considerations (and a host of others) taken into account, individual studies can *seem* to stand up—as can other studies with exactly the opposite conclusions. All in all, there just isn't sufficient support in the form of a good-sized "body of work" that Sander Greenland advises me to look for.

Below are a few factors getting in the way of that:

Drug forms tested are all over the map:
MPA, the drug tested in most hormone therapy research, is *individually* found to increase the risk of breast cancer and other harms, while OMP is not. Study results are typically reported in the media under the umbrella terms "hormone therapy" or "estrogen," obscuring the differing effects of the varying forms tested.

The WHI was an example of this, referring to a breast cancer risk-increasing CEE estrogen plus MPA combo drug as "hormone therapy," causing women to stop taking not just this combo but CEE alone, for which the WHI found no elevated risk.

Pre-existing cancer attributed to hormone therapy:
Researchers know breast cancer doesn't pop up like bread out of a toaster. Except for a rare and severe form, inflammatory breast cancer (which disproportionately affects black women), most breast cancers are slow-growing, with an average "doubling time" of 180 days (six months), the amount of time it takes for a single cancerous cell to "double" itself—to become two cancer cells.

This means a cancerous growth that is big enough to be detectable on a mammogram will typically have been present for many years. Studies looking at breast cancer risk from hormone therapy *should* take this into account to avoid falsely inflated findings of a causal link between hormone therapy and breast cancer. Yet, for example, epidemiologist Samuel Shapiro points out that the Million Women Study, among its many other methodological flaws, failed to exclude participants whose breast cancer was detected within four months of the start of the study.

The middle-aged white woman standard:
Studies and the news stories reporting their results refer to "women's" risk or this or that happening to "women." Well, *which women*? As we've seen, study participants are usually middle-class white women. In the WHI trial, 80.5% of the participants were white, 10% were black, 5.6% were Hispanic, 1.9% were Asian/Pacific Islander, and 0.5% were Native American.

Women aren't told that study results may not apply or apply all that well if "white woman" or "middle-class white woman" does not describe them. A breast cancer risk cited for white women may *underestimate* the risk for black women—a group more likely than any other to die of breast cancer—and it can also *overestimate* the risk for women in other groups. This may lead a broad population of women to make health-affecting decisions based on risks to the average white woman that they are led to believe apply to them.

These flaws and many more baked into so many research findings on breast cancer and in other areas distort our ability to make sense of the risks and benefits of hormone therapy, warping our ability to make informed choices.

"We need the definitive trial where women (given current knowledge) are treated with the correct hormones, for the correct indication, in the correct age group, to settle the argument once and for all" (of the effects of hormone therapy on breast cancer risk), writes International Menopause Society president, gynecologist Nick Panay, MD.

We have yet to see such a trial, so we and our doctors are left in a terrible position: needing to hazard an under-supported "best guess" about the risks and benefits of our using hormone therapy and the risks of going without.

Not a place any of us want to be.

THE SCIENTIFIC BIG NOWHERE ON PROGESTERONE AND BREAST CANCER

With all the complaints about the mess of inconclusive conclusiveness that the research on estrogen and breast cancer is, at least there's been a good deal of effort to fund and study it.

Not so for progesterone—as usual.

I was desperate to do better than I had above—to tell you something more definitive about progesterone and breast cancer risk. Disturbingly, I had come upon lab studies (on cells in petri dishes and such) in which progesterone *was* proliferative: made cells grow. Some of these studies were on breast tissue from breast reduction surgeries.

Dr. Prior explains in her work that there is initially a small, brief proliferative period by progesterone in the breast, but it's followed by decreased proliferation and then cell differentiation. Lab studies focus on short-term effects and typically don't last long enough for the decreased proliferation and subsequent cell differentiation to show up. Also, they investigate the effects on cells in a dish, as opposed to cells in their natural context—in a breast (acting in the presence of other hormones). The effects may be different from "in vivo" "within the living"—what happens in a woman's breast.

Still, though studies on women and mice find progesterone inhibits "carcinogenesis" (the growth of cancer), and though progesterone *deficiency* has been linked with breast and endometrial cancer, these findings required investigation. And investigate I did—without getting any sort of clarity on this sometimes-proliferative effect.

I spent a week chewing on my left pinkie finger—a sexy and sophisticated lifelong habit I absentmindedly engage in in the face of intractable problems. Somehow, it came to me—before I gnawed my finger to a nub. The answer, once again? Thinking small: going down to the cellular level.

For that, I turned to a pioneering breast cancer researcher, endocrine physiologist Kathryn Horwitz. In 2010, Horwitz received the Endocrine Society's lifetime achievement award for "exceptional contributions to the field of endocrinology."

Horwitz, back in 1975, right at the start of her career, filled in a vital missing piece in the science on breast cancer. Most breast cancers are estrogen-driven. They are estrogen receptor positive (ER+)—meaning they have receptors for estrogen that allow their growth to be fueled by estrogen.

It turns out there are also progesterone receptors in breast cancers. Horwitz discovered those receptors—as well as demonstrating that when progesterone receptors are present in ER+ tumors, the cancer is less aggressive and more responsive to treatment with hormone therapies.

"Even before her study was published, word of [her discovery] made waves in the scientific community," writes John A. Cidlowski, molecular endocrinologist and senior NIH researcher. "The news reached the White House, where First Lady Betty Ford was battling breast cancer. A sample of Ford's tumor was sent to Horwitz, who found it to be strongly PR-positive (progesterone receptor-positive); a good sign."

"In retrospect," writes Horwitz about Ford (who gave her permission to disclose this), "she would have been an excellent candidate for minimal surgery and hormone therapies; the standard of care today." Thanks to

Horwitz's discovery, "Since 1975, millions of patient tumor samples have been assessed" for progesterone receptors (as well as estrogen receptors), "which has spared many women extensive mastectomies in favor of lumpectomies and hormone therapies."

This was just the first of many important findings by Horwitz, now in her 80s, whose research continues to focus on the molecular biology of breast cancer and estrogen and progesterone receptors.

In a 2020 paper, Horwitz and endocrinologist Carol Sartorius "debunk the notion that progesterone 'causes' breast cancers," citing "considerable experimental and clinical evidence" that progesterone alone, at normal levels, "is incapable" of doing this. However—and it's a big however—they report that when animals were treated with a carcinogen, followed by estrogen plus progesterone, tumors developed.

In other words, once cancer is caused by a carcinogen, progesterone may feed and spread it. Referencing current evidence, they conclude: "It is our opinion that natural progesterone does not 'cause' breast cancer but can expand it" if it already exists in the body.

In contrast with their view, in a 2015 study in mice, oncology researcher Hisham Mohammed and his colleagues found that progesterone *inhibited* tumor formation in estrogen-driven breast cancers (ER+)—confirming findings in previous research. Progesterone also "significantly inhibited estrogen-stimulated proliferation" in estrogen-driven cancers. Other research on human breast cells likewise finds anti-proliferative effects.

Horwitz and Sartorius put these and other findings in context for women in and around menopause: "It is not unreasonable to propose that some women of menopausal age unknowingly harbor pre-existent minimal disease, which expands upon hormone supplementation leading to a diagnosis of breast cancer." They add that "Extensive research is required" in the lab and in humans to answer essential questions in this area.

What we're left with—besides the sickening observation that there's a sucking void where the clinical research on progesterone, progestins, and breast cancer should be—are the following two conclusions:

1. *If you don't already have breast cancer,* oral micronized progesterone seems likely to be either a neutral or preventive force—preventive

thanks to progesterone's jobs in the breast, such as differentiating immature "starter" cells into mature breast cells so they can't go wild making copies of themselves. Bonus: OMP will likewise protect you against estrogen-induced endometrial overgrowth and uterine cancer.

2. *If you do have some precursor cancer cells in you,* OMP could possibly trigger them to grow, divide, and proliferate.

Again, this is a complicated, crap set of facts. Where it leaves us is summed up by a quote I found through Dr. Bluming. It's from Siddartha Mukherjee from *The Laws of Medicine*: "It's easy to make perfect decisions with perfect information. Medicine asks you to make perfect decisions with imperfect information."

In this case, that information includes not just the imperfect information we have on breast cancer risk from hormone therapy but your individual health profile, including both your risk of breast cancer and heart disease.

For help making a decision, consider making an appointment with an oncologist—specifically one who specializes in treating breast cancer—as they are likely trained to calculate and assess risk in a way gynecologists and other doctors are not.

In a perfect medical world—no, in an *adequate* medical world—an oncologist would team up with a cardiologist and an osteoporosis expert and others experienced in menopausal and perimenopausal women's care and determine where the risks and benefits lie. By this, I mean, they'd look at the potential costs and benefits to you as *a whole woman*, with your individual health profile, to see where there's a trade-off needed, and what the wisest trade-off might be.

Probably few of us who aren't multimillionaires will ever have care like that. But if you can get referrals from your gynecologist or primary care doctor to these individual specialists, you can ask them to talk with each other.

— 22 —

DEM BONES

How to avoid smoking a hip joint

I'D BEEN SEDENTARY for years, planted in a chair at the computer all day writing my syndicated column and books.

I decided to walk up to Staples, half a mile from my house. I went almost one long block—not even a tenth of a mile—and my lower back hurt. *A lot.*

I was 52—maybe 53—and still in perimenopause. When I got home from Staples, the pain was pretty intense. Like there was a small fire down in there. I was terrified. Apparently, there was a piper to pay for this ass-in-chair thing, but he'd hired the world's slowest collection agency.

What if I'd ruined my bones forever? Would I be some elderly lady who couldn't get out of bed by age 55?

Fear, and especially fear that you're beyond repair, is a powerful motivator. With all the relaxed cool of a psychotic dog, I dug into the research on osteoporosis, the disease in which bones become progressively more porous, fragile, and breakable. Might there be some way to keep my skeleton from crumbling in old age (which leads to all sorts of other hideous medical problems)?

In fact, there was.

But I discovered something deeply disturbing. A monstrous medical scam is being perpetrated on women: the destruction of our health for profit in order to sell *supposedly* bone-preserving drugs. A raging flood of pharma money has tainted every facet of research, diagnosis, and medical treatment in this area, along with flooding medical and mainstream news sources with bogus "scientific" claims. These companies have been duping doctors and patients for decades—ultimately scaring healthy women at low risk of fracture into taking harmful medications they do not need: medications that will ultimately make their bones more fragile and breakable.

HOW OSTEOPOROSIS BECAME A DISEASE WHEN IT'S REALLY JUST A RISK FACTOR

There's a real problem for some women in old age: skeletal fragility. Upon reading the research, that's the term I came to use instead of osteoporosis. It reflects the actual issue: weak, fragile bones putting us at risk of fracture when we're elderly—typically in our 70s and 80s. In other words, it gets at what actually matters to us, which is simply this: Will we break bones?

"Osteoporosis" *is* the current medical term for the bone condition we're *told* predicts fracture, which it does not. The term *osteoporosis* is actually scientifically outdated—coined back in the 1820s before we had anywhere near the understanding of the components of healthy bone that we do now. It comes from two Greek words mushed together to mean *porous bones* (as opposed to more *densely packed* bones).

"Porous bones" sounds worrisome. However, less dense, more porous bones are actually not a disease in need of treatment but a *mere risk factor* for breaking a bone—and *not a very fracture-predictive one!* In fact, it's the *least predictive* of multiple risk factors for bone fracture—and may even be a meaningless indicator.

Here's the thing: Having bones that are more porous doesn't mean your bones will break, and having denser bones doesn't mean they won't! In fact, it can make you more likely to fracture! For example, despite bone density being lowest in Asians, white women, with generally higher bone density, have the highest rate of fracture. (Black women have the lowest rate of fracture.)

CREATING A DISEASE TO SELL DRUGS

Contrary to what we've been led to believe, while women's bones do decrease in strength and quality with age, this decrease is not necessarily cause for alarm—as in, it is not a medical fortune cookie telling us that we will break bones.

That's not what we're told—because it wasn't in the best interest of a drug company. Back in the 1990s, the pharma mega-giant Merck came up with a bone drug called Fosamax. It had a narrow market: treating elderly women at serious risk of fracture.

Hip fracture in elderly women—the group most likely to suffer it—is particularly devastating and can be deadly. This is not because hip fractures themselves are especially deadly, pharmacology professor Adriane Fugh-Berman, MD, explains. It is due to *contributing factors*, such as a pre-existing weakened immune system, heart disease, and diabetes.

What we call hip fracture is technically the fracture of the thigh bone right by the hip joint: the fracture of the "femoral neck" of the upper thigh bone, an inch or two from the hip joint. Hip fractures tend to happen when women fall—or, most disturbingly, a woman with particularly fragile bones might fall *because* she fractures: because her bone spontaneously gave way while she was standing or walking, causing her to crash to the floor. Younger women will sometimes break a hip, but their hip fractures tend to result not from taking a tumble at home but from car crashes, falling from high up (off a cliff or balcony), or some other traumatic injury.

In elderly women, death from breaking a hip comes in two forms: what I'll call "death-death," as in, you end up under a headstone, or the death of your independence and your way of life once you're too debilitated and frail to get out of bed at some care facility.

Fosamax had the potential to become a mega-seller—if only Merck could expand their customer base to a huge population of healthy younger women at low risk of fracture (and oopsy on the serious adverse effects they'd suffer from taking this drug they don't need). Merck just needed to come up with a disease to sell their drug. They decided "osteoporosis" and its defining characteristic, "low bone density," would do just fine. Marketing this weak risk factor for fracture *in elderly women* as an every-woman "epidemic"—a disease that could supposedly explode the bones of a healthy 50-something woman at any moment—was just the thing to turn Fosamax into a financial blockbuster.

This is a common practice by pharmaceutical companies. "First industry must sell you fear of a disease, then comes the drug to 'prevent' its most serious consequences," reports medical watchdog Maryann Napoli.

Napoli, from the nonprofit Center for Medical Consumers, notes that over 90 percent of hip fractures—the most devastating kind of fracture—occur in women *at age 80,* on average! In other words, if a 50-year-old woman at low risk of fracture takes the minor daily steps to keep her bones healthy that I'll lay out in this chapter, she'll have three decades of bone-health maintenance under her belt at the age she'd be at risk of fracture.

But check out how dishonestly fracture risk was presented by the heavily pharma-funded National Osteoporosis Foundation (now the heavily pharma-funded Bone Health & Osteoporosis Foundation): *"24% of women, aged 50 and over, die within a year of a hip fracture."*

Right. Die within a year of fracture IN THEIR 80s! That is... IF they spend three whole decades, from age 50 on, doing as I did before that painful wakeup call from my back—arrogantly assuming they can get away with living with slightly more daily mobility than a houseplant!

Getting healthy midlife women to believe their bones were on the verge of snapping like breadsticks took redistricting the medical boundaries of bone fracture risk—expanding them in an outrageously unscientific way so a huge swath of the younger, healthy female population could falsely be deemed at risk.

Normally, standards for diagnosis come out of careful consideration of a body of evidence that drives what the parameters should be: the dividing line between "You're healthy" and "Uh-oh..." and markers for increasing levels of physical decline and risk to the patient.

This new standard for diagnosing osteoporosis was created arbitrarily at a pharma-funded meeting in a hot hotel conference room in Rome when everybody was dying to get out the door. Some exasperated somebody drew an arbitrary cutoff line on a whiteboard (or other presentation board).

That cutoff—the line used to declare menopausal women's bones diseased? "The bone density of a woman at age 30, roughly the age when bone mass peaks for most people," reports Susan Kelleher in a *Seattle Times* exposé of the osteoporosis drug-selling scheme.

This standard—described as the bones of a healthy "20- to 29-year-old" woman—has tainted science in this area ever since. Healthy perimenopausal women and menopausal women in their 40s and 50s are declared sick because they do not have the bones of a 21-year-old or 29-year-old woman! Of course, there is no evidence that these women's bones will fracture due to the difference between their bones and a 21- or 29-year-old's, and there's plenty of evidence suggesting they won't.

RAGE AGAINST THE MACHINE
The scanners that turn healthy women into customers of drugs they don't need

Say, like me, you've been a bit of a slacker in the bone-fostering exercise department, and say you bring this concern to your doctor. Your doctor will sign you up for a bone X-ray called a "DEXA scan" (dual X-ray absorptiometry).

Afterward, you will be led to believe what your doctor has been led to believe: that a "bad" score from the scanner (reflecting "low bone density," also called "low bone mineral density") means you will fracture, and a "good" score means you won't. And unless you, at 48, have the bones of a 28-year-old, there's a good chance you will get a "bad" score—and walk out of your doctor's office with a prescription for Fosamax (a type of drug called a "bisphosphonate," now also available in generic form).

Endocrinologist Terence J. Wilkin notes that a "meta-analysis of 11 separate study populations and over 2000 fractures concluded that bone mineral density 'cannot identify individuals who will have a fracture.' So why do we measure it?"

These bone density scanners were the brainchild of a pharma marketing guy at Merck. They were already in existence but in a version too huge and expensive to be in use beyond major medical facilities. Merck got behind engineering them to be small enough for widespread use and subsidized them into doctors' offices and medical facilities in the 1990s. At the start of this massive scheme, in 1995, there were 750 bone-measuring devices in the United States, reports Kelleher. By 1999, there were between 8,000 and 10,000.

Merck put these things there for one reason: to apply that rigged arbitrary standard for bone health generated in Rome and create customers for the company's new bone drug, Fosamax—whether those customers need the drug or not.

The reality of scanning for bone density (aka bone mineral density)? Epidemiologist and pharma policy researcher Barbara Mintzes, echoing Wilkin, notes: "Bone mineral density testing is a poor predictor of future fractures, but an excellent predictor of start of drug use."

Bone density is a term for how much "bone stuff"—mineralized material, held together by collagen fibers in our bones—we have in a defined area (like a square of bone). The loss of bone density isn't unimportant. However, it's a measure of bone *quantity* rather than what we actually need to care about: bone *quality* and the properties that make it up, such as bone strength, toughness, and resilience. *Bone quality* is the meaningful determinant of whether your bones are likely to remain healthy and unfractured in old age.

However, these measures of bone quality—bone strength, toughness, and resilience—cannot be "read" in one of these bone scanners. They're largely ignored because there's no money in bone quality for pharma (as there's no pill to pop for it)—which is why the pharma-profiting siren song of low bone density is the only tune we ever hear.

Doctors believe they are helping their patients by ordering these scans and prescribing supposedly bone-saving pharmaceuticals—most commonly, bisphosphonates like the Fosamax my mother took and the drug Sally Field used to yap about whenever you turned on a TV. Generic versions of bisphosphonates include: alendronate (generic for mom's Fosamax), risedronate, ibandronate, and zoledronic acid.

These drugs may increase bone density, but they do not improve our bone health. In fact, in pretty short order, they cause our bones to become brittle and "microcracked"—riddled with tiny cracks throughout—making them more prone to fracture than before we took the drugs made out to be our pharmaceutical savior!

GOTTA DESTROY YOUR BONES TO (UM) SAVE YOUR BONES

The bisphosphonate Fosamax, the first brought on the market (in 1995, by Merck) and touted as *the* drug to reduce hip fractures does do that—reducing the risk of hip fractures by 1%, compared with a 2% hip fracture rate for women on the placebo!

These are results from the "Merck-sponsored three-year trial that won the drug Food and Drug Administration (FDA) approval," reports medical watchdog Maryann Napoli from the nonprofit Center for Medical Consumers. That measly risk reduction—"Hey, ladies, you can take this drug that will make you 1% less likely to break a hip!"—is not exactly the stuff pharma billions are made of.

Not a problem for Merck! Remember absolute risk—an individual's risk—versus the misleading use of relative risk (the comparison of one group with another)? The latter is what Merck went for: "A "50% reduction in hip fracture" is how Merck often portrayed the 1 percent reduction in risk, writes Napoli.

But that's not all you'll get from your bisphosphonate!

Bisphosphonates also come with some severe adverse effects (as do the drugs presented as alternatives). A common one from bisphosphonate use is gut eruption: gastrointestinal upset, playing out as nausea, stomach pain, acid reflux (aka heartburn), indigestion, and/or diarrhea or constipation in 40 or more percent of bisphosphonate users.

Thirty or more percent of patients experience the fun "Did I just swallow Barbie's barbed-wire fence?!" esophageal symptoms: an irritated, inflamed, and even ulcerated lining of the esophagus and difficulty swallowing. Finally, for between 1 and 10 percent of women, merely moving can be a suffer-fest, due to the severe and even debilitating muscle and bone pain triggered by bisphosphonate use.

Less common bisphosphonate side effects include...ZOMBIE JAW! Or—more formally—"osteonecrosis of the jaw": the rotting and death of your jawbone, leading it to protrude through your skin, horror movie-style.

This jaw ravaging occurs in maybe a half of one percent of patients, though the risk is greatest in women using high-dose injectable bisphosphonates like pamidronate and zoledronic acid. Osteonecrosis of the jaw is constantly referred to as a "rare" side effect, but let's get real: While it's rarer in *oral* bisphosphonate users, the risk of it from these injectables rises from over 1% at 12 months of treatment to 11% after four years, reports an NIH medical practice bulletin. And here's a nice big helping of terrifying: "Taking zoledronic acid alone increases the risk of osteonecrosis to 21% after the third year."

Another terrifying side effect starts with the sickening sound of your thigh bone cracking apart, signaling an "atypical femoral fracture." Particularly terrifying about these femoral fractures is how out of nowhere they tend to be. A woman may have aching thigh bones for a while—perhaps weeks or even months—and then, she'll be walking to the car or standing in a conference room at work when her thigh bone spontaneously breaks.

Cancer patients are especially at risk. Dental work can provoke this, so dentists tend to ask whether women are taking bisphosphonates—or should—because her doctor may need to pause her treatment to try to avoid this.

This fracture of the thigh bone affects 1% of women or slightly more who've taken bisphosphonates for more than three years (previously believed to be a five-year cutoff), report musculoskeletal researcher David Burr and his colleagues. That's a cumulative three years including any "drug holidays"—time off the drug for one year to several years—because there's an effect from previous exposure.

Granted, for some women whose bones fracture easily, and especially those in their 70s and 80s, initiating these drugs might be a worst-case scenario that's also their best hope of hanging on unbroken for a few years. Bisphosphonates are found to temporarily reduce fracture risk within the first three to five years of treatment, and possibly up to two additional years, per a massive observational study led by epidemiologist Monika Izano (though further research is needed).

However, bisphosphonates temporarily reduce fracture through making bones denser—but also weaker! They do this by inhibiting bone-cutter "osteoclast" cells from doing their important janitorial work: keeping bone elastic and resilient by clearing out decrepit old bone cells. A bisphosphonate that keeps a bunch of crappy bone still hanging around *can* reduce fracture risk... for a while—as it's causing that bone to become more brittle and breakable.

In other words, it's perniciously irresponsible to give younger menopausal women (in their 50s and 60s) who are at low risk of fracture a drug treatment that ultimately will make their bones more brittle and prone to fracture in decades to come. Few women break bones before the age of 65, endocrinologist Wilkin notes, "probably because they tend not to fall" (as do elderly women).

PRINCESS GRACELESS
Doctors should be prescribing rugs—rubber-backed rugs

Bisphosphonates and other supposed bone-protecting alternatives that we are scammed into believing are our pharmaceutical saviors from fracture do *not one thing* to prevent the single biggest risk factor for fracture in elderly women: taking a fall.

Elderly women fall for a number of reasons: often because they're dizzy from medications or medical conditions; because they need glasses or new glasses; or because they wear shoes with slippery soles instead of grippier rubber ones.

Another biggie behind fracture-risking falls? Being messy and inattentive—like me: walking to the grocery store while reading (and never mind the notorious broken sidewalks of Los Angeles) or inadvertently booby-trapping my bedroom floor with purple rubber gardening clogs and small piles of books. (Just the thing for any woman pining for a concussion while stumbling in the dark toward the bathroom.)

Though I feel your pain at corrective measures like swapping out Louboutins for Le Birkenstocks, randomized controlled trials suggest this can reduce falls in older people by 50 percent. Some other helpful measures are checking for and correcting visual impairment; assessing and managing cognitive function; and looking into other potential issues noted above, such as medications and medical conditions. And finally, for anyone like me with a decor style best described as "recently ransacked," consider whether getting a cleaning person is preferable to getting an orthopedist after breaking a leg.

THE BONE EATERS
*Corticosteroids, hysterectomies, smoking,
and other destroyers of healthy bone*

As evil as it is that we women have been turned into profit-driving prey by pharmaceutical companies, bone fragility and the erosion of bone that leads to it are a real problem. A genuine threat.

Take me. Before I started the daily weight heaving of "high-intensity training" or HIT (as I laid out in the previous chapter), my bones and I were on a seriously bad path—one they'd been on for quite some time. Bone erosion in women is largely a menopausal thing, meaning the results show up in menopause (and tend to be treated then). However, the breakdown of our bones gets its start in the decades before. Generally, bone loss tends to get going around age 35—gradually—though some women start losing bone in their 20s.

In perimenopause, though it's hard to lose the extra pounds we put on, we do manage to part company with a good bit of bone. Perimenopausal women experience a phase of rapid bone loss approximately two years before their final menstrual period, peaking in menopause, about a year and a half after the final menstrual period. Bone loss continues in menopause, but it's not as dramatic—that is, rapid—as in the late stage of perimenopause.

Remember my remark about our health, "It's all interconnected"? Research increasingly finds bone to be a regulator or helper in *many* bodily processes. These include healthy immune function, brain function, and energy metabolism. It's also found to influence insulin sensitivity, our appetite, and our fat storage.

Not surprisingly, when bone health falters, the functions it supports can go straight downhill. Take immune function—referenced in a research review by hematologist Noboru Asada, MD, and his colleagues. We've seen in the previous chapter that putting stress on bone by regularly lifting heavy weights maintains and may even build bone—maybe even in menopausal women. However, in bedridden patients and astronauts in a no-gravity environment, a continued lack of stress on their bones led not just to a "rapid progression of osteoporosis," but impaired immunity.

In addition to being sedentary, major contributors to bone erosion are smoking, heavy drinking, excessive dieting or anorexia, and unlucky genetics. Stress is yet another contributor through the inflammatory processes it triggers. There's also a bone-eating chemical compound: high doses or prolonged exposure to corticosteroid medications like prednisone, cortisone, and dexamethasone. In fact, even a very short-term prescription for corticosteroids can cause damage to bone.

Corticosteroids immediately inhibit bone metabolism—bone formation and the healthy removal of old bone—in a way that can erode bone strength. They suppress and deplete our skeleton's construction crew, bone-building cells called "osteoblasts," and jack up the number and lifespan of the bone-devouring cells called "osteoclasts."

These two kinds of cells, the builder osteoblasts and the cutter osteoclast cells are necessary for maintaining healthy bone. They work together in a paired process, with osteoclasts basically the sanitation workers clearing out old, past-its-prime bone. However, when the bone cutting outpaces the bone building, well, you can see the problem.

Oral corticosteroids tend to be much worse than inhaled or injected steroids, because the oral version has systemic effects, while the others—like inhaled corticosteroids targeting the lungs—remain more "local." And, again, even a short course of corticosteroids can adversely affect your bones, especially if you have inflammation already present in your body or your bones are already at risk of fracture.

Based on my experience over the past decade—conversations with people who've had corticosteroids prescribed—doctors do not tell patients how devastating these drugs can be to their bones. This is a major abdication of duty. Doctors should be letting patients know whether they have a dire need for one of these drugs, or whether there might be a safe, workable alternative: a drug that might not do the *same exact job* as the corticosteroid, but would do *enough of the job*.

Other circumstances associated with bone fragility are a lack or shortage of progesterone from anovulatory cycles (covered a few sections down). Hysterectomies (as well as oophorectomies)—removal of the uterus and the ovaries, respectively—are likewise enemies to maintaining healthy bone.

There was a belief that a hysterectomy without removal of the ovaries was a way to duck post-oophorectomy bone loss. In fact, research increasingly finds that women who had a hysterectomy and kept one or both ovaries are still at a higher risk of fracture.

SKELETON KEY
How to protect and maintain your bones

ESTROGEN

Long-term use of estrogen provides long-term protection for a woman's bones and overall health. In fact, "Estrogen is the only medication with evidence for a long-term reduction in fractures, especially when initiated within 5 years of menopause, as shown by observational studies of estrogen use for up to 34 years," reports osteoporosis researcher Susan Ott, MD.

"Every study about estrogen, from animal experiments to observational studies to clinical trials, has found that estrogen is beneficial to bone health, including a meta-analysis of 57 trials done before the Women's Health Initiative," adds Ott. "The bone(s) are stronger as long as estrogen is used."

However, there's near-religious belief to the contrary in the osteoporosis field. For example, "Many experts say that bisphosphonates could be used instead of estrogen in women with osteopenia, to prevent osteoporotic fractures," Ott observes. "This is based on wishful thinking instead of evidence."

Consider that we lose 30 to 50 percent of our bone density as we age. "It takes decades to reach 'the age of fracture,' and we don't know if any drugs except estrogen will work that long," Ott continues. "In my opinion, bisphosphonates should be used only if the risk of fracture within the next ten years is high enough to justify the potential risks."

By the way, the "osteopenia" Ott references is a scary-sounding made-up disease that is not a disease at all. Ott announces this in big bold letters on her website: "Osteopenia is not a disease!"

Osteopenia is a natural state—a slight thinning of bone density that happens to women with age—*not* a sign that a woman will break a bone. It is, however, ideal for scaring younger women, like women in their 30s and 40s, into believing they need to take a bisphosphonate. Bone health expert and former med school professor Steve Cummings, MD, sets the record straight: "Osteopenia is not a disease, does not indicate a high risk of fracture in the next five to 10 years, and is really almost a variant of normal."

PROGESTERONE

Estrogen and progesterone work together in a paired, complementary process to maintain healthy bone. Estrogen keeps the clearing away of old bone from outpacing the slower building process, which is where progesterone comes in.

Dr. Prior notes that "Most physicians and even some bone experts don't know" that progesterone is necessary to *build* bone to fill in the spots where old bone has been cleared away. Progesterone "sits on specific receptors" on the bone-building *osteoblasts* and "stimulates the formation of new bone."

In perimenopause, according to clinical research on *pre*-menopausal women—younger menstruating women—as well as petri-dish-in-the-lab studies, it seems OMP could be a powerful protector of bone. MPA is actually a stronger drug for this, but with MPA's strength comes MPA's harmful side effects.

You're likely to see MPA accused of being a bone eater, but there's an important nuance. MPA *is* shown to temporarily decrease bone density when administered in extremely high amounts, such as the 150-milligram dose used in birth control (Depo-Provera) or the 50-milligram dose used to treat some gynecological disorders. However, as menopausal or perimenopausal hormone therapy, MPA is prescribed in 5-milligram or 10-milligram doses.

Prior explains that the big blast of Depo-Provera "is strong enough to suppress the hypothalamus and thus to decrease estradiol." She adds that "When women taking Depo-Provera stop, their periods usually return and their bone density increases, not just to what it was before they started it, but to even higher levels because of the actions of MPA on the osteoblastic bone formation."

Studies of progesterone's effects in perimenopausal women have just not gotten funded. However, as I see it, the evidence we have that progesterone works to maintain and even build bone suggests you'll be doing right by your skeleton by taking OMP in perimenopause to make up for anovulatory or weakly ovulatory cycles that leave you short on progesterone.

Anovulatory menstrual cycles appear to be seriously problematic for bone health. Prior first showed this in 1990, in a yearlong observational study on menstruating women, ages 20 to 42. Those who were normally ovulatory or had just one month a year with a too-brief luteal cycle (to produce adequate progesterone) maintained their bone mineral density. However, those who had *any* cycles that were anovulatory or who had two or more inadequate-length luteal phases "significantly lost" bone mineral density at rates of 4 to 6 percent a year.

Likewise, in a meta-analysis, Prior and her colleagues saw that women, ages 18 to 42, with more frequent anovulatory menstrual cycles experienced a greater decline in "spine bone mineral density"—losing almost 1% of bone per year, on average. One percent might not sound like much, but Prior explains, "Over the 30–45 years of menstruating life," if you lose that much a year, you may reach late perimenopause—a time of rapid bone loss—thinking you have strong bones "but already having lost more than 10 to 20%" of your bone density.

We've seen that OMP is safe, without harmful side effects. So, it seems that taking OMP to make up for anovulatory cycles in perimenopause is likely to boost bone health—in addition to improving sleep, protecting you from breast and endometrial cancer, and alleviating hot flashes and night sweats.

For menopausal bone health and fracture prevention, OMP (or MPA) *must* be paired with estrogen. In menopause, taking either OMP or MPA alone—without estrogen—"is not effective therapy" for osteoporosis, gynecological endocrinologist Vanadin Seifert-Klauss, MD, and Prior explain. "It has no or little effect" for controlling the bone erosion of "resorption, the driving force in human bone loss and osteoporosis."

EXERCISE

We've heard over and over that a sedentary lifestyle is a major contributor to bone fragility (and all manner of ways our health can go south). If you are given only two options for exercise—walking or lying face-down on the couch—walking is better. However, there's not being sedentary and then there's not being sedentary in a way that improves your bone health. Walking is not one of those ways!

Dismayingly, many doctors treating midlife women recommend that women walk to prevent fracture. Medical providers' websites do, too—including my own provider, Kaiser Permanente. They even quote some noted bone doctor on their staff advising this, as if ineffective measures become magically bone-health-fostering when they're suggested by Dr. Famous.

Why is walking useless for strengthening your bones? Because you're most likely walking carrying just a small purse or your phone—as opposed to a baby elephant! It takes putting significant weight on your bones to signal them to adapt: that is, prepare themselves to carry heavy weight through biochemical and physiological changes, including remodeling themselves to be stronger and more fracture-resistant. In contrast, if you leave your bones unchallenged, you send them a different chemical message: telling them they aren't needed—a message they heed by progressively eroding.

Keeping our *bones* strong and healthy starts with keeping our *muscles* strong and healthy. In short, what we do for muscle, we do for bone. That's why the single best exercise we can do is that intense, slow-speed, high-intensity training, challenging our muscles by lifting weights heavy for us till we get to "muscle failure."

Perimenopause is generally said to be the last stage at which women can build bone, because without the inhibiting effects of estrogen on bone-cutter osteoclast cells, bones break down faster than they can be built by osteoblasts. However, though it's often claimed that women *cannot* build bone in menopause, that might not be true. Research by exercise scientists Kerri Winters-Stone, Christine M. Snow, and Gianni Maddalozzo suggests that slow-speed, muscle-challenging weightlifting can preserve and maybe even build bone in menopause, when it's most difficult (or even near impossible).

It may also be a way to avoid needing any medications at all. These three scientists conducted a study comparing spinal bone mineral density in women in early menopause given hormone therapy or hormone therapy plus resistance training or resistance training alone. They and their colleagues found that resistance training alone was *as effective as hormone therapy* in preventing bone loss at the spine, and was *more effective* in reducing bone loss in that area. Other research has similar findings—not just for spinal fractures but also hip, leg, and wrist fractures.

THE CALCIUM MYTH

There has been a longstanding harmful myth that if you don't choke down horse-sized tablets of calcium or gobble dairy products, your bones will turn into dust and you'll end up a big fleshy blob a caregiver totes to medical appointments in an extra-large beach pail.

Researchers and doctors seem to have confused osteomalacia, a disease marked by calcium deficits in bone tissue, with osteoporosis, reports medical historian Gerald Grob. I'll add that they failed to consider bone engineering—how bones are actually built and maintained. Your body doesn't have a rubber hose from your gut to your bones that pours sparkling calcium crystals into your skeleton.

Calcium recommendations widely made to women that supposedly maintain healthy bones are actually excessive and unhealthy, explains endocrinologist and metabolism researcher Terence J. Wilkin, MD—among others. "Calcium intakes of between 1 g and 1.5 g daily [1,000 to 1,500 milligrams] commonly recommended in postmenopausal women, are associated with an increased rather than decreased risk of fracture." And note that this is an amount few women can hit without opening their wallets to Big Supplement.

Wilkin adds that "excess calcium supplementation will suppress the secretion of parathyroid hormone" (vital for bone health) "and slow the natural turnover of bone." Additionally, taking a big bolt of calcium—even in "lower" spread-out single doses like 500 milligrams—may cause elevated calcium levels in the blood that last for several hours and raise the risk of heart attacks and stroke.

Research suggests we need far less calcium than we've been led to believe. Populations in Asia and Africa maintain good bone health on roughly 300 milligrams of calcium a day. Harvard epidemiologist Walter Willett, per an 18-year-observational study on menopausal women, recommends 500 to 700 milligrams of calcium a day, and other researchers' work (endocrinologists Ian Reid and Mark Bolland, for example) supports that.

BONE HEALTH-HELPING SUPPLEMENTS

There *are* a few supplements that are vital for bone health and strength—as well as overall health: magnesium, vitamin D3 (cholecalciferol), vitamin K2 (in MK-4 form), and also boron. Taking all of these makes them more than the sum of their parts, as they work synergistically—more powerfully and helpfully together than they would alone.

DIETARY PROTEIN

What really matters for healthy mineralization of bone is eating enough protein. And "enough" is not the 0.8 grams per kilogram of body weight the NIH website recommends. To have sufficient protein to support bone health, you need at least 1.2 grams per kilogram of body weight, reports bone biology researcher Robert P. Heaney. (Look for grams-to-pounds converters online to do the math for you.)

It's also a myth that protein will destroy the kidneys of a healthy person. That notion comes from an unwarranted stretching of the effects of high protein intake on people with chronic kidney disease (CKD), wrongly applied to all. In a person with CKD, weakened kidneys can struggle to process protein, causing waste products to build up in the blood. A healthy person's kidneys efficiently process the waste products from protein metabolism and get rid of them in urine.

Accordingly, in studies comparing people eating high-protein diets versus those on lower- or normal-protein fare, there was no difference in kidney function, according to a 2018 meta-analysis of 28 studies involving 1,358 participants led by kinesiologist Michaela Devries. There is simply no evidence linking high protein intake to declines in kidney function in healthy people, the researchers conclude.

THE COLOR OF BONE HEALTH

Check out the data in a 2015 paper on older women—13,550 women, ages 65 and up—who'd fractured a hip: 84.6 percent were over 75 years old. Not a surprise. However, results from that study that osteoporosis researcher Joan C. Lo, MD, and her colleagues broke down by race are a stark reminder of why so much of the research done on a bunch of middle-class white ladies needs to be rerun in other populations.

In the Lo study, a whopping 83.6 percent of the women who'd suffered hip fractures were white. To put that in perspective, picture 10 women with broken hips. Eight are white. Black women and women of other races had significantly lower rates of hip fracture than white women.

Only 2.8 percent of the hip-fractured women were black, 5.6 percent were Hispanic, 4.5 percent were Asian, and 3.5 percent had their race listed as "other/unknown." In other words, when there's a universal-sounding result announced about "women's" risk of osteoporosis or other conditions, there's a good chance it isn't universally applicable at all. It's also important to remember that our individual differences could make us outliers—atypical of the group we otherwise fit into.

A black woman should not assume that a low hip fracture risk, on average, for black women as a group means a low fracture risk for her as an individual. Though black women *are* found to have a lower incidence of osteoporosis and fracture than women of other races, black women are more likely to have sickle cell and lupus, and are prone to diabetes and hyperthyroidism (excess thyroid hormones)—diseases associated with an increased risk of osteoporosis.

Likewise, the high percentage of white women who break their hip isn't a sign that being white means you will break bones. You could be a white woman like my friend Catherine Salmon, who squat-lifts barbells with weight discs the size of pool floats on either end—and, in her 40s, had a doctor tell her she had the bones of a 20-year-old.

Chances are, however, you're like a whole lot of other white women, whose "lifting" involves glasses of Chardonnay and this and that around the house—and because of that (and perhaps genetic and other reasons), you should be concerned your bones could be in trouble.

Interestingly, while Asian women's bone density is similar to or lower than that of white women, this does not seem to result in the fractures that lower bone density is *said* to lead to—including hip fractures. Research led by Steve Cummings suggests that Asian women's low levels of hip fracture may be related to their shorter hip axis length—a measurement from the hip to inner pelvis associated with a lower risk of hip fracture—along with other differences between their skeletons and white women's.

Do Asian women hear any of this from their doctor—that is, *does their doctor apply the appropriate information in calculating their level of fracture risk*—or are they told they need a bisphosphonate based on research on white women's skeletons, blindly applied to them?

In other words, will their doctor follow through on their duty to determine the optimal choice for them, as *individuals who are Asian*? Or...will they be victims of knee-jerk, one-size-fits-all medicine—or what might better be termed "one-size-sickens-all"?

In light of the current state of "evidence"-based medicine, I am under-optimistic.

Personally, I'm erring on the side of "Holy crap, look at all the crumbly white women in that study!" Not *just because I'm a white woman,* but because my big white butt spent the better part of a decade practically Krazy-Glued to my desk chair. This—plus my low individual risk of gallbladder disease and other risks that might make estrogen a no-go—suggests I'd be wise to protect my bones with estradiol and OMP. And not just to protect myself for five or 10 years but for decades—into my 80s and beyond: the age we're prone to break a hip (while doing some strenuous activity like reaching for a teabag).

PART 4

HOW TO HELP YOUR DOCTOR GIVE YOU EVIDENCE-BASED CARE

PART 2

— 23 —

CLUELESS-CARE FOR MENOPAUSE AND PERIMENOPAUSE

Is your gynecologist qualified to treat you—or required to act the part?

THERE'S A HORRIBLE secret ob-gyn departments across the US have been keeping: Most ob-gyns are what I call "baby doctors"—maternity specialists who know next to nothing about menopause and perimenopause and have had zero training in treating either.

This seems impossible. Insane! Like something I just made up.

I wish it were.

A 2013 survey of American ob-gyn residents found that a mere 21% were in programs that included a menopause curriculum: lectures, readings, and case presentations. Only 16% had training in treating menopausal patients. And 66 to 79% of ob-gyn residents "reported needing to learn more regarding key menopause issues or knowing nothing" about them.

Knowing NOTHING.

This means they cannot responsibly diagnose and treat menopausal and perimenopausal women. "Responsibly," as in, it's a violation of medical ethics to do anything but refer you to a doctor who has the knowledge and expertise they lack.

This is not just my opinion. Cardiologist and bioethicist Sarah Hull, MD, explains that it's "obligatory" for doctors to refuse care "when the treatment requested is outside a doctor's scope of practice." For example, it would be outside of her scope of practice if one of her heart disease patients asked her for pain meds for a lower back strain or antibiotics for an ear infection.

Referring a patient back to his primary care physician "may be an inconvenience to my patient," she writes, but "my providing non-cardiac treatment without being up to date on current guidelines and practice standards presents a real potential for harm. My prescribing the wrong antibiotic, for example, might delay him from getting the right treatment and put him at higher risk for infectious complications, which would violate my duty as a physician to do no harm."

WHEN MEDICAL IGNORANCE AND NEGLECT BECOME THE STANDARD OF CARE

It's probably the very rare ob-gyn (if any) who does the ethical thing and discloses something like, "Really, I have not a clue about perimenopause. Go find someone else to treat you."

Instead, ob-gyns in this position keep mum. Their treating menopausal and perimenopausal patients who are very much outside their baby doctor expertise is just what's done—what's *expected* in their department, at their institution, in their field. Of course, that is no excuse for going through with it, as we see from Hull's remarks on the potential harms. Borrowing from historian and philosopher Hannah Arendt's description of evil gone routine—"the banality of evil"—there's a banality of negligence here: negligence that's become a routine part of the job.

The results of this filled me with rage pretty much every time women in menopause and perimenopause told me about their medical experiences. There they were, expecting to get medical *care* from their gynecologist and instead getting misdiagnosis and mistreatment or no treatment at all. A woman I'll call "Ruby," my favorite bus driver, is one of them, and Amy Dresner is another.

When I started riding Ruby's bus route, I liked her immediately. Strong, smart, stylish, and a kind person without being a pushover. I sit at the very front of the bus so I don't get carsick, and we got to talking on Wednesday evenings as I rode it to my extreme-nerd meetup group.

She told me she'd spent a big chunk of perimenopause seriously uncomfortable—blasted with wicked hot flashes and night sweats, which wrecked her sleep and stuck her with downer moods. She went to her gynecologist to get care. Chances are she should've been prescribed the 300-milligram dose of OMP that gave me my life back. Instead, she was "prescribed" the brush-off by doctors: told she'd *eventually* be in menopause, so she should "just wait out" her symptoms. Translation: "Suck it up, and keep suffering, lady."

Outrageous. And all too common. She was still in the middle of this suffering, so I offered to do what I've done for a number of my friends: help her fight for a prescription for OMP. I told her I could give her four or five bullet points from the research I'd been telling her about ride after ride (like the evidence of sleep benefits), plus give her the study citations for them. That information should make it hard for her doctor to have a case for refusing to treat her, I told her. I'd pull them together, print them up on a page or two, and bring it to her.

However, she was just *done*: fed up with doctor after doctor who left her suffering and feeling very much not up to the task of trying to use a bunch of secondhand science on a pad to get doctors who denied her care to mend their ways.

I completely get it—and I'm completely disgusted it came to this and comes to this for so many women: left to suffer, not just from symptoms of perimenopause and menopause but ignorance-driven medical abdication in place of medical care.

Doctors often become irritated and angry when women push and keep pushing for the treatment they'd come for, as did the intrepid "Dres"—Amy Dresner, author of *My Fair Junkie*.

Dres came into my life because I hire a part-time editor to "yell" at me for my writerly shortcomings, which allows me to fix them rather than publishing them. For six years, she was that person, editing my weekly syndicated column and early drafts of this book. Editors' comments tend to be useful but dull; however, Dres is a former professional comedian, and I lived for her edits-slash-insults:

TRY NOT TO MAKE THIS THE LONGEST SENTENCE IN FUCKING HISTORY, MADAME BLOWHARD

THIS LINE IS AN ABOMINATION!!!

I write and rewrite (and then some), so Dres got an education (and re-re-re-education!) in the science on perimenopause and menopause. She put this less politely—accusing me of trying to give her a brain bleed. However, the knowledge came in handy several years later, when perimenopause hit her hard, bringing on the full funpack: hot flashes, mood swings, and sleeplessness.

She asked her gynecologist for OMP. Her doctor refused. And refused.

There's a point at which a reasonable person gives up. Dres and that point remain unacquainted. She wore her doctor down—but only to the point of prescribing 100 milligrams of OMP a day: too little to alleviate her symptoms or provide protection against endometrial hyperplasia—that estrogen-induced overgrowth in the uterine lining that can lead to cancer.

Dres eventually tormented her doctor into upping the amount. Though she'd asked for 300 milligrams, her doctor would only prescribe her 200: a partial dose that did a partial job. Dres emailed me: "So last night was my second night on 200 and my sleep was totally fucked. I woke up feeling like I was on fire and then just kept waking up all night. It was awful. I'm exhausted. Fuck."

She explained this to her doctor and kept begging for the full 300 milligrams. I'd sent Dres a bunch of studies demonstrating OMP's safety, including papers detailing how it's been prescribed in France since the 1980s in doses of 300 milligrams (or more!) without ill effects. The doctor, who gave no sign to Dres of having read a word of this research, refused to budge and trotted out the same nonsensical argument the Kaiser ob-gyn boss used with me: 300 milligrams is "not the standard of care in the US."

Hello?! French women are not Martians! They are *women*, just like us—they just dress better and eat better food! So this 300-milligram dose that has been shown—over a 40-year period!—to be safe and helpful for French women is sure to lead to only one thing in American women: relief from menopausal and perimenopausal symptoms!

Dres explained this to her doctor, who was unrelenting—but messaged Dres: "Maybe you can try adding some transdermal [progesterone] from the homeopathic pharmacy to see if that will top it off."

Ugh. Unbelievable.

Rotten, baseless denial of the safe, protective, symptom-alleviating FDA-approved OMP Dres kept asking for—paired with scientifically unsupported, harmful advice to use "transdermal progesterone." That's the progesterone cream you can buy without a prescription—meaning it's part of the Wild West of cosmetics and supplements the FDA doesn't regulate or test.

Again, whether a bottle of the stuff contains the amount of progesterone claimed on the label is anyone's guess, though it might contain unlisted bonus ingredients: bacterial endotoxins, industrial solvents, Viagra, and manufacturing byproducts—like male hormones.

The dosage of these creams is inexact—"one pump" or "a dime-sized dollop"—and varies from product to product. Users have not the slightest idea how much progesterone makes it into their system as an active drug—in contrast with standardized, highly regulated and tested FDA-approved OMP. But the single biggest problem is what research finds this cream *can't* be trusted to do: protect your endometrium, the uterine lining, from estrogen-induced overgrowth and cancer.

Medical care is not supposed to veer into the absurd. But there was Dres, begging her doctor for the safe, FDA-approved form of oral micronized progesterone, in a dose adequate for alleviating her suffering. And there was Dres's doctor, advising her to take her chances with a sketchy, unregulated cream that could turn her uterus into an open house for cancer cells.

As Dres saw it, she had two choices: accept the suffering and elevated cancer risk her doctor had effectively prescribed by denying her a scientifically valid dose of progesterone—or find a way to get it. By this point, her symptoms had become way worse. She was a hot mess—a hot, sweaty, angry, very determined mess—so she went with door number two and ordered OMP from an online pharmacy: the dicey sort that lets you buy prescription drugs without a prescription.

It finally came in the mail, and she texted me a photo. Uh-oh. It was a generic version—from India. I'd just finished reading *Bottle of Lies*, science journalist Katherine Eban's great exposé on the corrupt Indian pharmaceutical industry killing patients around the globe with tainted versions of generic drugs.

"You CANNOT take this," I told Dres. "I hope you can get your money back."

This happened mid-COVID, and the world, including the world of medicine, had gone remote. Telemedicine turned out to be the answer. One 20-minute Zoom appointment with a nurse practitioner later, Dres got a prescription for that elusive 100 milligrams of OMP to bring her dose up to 300 nightly.

Money was tight for her—as it is for many of us authors who are not named Stephen King. However, she was forced to pay out of pocket—for a drug that would've been covered by her insurance—to keep it from showing up on her patient record and alerting her doctor.

There was major irony in Dres's struggles to get a legal, FDA-approved drug. (Recall the title of her book: *My Fair Junkie*.) Dres, sober for the better part of a decade, ranted: "Right now, I could get any illegal drug I wanted! Meth! Oxy! Molly! Meet some dealer at Jack in the Box who'd hand it through the window of his '87 Honda! But progesterone, this drug made of yams? 'Forget you, lady...can't score you that!'"

> **BONUS POINT**
>
> ### THE "USP" PROGESTERONE CREAM SCAM
> *Misleading consumers with "USP" in online product listings*
>
> These non-prescription progesterone creams are sold on Amazon and other online sites. On Amazon, for example (as of August of 2024), many of these creams have "USP" in their listing or product name; for example, "USP Progesterone Cream."
>
> There's no such thing.
>
> USP is the United States Pharmacopeia, an independent nonprofit that tests dietary supplements for "quality, purity, potency, performance, and consistency." Those that pass their tests can include the circular "USP-verified" logo *on their package*—a selling point for consumers hoping to protect themselves from unsafe and ineffective products.
>
> These creams with "USP" *merely in the listing* are *not* USP verified, meaning the USP has *not* checked that their product contains the listed amount and contents and that it is without contaminants. A cream, in fact, is not even eligible for USP verification, since it is considered a cosmetic and they only verify dietary supplements.
>
> *Ingredients* used to make the cream—such as the progesterone the company purchases from a supplier—are substances the USP does verify. Of course, the company could just say the progesterone they used is verified. And even if it is, *anyone* can fork over for an ingredient that meets USP standards—and then, in their brother's dirty garage, mix it with a bunch of cheap goop they bought at the 99-cent store: duping their way to bigger profits.

THE LITTLE SEARCH ENGINE THAT COULD
How to find a doctor familiar with menopausal and perimenopausal medicine

There's an upside to understanding the depressing abdication of the duty of care that menopausal and perimenopausal women are subjected to—sometimes from gynecologists we've trusted throughout our adult lives—and it's being aware of the need to seek out a gynecologist with at least basic knowledge in these areas.

How would you find such a doctor near you?

You can ask a search engine—the one at menopause.org, the website of The Menopause Society (formerly The North American Menopause Society until July 2023). At the top of their home page, there's a clickable link: "Find a Healthcare Practitioner."

That will get you to a list of "Menopause Practitioners," including "Menopause Society Certified Practitioners" (MSCPs) who have passed a "competency examination" reflecting knowledge "in the field of menopause and healthy aging." Presumably, perimenopause is included in "the field of menopause," but even The Menopause Society sees it as unworthy of mention.

Unfortunately, the exam is just a multiple-choice test given remotely, but a practitioner who has passed *has* demonstrated basic understanding of the subject matter. Note that not all practitioners on their "Menopause Practitioner" list have taken and passed this test. Some are merely Menopause Society members who have asked to be included on the list. Only the members who are certified have MSCP by their name.

Again, you'll have more options if you live in some huge urban area. Here in Los Angeles, there were 13 Menopause Society-certified doctors within 10 miles of my house. But even states that have more tumbleweeds than people at least list certified doctors available for "Telehealth" appointments.

Though the organization *was* previously named The *North American* Menopause Society, they've long had a search engine for countries beyond the US and Canada. If you're in Belize, Greece, or Bali, you're out of luck. But, as of October 2024, there *is* one doctor in Belgium. One in Japan. Three in Brazil and three in Mexico.

The grim reality: Even a doctor with menopause education and expertise may not be knowledgeable about the huge mass of science in this area—especially the findings that run contrary to practice standards and entrenched beliefs in the field. If you don't feel you're getting respectful, expert care, and you can't get the doctor to consider the science, take care of yourself by going to another doctor.

Seeing another doctor would not be free—nor would seeing another after that if this doctor, too, is a disappointment—so my suggesting this might make me sound like some trust-fund chick who's never had the slightest worry about money. (If only! And I am a major frugalista!) However, one thing I *do* know is that some expensive things are, in the long run, worth investing in or—if you've got generous friends or relatives—getting help paying for.

It is vital that you get diagnosed and treated by an expert—at least initially (and possibly later, should new issues arise). However, once you get a diagnosis and prescription, you can default to using a doctor covered by your insurance—including one of those baby doctors whose med school shorted her on menopause education and training. She would be giving you what I'd call menopausal or perimenopausal "healthcare maintenance." The science-based heavy lifting is done, so she just needs to sign to refill your existing prescription from the menopause and perimenopause expert when it comes due. (Should you have concerns she can't address, you could go back to the menopause and perimenopause expert.)

Women who can't afford or get to one of the doctors on the certified menopause practitioner list might ask friends for recommendations. This is less than ideal. You're relying on "people's opinion-certified" practitioners, and chances are their recommendation is based on something other than an ability to comprehensively assess a doctor's knowledge and expertise. As medically unqualified as some ob-gyns can be to treat women in menopause and perimenopause, Dr. Healing Hands, the vibe fixer some lady on Twitter swears by, is vastly less so.

A better option is hitting up somebody more in the know: the nurse with the longest tenure—who's been there *just forever*—in the ob-gyn department at the healthcare institution that treats you. Ask her if there are any docs at the facility who specialize in menopause and perimenopause and really know their stuff. They may or may not be paragons of menopausal treatment excellence, but if you're locked into the institution due to insurance restrictions, it's better than taking your chances with the baby doctor the computer assigned you.

— 24 —

THE KEY TO THE GATEKEEPER

Shifting the doctor-patient power imbalance

KNOWING DOESN'T CONTROL doing," Yale clinical psychologist and child behavioral researcher Alan E. Kazdin explained on my former science podcast. In fact, "knowing has very little relationship to doing."

We were talking about instilling "intrinsic motivation" for positive behavior in kids, but his remark also applies to menopausal and perimenopausal medical care. *Knowing* what evidence-based care would be is only the first step. There's a major hurdle to getting it, and it's that doctors hold all the power. This doctor-patient power imbalance shows up in two ways.

First, there's "information asymmetry"—unequal access to important information about our doctor that has bearing on our health. More simply put, we don't know what our doctor knows or doesn't know: whether they have expertise and training in menopausal and perimenopausal medical care, whether they keep up on the science—a little or *at all*—and whether they have any training in how to read and assess it.

They likewise don't disclose whether they are among the many doctors who lack training in diagnostic reasoning and whose treatment decisions are based on assumptions, leaps to conclusions—or maybe just a recent lunch with a pharma rep.

That last bit might sound unfair. I wish it were. In one study, a pharma rep spending just $13 on a doctor (perhaps the cost of soup, sandwich, and a cappuccino in the hospital cafeteria) was associated with 94 days of brand loyalty—94 days of the pharma rep's drug being prescribed instead of the generic.

Second, doctors are the gatekeepers to treatment. There's good reason for this—in concept. They went to med school and are experts compared with patients. That means *their* opinion about how to treat us (which may amount to leaving us untreated) trumps ours—even if their opinion is based on some degree of medical ignorance.

We patients—we perimenopausal and menopausal women—deserve so much better. And we can get it—and *you* are especially equipped to get it. My intent with this book has been to arm you not just with knowledge—about your body, the science, and our medical care—but with *strategic knowledge*: ways to shift the doctor-patient power imbalance and get the evidence-based treatment you and all women have every right to expect.

Three tools are particularly vital for doing this. These appear individually in some form in various chapters, but are most powerful when used as a set:

1. **The Power of Knowledge**
2. **The Power of Data**
3. **The Power of Assertiveness**

1. THE POWER OF KNOWLEDGE

Having read this book, you aren't going to the doctor in a state of blind trust. You know the possible gaps in doctors' education and training in menopausal and perimenopausal medical care. You know the scientific shortcomings of medical practice standards in these areas. You understand what goes on in our bodies in menopause and perimenopause. And you know what evidence-based diagnosis and treatment is.

In short, you've given yourself the background you need to protect yourself, which you do by asking questions—starting with asking your doctor whether they specialize in menopausal and perimenopausal medical care or whether they're more of a specialist in other areas. (Including that latter bit is important, as it gives them an ego-saving out.)

You may be most comfortable asking via email or whatever messaging system your provider uses. You could also call without giving your name (just saying you're a patient) and ask a head nurse or senior nurse in the department which of the doctors, if any, specialize in these areas. If the answer is none, you could ask whether they know of any in your area. Ideally, if your medical institution or insurance group is big, and you don't live in an out-of-the-way rural area, you could perhaps be referred to someone at a nearby facility. If none of that works, and you can't see a doctor from The Menopause Society list of certified menopause providers, the fact that you're walking into a provider's office informed rather than naive is a major means of both protecting yourself and advocating for your health.

At your appointment, you have a right to know the basis of your doctor's diagnostic and treatment decisions—including whether they made an accurate assessment of your risk (or any assessment) or are just crossing their fingers and hoping everything turns out okay. Discovering this takes just three essential words: "Can you explain..." and then, for example: "why you think I should take this drug?" or "why you think this is the wisest course of action?"

If you're like me and your memory goes into hiding when you're under the slightest bit of stress, it might help to have this list of questions I came up with—perhaps saved as a photo on your phone to refer to during your appointment.

SIX QUESTIONS TO ASK YOUR DOCTOR
BEFORE AGREEING TO TREATMENT

1. Can you lay out your reasoning behind your diagnosis and the treatment you're recommending?
2. Could there be other conditions that are causing my symptoms?
3. What are my risks from this treatment?
4. Are there safer, less invasive alternatives?
5. What can I expect during the treatment and what sort of recovery?
6. Do I need to do this now or could I wait—or go without the treatment?

If your doctor isn't explaining things understandably, ask them to re-explain (and re-explain) until you *do* understand. If they're talking in medical-speak, ask them to clarify what they're saying "in plain language," advises Debra Roter, a Johns Hopkins professor of public health. "It's perfectly fine to say, 'Sorry, I'm just not following you. Can you explain that in another way?'"

If a doctor is dismissive in response, there's a tendency to feel shamed and to let that drive our reaction: allowing ourselves to be dismissed. Keep in mind that you *deserve* to be heard and to be treated with the respect of real answers—as opposed to the flippant reply my friend Stef recently got from a doctor when she asked about a drug's side effects: *"Everything* has side effects!"

Having your concerns blown off like that is a red flag. However, circumstances sometimes make it more costly to leave a certain doctor than to stay, like if you lack other providers to choose from. Consider an outburst like that in the grand scheme of your experience with them and then consider whether there's any pattern. If you want to stick with them, let them know you expect better. The most productive way to do this is to evoke their empathy: "I felt bad when..." or "I felt unheard..." Wait for them to respond, and if they don't simply double down on their previous behavior, tell them how you'd like your questions answered in the future—that is, what sort of reply would make you feel respected, answered, and *heard.*

Having a doctor explain their reasoning for the treatment they're advising might make you feel you're in really good hands—or it might suggest otherwise, like if it amounts to "Because that's what we do around here." Or, in the words of my (of course former) primary care doctor, whom my friend Susan sarcastically nicknamed "Dr. God": "Because I'm the doctor, and that's my clinical judgment!"

With any doctor you see, you shouldn't be bashful about going for a second opinion (or telling your doctor you'd like to get one before deciding on treatment). And feel free to get a third, a fourth, and so on. This isn't disrespectful. It's a normal, expected part of medical care—and your right.

Finally, doctors at major institutions often have a limited amount of time they're allotted to give each patient in an office visit. You might not get through all of these questions—or other questions you might have. Don't be rushed into making a decision without information. You can ask to make a phone appointment to go through your other questions. And then make another phone appointment if you still need more answers.

Asking for more of your doctor's time might feel like an imposition or princess behavior. It's anything but. Medical care—save for emergency situations—requires patient's "informed consent." If you're giving your "kinda confused consent" or "half in the dark consent," you're gambling with your health. You matter. You owe yourself better. Don't be afraid to ask for it—and even demand it, if that's what it takes.

2. THE POWER OF DATA

You don't have to be a researcher to collect valuable scientific data that can determine the course of medical care. You can be a woman in menopause or perimenopause who logs her daily symptoms on a calendar or calendar app (including the intensity, frequency, duration, and other facts).

Consider the difference from a doctor's point of view between a general complaint of "I'm not sleeping very well" and a detailed log, spanning a week, two weeks, or a month, that shows in color bars how you slept in occasional shards throughout the night (for example, two hours and change on Wednesday, three hours on Thursday, and so on). In terms of the effect on your "audience," the first claim is a pity. The second is a sleep emergency.

Knowledge "is power" but knowledge powerfully presented—visually, over weeks or a month, with detail—can evoke empathy in a doctor (and motivation to alleviate your suffering) in a way a passing remark lacking detail does not.

By the way, those color bars can simply be lines you color in with marker on a paper calendar you print out with spaces for the hours. Google "blank weekly calendar with hours." Giving your best honest guess on what the hours were will likely do the job as data for your doctor.

It's likely impossible to time your own sleep accurately, and you will not be able to assess your sleep quality. Wearable "smart" devices like an Apple Watch or Oura Ring are helpful for this, using sleep apps. These devices are expensive, but you might be able to borrow a friend's older model, and there are sites (look for the legit ones!) that sell used and refurbished versions.

Take care to get one that's recent enough to be compatible with sleep apps. A number of these apps are pricey, requiring a monthly fee. I use AutoSleep because it was well-reviewed on a Mac site and because it required just a one-time fee of $3.99 when I bought it.

Few of these apps are evidence based or validated for accuracy—as in, only three out of 73 in a recent systemic review were assessed using the gold standard, polysomnography—and those that claim to measure REM (rapid eye movement) sleep probably can't.

Despite this, I would guess many or most do the job you need for data for your doctor: accurately showing the hours of sleep you're getting nightly. I base that on downloading not just my $3.99 app, but also the pricey apps (those that charge you a chunk o' change monthly) and using them on the free tier, where they basically just show you the hours and their guess at sleep stages. For a while, I had five of them on my phone for comparison, and they all came up with pretty much the same hours and minutes slept, give or take 20 minutes or so.

In perimenopause, the other vital way to collect data is with a $9.99 digital thermometer. Using that and the Quantitative Basal Temperature (QBT) measurement tool, created by Prior and her colleagues (©CEMCOR), will show whether you might be experiencing the anovulatory menstrual cycles that leave us deficient in progesterone. (Unfortunately, this tool can't be used by women on hormonal birth control, which suppresses ovulation.)

QUANTITATIVE BASAL TEMPERATURE (QBT)
Your fast, easy, DIY perimenopausal progesterone level checker

"Basal" temperature (aka "resting temperature") is your body's temperature immediately upon opening your eyes, before you get out of bed. It's the lowest temperature your body hits after you fall into deep sleep—extending to the moment you wake up in the morning.

Why is basal temperature important? Well, Swiss menstrual cycle researcher Rudolf Vollman, MD, discovered that, upon ovulation, a woman's usual basal temperature rises by a half-degree to one degree Fahrenheit (or 0.2 to 0.3 degrees Celsius). It remains elevated for a period of days (the "luteal" or progesterone phase of the menstrual cycle) and goes back down when her period comes.

The temperature rise indicates that progesterone is active in our brain (in the hypothalamus). Tracking basal temperature over a month is a reliable way to determine whether we've ovulated and for how many days the ensuing progesterone-rich phase of our cycle lasts.

Though "quantitative" might sound like a code word for "complicated," it simply refers to data that can be measured and expressed numerically; for example, using the numbers from daily temperature readings—ideally taken over multiple months.

Having a month's worth allows you to learn your average temperature and can help you determine whether you're ovulating *at all*. However, a single month's reading might not represent your typical cycle, so it's important to keep measuring for at least one or two more months to get a clearer picture and see patterns.

Normally, if you are robustly ovulating (before the "runt" follicle stage of perimenopause, for example), Prior says you should have higher temperatures for 10 to 16 days—all the way through the day before your period returns. If you have only three to nine days of elevated temperatures, your "luteal phase," the progesterone part of your cycle, is too short. This means it lasts for too little time to do its work: to keep you feeling well (as opposed to moody, sleepless, and besieged by hot flashes), protect your cardiac health and your bones, and decrease your risk of breast and pelvic cancers by counteracting estrogen's proliferative effects.

QUANTITATIVE BASAL TEMPERATURE (QBT)—THE HOW-TO

1. **Shop:** Get a digital thermometer that shows you your temperature in tenths of a degree. (The part after the decimal point, the .6 in 98.6 is tenths.) There are specific "basal thermometers," but any digital thermometer should do just fine. Either can be bought at the drugstore or online for $10 or $15.
2. **Measure:** Take your temperature orally every morning of the month as soon as you open your eyes—and while you're still in bed. This is your resting or "basal" temperature: again, the lowest temperature your body hits after you fall into deep sleep, extending to the moment you first wake up in the morning.
3. **Record, Add, and Divide:** Figure out your average temperature by recording your waking basal temperature on a calendar every day for a month or however long your cycle is (and then the following cycle—at least one, but ideally more).

    Day 1 of your calendar is the first day of your menstrual flow, even if it happens on, say, day 12 of a particular month, making your "month" extend into the next calendar month. You'll only know the last day of your cycle when your period starts again. (It's the day before.)

    Once you've collected your data for a month, add up all the temperatures you have for the month and then divide them by the number of days. The temperature you come up with is your average temperature.

Dr. Prior advises that you also "record any events that may affect your morning temperature" (such as sleeping in, having the flu, or staying out really late). She has calendars (diaries) you can download for free on her CeMCOR.ca site (search: "Daily Perimenopause Diary"). In addition to a space to record your daily basal temperature, they have checkboxes for all sorts of data you can record to track other changes (such as "breast soreness," "sleep problems," and other issues).

4. **Total Up:** Check how many days per month your temperature is higher than average. Again, 10 or more days of higher-than-average temperatures indicate that you've ovulated—a sign that your menstrual cycle is normal, with sufficient progesterone produced.

    If, on the other hand, you have only three to nine days that are higher than average, chances are you have ovulated but have too few days of progesterone post-ovulation. If you don't have a temperature jump, you haven't ovulated.

Explaining to your doctor that you're low on progesterone with the weight of QBT data behind it—handing your doctor pages of evidence you've collected about your own body—makes what you're saying hard to dismiss.

It can also open the door for you to explain that you've "learned"—important wording so you don't come off as an arrogant know-it-all—that being short on progesterone leads to all sorts of symptomatic suffering and is associated with lasting harm (to our bones, our cardiovascular system, and more). And explaining that opens the door to asking for treatment—a data-based, science-based request. That kind of request is much harder for your doctor to turn down.

3. THE POWER OF ASSERTIVENESS

I was going to call this "The Power of Reddyness." No, menopause has not trashed my spelling along with my vagina and my ability to wear long sleeves in climates beyond the North Pole. It's a reference to Helen Reddy, who wrote and performed the 1971 song with the line that became an anthem for women at the time: "I am woman, hear me roar."

To me, it's a reference to a resource you have or *can have*—simply because you decide to have it, and then, fears be damned, put it out there. That resource is assertiveness.

Assertiveness is the active form of self-respect: the sense that you have value and deserve to be treated accordingly. Being assertive means sticking up for yourself and your needs in your interactions with other people. "You do this by being direct and honest about how you'd like to be treated," I explained in my advice column. "State your needs calmly, using respectful language, and do it in a timely way—as soon as possible—instead of endlessly festering with resentment that someone hasn't read your mind and changed their behavior accordingly."

You aren't dumb, and if a doctor treats you like you are—if they try to shame you into shutting up when you ask them to clarify what they're saying—they're a disrespectful jerk who's perhaps trying to pass off baseless reasoning by hiding it in a thicket of complicated verbiage. Remember, they aren't done explaining till they explain so you understand what they're proposing.

You have a right—and actually, an obligation to yourself—to assert yourself to get medical care based on the best current evidence. You deserve to have a highly trained expert in menopause and perimenopause treating you—not a doctor taking a break between pregnant ladies to hazard a guess at your care. You deserve to have your doctor truly listen to you and take your values and concerns into account in treating you—and if they aren't listening, to (politely but firmly!) call them out and tell them that's what you expect. And you deserve to have your doctor's decisions explained to you so you fully understand the reasoning behind them (even if they have to explain something 26 times).

In short: "I am woman, hear me roar."

"Roaring" might not come naturally to you. In fact, what comes naturally might be "I am woman, watch me muffle myself"—and you're not alone. We women tend to be high in "agreeableness," the "pleaser" personality trait that plays out in kindness, warmth, and concern for others—including a strong motivation to avoid being a bother or hurting others' feelings. These are wonderful qualities in a whole lot of situations, but they have a dark side: motivating us to throw our obligations to ourselves under the bus.

To quit automatically putting your own needs dead last, you might borrow the thinking I use to make myself exercise: "Your feelings are not the boss of you." In other words, you might feel terribly uncomfortable asserting yourself—queasy and afraid—but asserting yourself doesn't take feeling brave. It just takes acting brave. Flip the bird to the fear and other feelings holding you back and stand up for yourself—at the doctor and beyond.

"At the doctor" is actually the key to the "beyond." Once you get perimenopausal and menopausal suffering under control, you can get on with being—with carving out who you're going to be and the life you're going to have with all you've developed yourself into so far.

— 25 —

HOW TO TALK TO YOUR DOCTOR

How to partner with your doctor to get evidence-based care (despite their institution's myth-based practice standards)

BEING RIGHT—HAVING THE evidence from this book or elsewhere to back up the menopausal or perimenopausal treatment you're asking for—isn't enough.

Like all humans, your doctor has a built-in psychological defense system that can block them from considering your request—and any request that conflicts with their practice standards or previous practice. A powerful factor in this is confirmation bias—that tendency we have to cling to information that confirms what we already believe and to dismiss new and conflicting information that suggests our beliefs (and any actions they led to) might've been wrong.

In other words, for your doctor, going with the treatment you're asking for comes with some ego baggage. It takes a person with some strength of character to not just fall in with confirmation bias and let that be that. Take the gyno boss who eventually okayed the 300-milligram dose of OMP for me and my gynecologist who stuck his neck out to bring my (many annoying!) requests to her. As I noted about them, their doing this, "in effect, saying I was right, or might be—was a tacit admission that they might be wrong."

My work as a mediator has helped me understand the approach we can use that's most likely to help others open their mind to what we're suggesting or asking for. We need to create an interpersonal environment in which the other person doesn't immediately steel up and defend their beliefs and actions. This approach tends not to come naturally to most of us. When we and another person have conflicting beliefs, we are actually predisposed to motivate them to refuse to see things our way—though that's not our intention.

We immediately get off on the wrong foot, going in "ready to do battle, hammering the other person with how right we are," I explained in a 2022 TEDx Talk. This is the "facts or nuthin'" view, and it *is* successful—typically in getting the other person to do whatever they *were* doing, but longer, stronger, and louder.

The key to getting a person to listen to *us* is listening to *them*, or, as I put it in my talk, "Listening to learn instead of fighting to win." We want to persuade the doctor to see things our way, give us the treatment we see all this evidence supports. Because of the power imbalance I talked about in the last chapter—and how your doctor has all the power to say no—we tend to go in feeling threatened. Afraid. And fear tends to come out as anger. Angry disrespect.

Our fight-or-flight system reads anger as an attack, and it sets them physically, chemically, and psychologically on the defensive—making it impossible for them to listen to you. To prevent this, go into your appointment prepared to make space for your doctor to express their views about what you're telling them—including asking them what they think.

When they tell you, really listen to them and consider what they're saying—even if you immediately know they're getting the science wrong. And don't think you can get away with being sneaky—simply affect the look that you're listening (a behavior I have been guilty of!—à la the Fran Lebowitz crack, "The opposite of talking is not listening. The opposite of talking is waiting"). Humans evolved to have an ability for "cheater detection"—spotting the ways other humans have been prone to scam us throughout human history. Because we also evolved to engage in reciprocity, you are likely to get what you give: the respect of real listening.

By "consider what they're saying," I don't mean "pretend unsupported claims are supported." In line with reciprocity, it involves engaging in an act of generosity—in this case, generosity of spirit: making an effort to understand where they're coming from, recognizing that they mean well, and seeing them as a cog in a massive system they don't control—which they are.

Chances are they will be able to read your attitude. No doctor wants to feel like a prescription pad with legs. Listening to them not only prevents that, but it also allows you to benefit from the wisdom and experience they do have.

No, you absolutely *should not* have to do any of these psycho-behavioral acrobatics to get the evidence-based care that medical institutions profess to be giving us. However, as Dr. Albert Ellis, the late founder of rational emotive behavior therapy (REBT), used to say: "There's no such thing as 'should'"—only what is and what isn't and what you'll do about it.

To contain the fear that can come out as anger or angry desperation, go into your appointment recognizing that this particular doctor's answer isn't your only option—the last exit on the road to suffering forever. Other options—seeing another doctor or other doctors—might be annoying, difficult, and expensive. The point is, there *are* other options if your doctor simply puts her foot down and refuses to treat you in alignment with the science.

That said, by approaching your doctor in ways that lead them to feel respected and needed, you ultimately give yourself the best chance to motivate them to listen to you and help you: to *partner* with you—as opposed to doing whatever they can to shoo you out of their exam room as quickly as possible.

PERIMENOPAUSAL SYMPTOM RELIEF
How to get a prescription for oral micronized progesterone

If you are suffering perimenopausal symptoms and want to take OMP to alleviate them, you'll need a prescription for it. Unfortunately, there are five major stumbling blocks to getting your doctor to give you one. (These same stumbling blocks apply to women seeking an OMP prescription in menopause.)

I've laid these out throughout the book, but I'll sum them all up here, because they're vital to keep in mind in asking for evidence-based treatment, in order to have your best chance at success.

First, there's your doctor's *fear* they will harm or kill you, leading you to sue them, and they will lose everything and end up living in a tent on the street corner.

Second, there are the *medical practice standards of their institution*, which they are required to follow. They can get in big trouble and lose their job and professional standing if a patient accuses them of harm and it turns out they've deviated from the institution's practice standards.

Third, *medical myths about menopause and perimenopause* have long crowded out the science. It's probably hard for your doctor to believe they aren't supported by evidence, especially when the person suggesting it is merely a patient. Of course, the government—via the FDA—doesn't help matters with their drug "fact" sheets.

Fourth, as Dr. Prior has explained, *many doctors have little or no knowledge about oral micronized progesterone* or how to treat patients with it. Many have no understanding of how it differs from the synthetic knockoffs, progestins (or that it differs at all), and the FDA-approved "fact" sheet for OMP is no help, as it lists the awful side effects for an entirely different drug, MPA!

And Fifth, *most doctors are strangers to the research.* Recall from Chapter Two that few doctors have time to read research in any comprehensive way—meaning read more than a newsworthy paper here and there. Many aren't trained to read research or assess it.

This chapter focuses on breaking through a doctor's objections to giving you OMP in perimenopause because getting estrogen (with or without OMP) in menopause tends not to be anywhere near as difficult. You just need to find a doctor who isn't still riding on the circa 2002–2003 panic from the WHI announcements. From my regular reading of the menopause Reddit, a disturbing number still are. However, because menopause and perimenopause have been in the news starting in 2023 and 2024 in a way they never have been, getting a prescription for estrogen should become increasingly easier.

HOW TO HELP YOUR DOCTOR HELP YOU

Honestly, getting your doctor to prescribe OMP for you might be a long shot. They are likely to see you as yet another patient who spent five minutes in the Google School of Medicine. To chip away at their reticence, it helps to have steel-belted arguments to present to them—those they find hard to justify saying no to.

There are two: Sleep and Post-Appointment "Me-Search."

Sleep: We all need sleep. Impaired sleep has terrible effects on long-term health—yours and others' if insomnia leaves you drowsy behind the wheel.

Your single best shot at getting your doctor to prescribe progesterone for you is telling your doctor that your sleep has been messed up in perimenopause or menopause. Say, for example, "I have terrible insomnia and brain fog, and progesterone is the only drug that increases sleep without harmful side effects."

Post-Appointment "Me-Search": In addition to the data on your symptoms and experiences that you collect prior to your appointment (in QBT and symptoms logs), it may be helpful to collect data in the wake of it.

If your doctor is reticent to give you OMP, you can suggest a compromise: letting you try it for a limited period of time. Prior told me that she advises saying to your doctor: *"Let's do a small trial*—I'll keep the Menstrual Cycle Diary (or Perimenopausal or Menopausal) and record what I experience, and you provide me with a three months' supply of oral micronized progesterone. Then we'll both learn if it is right for me and what progesterone does."

This "Amy on OMP show 'n' tell" is basically what I did in my meeting with my gynecologist and the gyno boss—pretty much spewing sonnets about my improved sleep, cleared brain fog, and other relief I was getting from OMP. My battles with them aside, they're nice people and they're in medicine to help women. What were they going to do, take all of that away?!

You can also present other benefits for OMP from throughout the book—as well as the lack of detriments, or as they're referred to in medicine, a lack of "adverse effects."

For example, French endocrinologist Bruno de Lignières, MD, points out that OMP has been used in France since 1980, and "widely in Europe," in a 300-milligram dose. "Widely"—and safely. Higher doses—including 600- and 1,200-milligram doses—have not been found to have adverse effects, save for the predicted sleepiness: fatigue and drowsiness in a few of the research participants given the 1,200-milligram dose by endocrinologist Ellen W. Freeman.

However, sometimes less is more. The strongest argument—the sleep argument—should be the only one you need. (After all, what counter-argument could your doctor give you—"I think you should keep an open mind about the possible benefits of insomnia"?!)

A FEW CAUTIONS ABOUT OMP

Not to worry—this isn't like one of those side effects disclosures where they casually list "and death" right after "may cause a temporary case of really bad sniffles." However, there are individual differences in how drugs affect us, and the following are a few things to be aware of about OMP.

WHO CAN AND CAN'T TAKE OMP

Gynecological endocrinologist Pedro-Antonio Regidor, MD, notes that there are a few women who might not be able to take progesterone—for example, women with rare autoimmune allergic reactions. He adds that progesterone may be less effective in women taking anti-epileptic drugs or drugs for tuberculosis, as these drugs ramp up metabolism in the liver.

Prior adds that "Women with liver failure (jaundice, fluid in the abdomen called ascites, and very abnormal liver blood tests) should avoid Oral Progesterone." Finally, women with PMDD—premenstrual dysphoric disorder, a severe form of PMS—may either be helped by OMP or find it makes their symptoms worse. *(See the PMDD section in Chapter Fifteen.)*

ORAL MICRONIZED PEANUT ALLERGIES

In the US, Prometrium, the oral micronized progesterone brand drug, is made with peanut oil (also called "arachis oil"), as are *all* of the available generics. In April of 2024, I checked the generics from Amneal, Bionpharma, Dr Reddy's (RPK), Eugia (Aurabindo), Sofgen (Akorn), and Xiromed, and *every one* uses peanut oil.

In Canada, as of 2021, the *brand drug* Prometrium is now made with sunflower instead of peanut oil—*though all five generics currently available in Canada contain "at least some peanut oil."*

Women with peanut allergies who cannot have even a tiny amount of peanut oil can get OMP made up with sunflower or other oil from a compounding pharmacy. Vitally important for safety purposes: ONLY use compounding pharmacies certified by the Pharmacy Compounding Accreditation Board (PCAB) to have the best chance that the OMP you get contains the correct amount of micronized progesterone, as claimed on the label, without contamination or formulation errors. If it is improperly compounded, degraded, or contaminated, it could be ineffective, harmful, or even toxic.

THINGS TO WATCH OUT FOR WHILE TAKING OMP

Prior explains that, in menopause, it "is highly unusual to have vaginal bleeding or spotting on progesterone or medroxyprogesterone taken without estrogen." She adds that OMP is "an effective treatment for endometrial cancer" (as is MPA) "and does not cause it." Again, however, *any* bleeding after menopause is reason to go see your doctor *ASAP*—on the better-safe-than-sorry principle, to get checked out for cancer.

Let's say you do encounter some bleeding, and—huge relief!—there's no cancer. Prior points out that it's possible the bleeding occurred because the endometrial lining of your uterus was thickened (from past estrogen treatment, being overweight, or due to type 2 diabetes). "If any of those factors might apply to you, and you are just starting Oral Progesterone, take it for 14 days and then stop it for three to five days," Prior advises. "If there is any lining to shed you will have some flow during those first days off Oral Progesterone. You can re-start Oral Progesterone with an extremely low risk for further bleeding."

GIVE "P" A CHANCE

I've learned from my psychiatrist to be a little bit patient when I start a new drug. Initially, your body may experience what I describe as a "What the hell...?" effect—meaning it isn't used to the new substance and reacts more strongly at first than it will once you get used to it.

Prior explains that when you first start taking OMP, "You may notice some changes in your breasts" or feel a little warmer overall. This is evidence of progesterone acting normally and not anything to worry about. However, "If you get moody, feel bloated and have very sore breasts it means progesterone is temporarily stimulating your body to make higher estrogen levels. This improves after one cycle." (Menstrual cycle, that is.)

SEE SICKNESS

If your perimenopausal world suddenly starts spinning, progesterone is not to blame. Progesterone does not cause nausea. Estrogen is the culprit, Prior explains—"high estrogen levels that are often present in perimenopause." She adds that, "For some women, for reasons that are not entirely clear, nausea is worse in the first few days after starting progesterone. This subsides within a week or so. I don't believe it is the progesterone that is causing the nausea but rather some cross-talk with our own high estrogen levels."

— 26 —

DIY MEDUCATION
What your doctor doesn't know can hurt you

THIS CHAPTER SHOULD not exist.

You should be able to go to your gynecologist with your menopausal or perimenopausal symptoms and trust them to know the exact treatment you need, the precise dosage, and how and when you should take it. However, since few doctors have training or expertise in menopause and perimenopause, it's important that *you* have this information.

This chapter lays it all out.

Some of this you've seen elsewhere in the book, but I wanted you to have the prescribing essentials all in one place so you don't have to go off on a hunt to find them.

ORAL MICRONIZED PROGESTERONE DOSAGE
Amount, timing, and frequency

It's unlikely prescribing standards for oral micronized progesterone were covered in doctors' standard med school curriculum before 2020. Research papers and medical practice organizations now call for using OMP instead of MPA (medroxyprogesterone acetate)—but it may take a while for this advice to trickle down to the medical practice of doctors who don't read the research or pay close attention to news in the field.

Dr. Prior, from her experience treating patients throughout much of her career, offers guidelines on OMP dosage, which I've included below. You can also suggest your doctor verify the information below by consulting Prior's advice on her CeMCOR.ca website or in her published papers (available on Google Scholar and PubMed). The same applies to any questions your doctor may have about using OMP to help sleep or alleviate other symptoms.

HOW MUCH PROGESTERONE TO TAKE AND WHY

In both menopause and perimenopause, the correct dose of oral micronized progesterone (OMP) is 300 milligrams at bedtime, explains Dr. Prior—that dosage that French endocrinologist Dr. de Lignières notes has been used widely (and safely) in Europe since 1980.

The 300-milligram dose helps sleep and seems to be "optimal" for alleviating hot flashes and night sweats, Prior explains. She adds that she uses 300 milligrams of OMP in part because it "has an independent positive effect to promote bone formation."

Regarding safety, in two randomized controlled trials by Prior and her colleagues, they found no "adverse events" greater than those in the placebo group and none that were serious in menopausal and perimenopausal women who were given 300 milligrams of OMP nightly, at bedtime.

Reproductive endocrinologist Petra Stute, MD, head of the menopause clinic at Bern University Hospital, led a 2016 research review on the impact of OMP on the endometrium. The conclusions: 1) OMP protects the endometrium at a 200-milligram dose if applied for 12 to 14 days a month for up to five years. 2) "Vaginal micronized progesterone may provide endometrial protection if applied sequentially for at least 10 days/month at 4% (45 mg/day) or every other day at 100 mg/day for up to 3–5 years." 3) "Transdermal micronized progesterone does not provide endometrial protection."

Prior counters that in the KEEPS cardiovascular study, a few women on the 200-milligram dose had "endometrial hyperplasia," an overgrowth of the endometrium. She adds that some women on estradiol and progesterone in the E3N study—a massive, long-term French observational study—had endometrial hyperplasia or even cancer. "Unfortunately the doses and durations were not carefully tracked," she told me, "but usually they list 200 milligrams as the dose."

My take—because of the safety profile we've seen for progesterone throughout these pages and because each of us metabolizes drugs differently—is that the 300-milligram daily dose of OMP (taken at night, before bedtime) is the "be-on-the-safe-side" amount. Especially for the endometrium.

WHY BEDTIME IS PROGESTERONE TIME

"OMP *must be taken at bedtime*," emphasizes Prior, "because its beneficial sleep-enhancing effects would cause drowsiness or almost 'intoxicated' feelings if taken when awake." (I take my OMP about a half-hour to an hour before I get in bed to give it time to start making me drowsy.) If you are sleep-deprived and/or thin, Prior recommends you wait to take OMP for the first time on a night when you can sleep in the next morning. Otherwise, she says, "catch-up sleep" may make you feel OMP caused a 'hangover.' Should that happen, it won't last. These morning sleepy feelings... do not persist more than a few days."

DAILY PROGESTERONE FOR WOMEN
IN MENOPAUSE AND PERIMENOPAUSE

Prior recommends daily progesterone (that 300 milligrams taken at bedtime) for menopausal women and for perimenopausal women with daily symptoms, such as night sweats, hot flashes, and insomnia—especially if they have irregular or skipped cycles.

CYCLIC PROGESTERONE FOR REGULARLY
MENSTRUATING PERIMENOPAUSAL WOMEN

"Cyclic" progesterone is progesterone timed to a woman's menstrual cycle—300 milligrams taken at bedtime on the days when progesterone would normally be elevated during a woman's menstrual cycle.

Back when Prior was still practicing medicine, if regularly menstruating women were suffering daily perimenopausal symptoms, she might've ended up prescribing daily progesterone for them, but she would start by prescribing cyclic progesterone. (See below for the set of days it should be taken.)

The exception is regularly menstruating women who suffer migraines, who need daily progesterone. Though OMP does not *cause* migraines, stopping it (for 14 days each cycle, per the "cyclical" dosing detailed below) can trigger them. If the migraine sufferer taking daily progesterone has regular cycles, OMP will make her menstrual flow lighter, Prior explains, "but usually doesn't entirely prevent periods."

WHEN TO TAKE CYCLIC PROGESTERONE

Day 1 of the cyclic progesterone calendar is the first day of your menstruation—that is, Bleeding Day 1.

If your periods are regular (with cycles lasting 27 to 30 days):
Prior says to start cyclic progesterone on day 14—the 14th day after your flow began—and take it for 14 days (or until day 27 of your cycle).

If your periods are regular but shorter (for example, if your period starts every 21 to 26 days):
Start cyclic progesterone on day 12 of your cycle—the 12th day after your flow began—and continue it for 14 days "or until cycle day 25."

PROGESTERONE WITHOUT ESTROGEN
An option not just for perimenopause but for menopause

As Dr. Prior points out, women in perimenopause *should not* take estrogen (because their own levels are likely spiking, and piling on with more can lead to overdose amounts in the body). In menopause, some women can't or won't take estrogen. Without it, OMP is not effective for bone protection.

However, it does offer relief from hot flashes and night sweats, according to a randomized controlled trial on menopausal women by Prior and research psychologist Christine Hitchcock—deemed to be "high quality evidence" per a methodology assessment tool called GRADE. Over a three-month period, 300 milligrams of OMP was found to be a highly effective treatment, leading to a 55 percent decrease in hot flashes and night sweats.

Though this is a study on menopausal women, research on progestins in perimenopausal women, along with Prior's decades of clinical experience with OMP, strongly suggests that OMP alone is an effective treatment for perimenopausal hot flashes and night sweats.

I strongly, but anecdotally, second that!

ESTROGEN: BE CAREFUL WHAT YOU ASK FOR
The limited menopausal symptoms doctors are allowed to prescribe estrogen for

Medical practice standards are like France, where bureaucracy rules. Say you don't have the right stamp from the right office on your document—which no one will give you because it's August and the entire country is on vacation. You could be Napoleon reincarnated, and some stone-eyed French government bureaucrat would deny you entry to your own tomb. Likewise, if you want a prescription for estrogen, you need to know the passwords: the symptoms your doctor's medical practice standards will allow them to prescribe it for.

Per the guidelines of the major women's health medical societies and the FDA, estrogen is to be prescribed *only* for three menopausal symptoms and issues: vaginal symptoms (and other issues in that "neighborhood," like bladder and urinary problems), hot flashes and night sweats, and prevention of bone loss in women at risk of fracture.

Beyond these common menopausal symptoms, hormone therapy is also FDA-approved for women who are prematurely lacking in estrogen due to surgical menopause prior to natural menopause, early menopause (before age 40), or conditions like hypogonadism, in which a woman's ovaries produce little or no estrogen.

You, like me, can hope estrogen will help you with symptoms beyond the gates of the current prescribing standards, but it's best to keep those hopes on silent and ask for estrogen only for symptoms your doctor is allowed to prescribe it for. (Why raise red flags when you can turn them into spiffy throw pillows?)

ESTROGEN TYPES, DOSES, AND ALTERNATIVES

As I explained in Chapter Nine, systemic estrogen is estrogen that's absorbed "globally": throughout the body (our "system"). It helps alleviate the various symptoms of menopause—including vaginal symptoms. Sometimes, doctors will prescribe both systemic and vaginal estrogen if the systemic dose isn't doing enough for the "down there" issues.

Vaginal estrogen, in contrast, is "local." Its effects seem to be limited, meaning contained to the area it's applied to: the vagina and its neighbors, like the bladder and the urethra, though there may be a small amount of systemic exposure, especially at first.

One kind of vaginal estrogen is also systemic: the "Femring." This is an estradiol-releasing ring you insert in your vagina every three months. It alleviates genitourinary symptoms but also affects your entire system because it provides a higher dose of estradiol than another ring that remains "local." This means it has the accompanying risks and potential side effects of systemic estrogen, like the patch I use, along with the systemic benefits, like alleviating hot flashes and night sweats.

TYPES AND DOSES OF SYSTEMIC ESTROGEN

The safest type of systemic estrogen—estrogen that affects your entire system—is FDA-approved bioidentical (aka body-identical) transdermal estradiol. This stick-on skin patch provides the most consistent dose, avoiding the "peaks and troughs" of both oral estrogens and other transdermal forms (cream, gel, and skin spray). Avoiding these highs and lows might be especially important for a woman who is prone to depressive symptoms.

For many years, the standard type and dose of estrogen has been 0.625 milligrams of CEE (conjugated equine estrogen). Its oral estradiol equivalent is said to be 1 milligram. The equivalent transdermal estradiol dose is said to be 0.050 milligrams.

"Said to be" reflects how estrogen is metabolized differently by different bodies. The form it comes in may play a role. For example, some women's skin might be better or worse in allowing estrogen into their tissues.

The goal in taking estrogen in menopause is not to match your levels as a fertile young woman—described as premenopausal luteal levels—but to achieve the levels needed to have positive and protective effects on your bones, vaginal tissues, cardiovascular health, and mental health, as well as alleviating hot flashes, night sweats, and other symptoms.

Transdermal estradiol patches tend to come in doses of 0.025, 0.0375, 0.050, 0.075, 0.100 milligrams. A patch with 0.025 milligrams of estradiol is considered low-dose; 0.050 milligrams is considered standard; and 0.1 milligram is considered high (meaning, in some tests, it's found to elevate your estrogen level to those typical of a premenopausal woman).

Recall that estradiol—and especially transdermal estradiol—can vary in how much of it manifests in our system, with some women given a 0.050 milligram dose ending up with severely low estrogen levels: just 9 to 11 pg/mL (picograms per milliliter). Compare that with the projected levels in menopausal women in transdermal "E" pharmacology charts (in picograms per milliliter, pg/mL): maximum, 99 pg/mL; average, 72 pg/mL; and minimum: 41 pg/mL.

Researchers measure these with sophisticated technology, not available to doctors running medical tests. Some doctors will special-order a pricey "free" or "unbound" estradiol test, but there is no widely available, precise test right now that can tell us how much estrogen is active in our tissues.

Because of this, doctors tend to prescribe according to symptoms, typically starting out with a low dose and adjusting based on a patient's response. In research, including meta-analyses and systematic analyses, the 0.025 transdermal dose was found to work for hot flashes and night sweats as well as improving urogenital symptoms (vagina, bladder, and other "down there" problems). Studies on bone find the 0.025 dose works for increasing bone mineral density, but there's a lack of research on what dose might prevent fracture. The 0.025 dose was also found to improve other menopausal symptoms, such as depression and anxiety, muscle and joint aches, and sexual problems (after three weeks, compared with placebo). That said, three weeks is a very short time and some of this could be the placebo effect.

Though I'm laying out these numbers, I have to say I have very low confidence in them. Much of the research is low-quality. Most importantly, we really have no idea at this point how much estradiol is needed to protect our cardiovascular system.

Recall Dr. Hodis and his KEEPS study colleagues explaining that "the arterial wall is dose-responsive to estrogen." (A dose-response relationship is the amount of a drug that's needed to make a change in your body.) While I can do a detailed monologue on the frequency and intensity of my hot flashes and night sweats, I can't feel whether my estradiol patch is doing the job on my endothelium.

Various pharmacology papers report the *minimum effective dose* of oral CEE for most women—enough to have a systemic effect—is 0.625 milligrams daily. The transdermal dose of 0.050 is supposedly equivalent to the 0.625 CEE found to have an effect in Hodis and Mack's clinical research.

Until more research is done—both on the effective dose and on a method for measuring the estrogen active in our tissues—we'll be in guessing-game territory. Because cardiovascular protection is the most vital in terms of our long-term health and well-being, my personal belief is that it makes sense to prioritize that in decision-making about the amount we should take, despite the uncertainties involved.

"LOCAL" VAGINAL ESTROGEN

Recall that vaginal estrogen is delivered into the vagina and alleviates only genitourinary symptoms; it will not help with hot flashes, night sweats, and other symptoms that systemic estrogen addresses.

There are four forms of local vaginal estrogens: creams, tablets, gel capsules, and vaginal rings. (Alternatives to vaginal estrogen, such as the SERM ospemifene, are detailed in Chapter Fourteen.) There are six FDA-approved vaginal estrogens available by prescription and applied directly to the vagina:

Creams: Estrace and Premarin
Tablets: Vagifem and Yuvafem (inserted with a tampon-like applicator)
Gel capsules: Imvexxy
Vaginal ring: Estring

And no, they couldn't be bothered to name the local-estrogen-delivering Estring vaginal ring something that is not completely confusable with the systemic-estrogen-delivering vaginal ring, Femring.

These vaginal estrogens tend to be terribly expensive—hundreds of dollars a month.

The exceptions: Generic Estrace can be had for around $30 a month—in contrast with the Estrace brand drug, which could run you around $350 (as of March 2024). Vagifem tablets also come in a more affordable generic version (around $49 for a month of maintenance doses—two per week—after the initial week of daily doses).

ANTIDEPRESSANTS FOR SYMPTOMATIC WOMEN WHO CAN'T TAKE HORMONES

Low-dose paroxetine, an SSRI antidepressant, is an FDA-approved option for women who cannot use hormones, like cancer survivors and women at high risk of breast cancer. Research finds it reduces hot flashes and night sweats, though not as effectively as estrogen. Because it's an antidepressant, it could possibly improve mood symptoms, too. However, paroxetine might work better in perimenopause than in menopause because SSRIs tend not be as effective in alleviating symptoms in menopause.

The special low dose of paroxetine for hot flashes and night sweats is 7.5 milligrams, while the lowest dose typically prescribed for depression and mental health symptoms is 10 milligrams, with doses going up to 40 milligrams. Though paroxetine and another medication, venlafaxine (different from desvenlafaxine), can cause nausea, headaches, and dizziness, gynecologist Andrew Kaunitz reports that these side effects are less common at the lower menopausal dose and "often subside within several weeks of initiating treatment."

However, psychiatrists may sometimes increase your dose if you aren't getting adequate symptom relief or if you're experiencing depressive symptoms. At higher doses (such as the 20-milligram dose), trying to stop taking paroxetine can lead to "discontinuation syndrome," the persistent, debilitating withdrawal symptoms from SSRIs (mentioned in Chapter Ten), including dizziness, nausea, fatigue, vomiting, and insomnia. If you are taking it and want to stop, it must be done with the guidance of your doctor.

Desvenlafaxine, the SNRI (selective norepinephrine reuptake inhibitor) covered in Chapter Fifteen, also alleviates menopausal symptoms; but it is "off-label"—not approved by the FDA for this purpose. It is, however, approved for treating major depressive disorder in both perimenopausal and menopausal women.

Like higher-doses of paroxetine and the SSRIs that can be hard to taper off, desvenlafaxine is associated with severe withdrawal problems. These can include visual disturbances, coordination difficulties, sudden loss of muscle control, delirium, mania, and psychosis. Again, if you are taking it and want to stop, it's imperative you do this with the guidance of your doctor.

In either of these cases, if you have been prescribed these drugs by a primary care doctor or gynecologist, it's wise to ask for a referral to a psychiatrist, who will have had experience and training in tapering patients off antidepressants. (I also think it's wise to ask for a referral to a psychiatrist any time a non-psychiatrist prescribes a psych med for you—a drug outside their area of training and expertise.)

It's important to take this tapering thing very seriously. Some of us have a tendency to think we can just tough it out and manage in any situation. However, when a drug is chemically altering you in some pretty awful ways, you may end up endangering yourself, and because you're altered, keep endangering yourself—while insisting to yourself and others that you're just fine.

— 27 —

GENERIC DRUGS ARE THE SAME AS BRAND DRUGS (EXCEPT WHEN THEY'RE NOT)

How to know when you've gotten a bum generic and get it replaced

YAMS. THEY'RE BASICALLY fashionable potatoes.

They should not cost $1,000.

But if I'd been taking the brand form of OMP, Prometrium—basically finely mashed yams turned into a drug stuffed into an itsy-bitsy capsule—I would've shelled out over $1,000 a month, as opposed to a $30 co-pay for the generic.

Because brand drug prices tend to run outrageously high, I'm grateful for the existence of generic versions. Apparently, gratitude makes you gullible, because I completely bought into the FDA's story to the public that—as the agency's website puts it in their headline—the "FDA Ensures [the] Equivalence of Generic Drugs."

In that FDA article, an agency honcho reassures us that cheaper doesn't mean crappier. "Most people believe that if something costs more, it has to be better quality. In the case of generic drugs, this is not true," says Gary Buehler, director of FDA's Office of Generic Drugs. He tells us that "FDA-approved generic drugs are bioequivalent" to their brand drug counterparts.

"Bioequivalent," the FDA's website explains, means the generic "performs in the same manner" as the brand drug. "People can use them with total confidence," Buehler says.

Sounds good, huh?

In fact, investigative science journalist Katherine Eban explains generic drugs as more of an "approximation rather than a duplicate of the original."

She writes in *Fortune* that the generic drug producer has to guess at the brand drug's formulation (after its patent runs out or is challenged). "It's not as if the maker of the original pharmaceutical hands over its manufacturing blueprint."

Though the FDA requires the generic to contain *the same active ingredient* as the brand drug, the binders, the fillers, and coloring that make up most of the content of pills can be very different, explain the pharma watchdogs behind "The People's Pharmacy" column and radio show, pharmacologist Joe Graedon and medical anthropologist Teresa Graedon.

This leeway on drug composition allowed by the FDA means that a patient could be allergic to one formulation of a generic even though they do fine with the brand drug or another generic. Additionally, the Graedons explain, "the way pills are designed to release their active ingredients can also differ substantially from the brand to generic drug," as well as between different generics for that brand drug.

Patients are put at risk when they are flooded with a big blast of a generic drug that would be released slowly into their bloodstream by the brand drug, as was the case with Budeprion XL 300, the 300-milligram generic for the extended release antidepressant Wellbutrin XL 300, approved in 2006. People taking it suffered symptoms including "headache, anxiety, irritability, nausea, dizziness, insomnia, tremor, mood swings, panic attacks, depression," and suicidal thoughts, among others, report the Graedons.

Few of us have any idea about this—or why it's allowed to happen. "We suspect that most physicians, pharmacists, and patients do not realize the FDA sometimes approves drugs for which it has not required actual test results," explain the Graedons. Starting in 2007, the couple spent five whole years pushing the FDA to acknowledge the problem. Finally, on October 3, 2012, the FDA ordered Teva Pharmaceuticals to withdraw its generic, Budeprion XL 300, from the marketplace, deeming it "not therapeutically equivalent" to the brand drug, Wellbutrin XL 300 mg.

WANE, WANE, GO AWAY
When a generic seems to be lying down on the job

In perimenopause, I got my progesterone prescription refilled and the pharmacy gave me a different generic, produced by a company called Bionpharma. I had been taking the Virtus generic, which worked to alleviate my symptoms, as did the Prometrium, which the pharmacy once gave me when the Virtus was slow to come in. Actavis, too, worked just fine.

However, on the Bionpharma generic, my hot flashes, which the Virtus had largely dialed down to intermittent muggy annoyances, punished me with constant sweat baths throughout the day. I also suffered soaking night sweats that ate my sleep and left me pondering whether I could replace my bottom sheet with a giant diaper.

I started to wonder whether the Bionpharma generic might be some sort of "weak tea" version of the brand drug and the other generics. To be fair, I don't know that it is or was: The rerun of my symptoms might've had some other cause—or maybe I wrongly perceived my symptoms as worse when they really weren't. But knowing about the problems with generics armed me with the right words to ask the pharmacist to swap the Bionpharma generic for the generic they'd given me previously that had worked to alleviate my symptoms.

"I know generics aren't always the equivalent of the brand or each other," I told the pharmacist. "This generic I just got is not working on my symptoms like the previous generic—and like I know progesterone should." (I gave her some details—the symptoms I mention above.) "Could I bring this drug in, and would you swap it for the generic you gave me last time?"

The pharmacist agreed, and I got the Virtus generic I'd been taking before. And once again, my hot flashes were tamped down and I got my sleep back. I was relieved—and then enraged. Because I had done all this reading about the issues with generics, *I* knew to ask for a replacement prescription. How many women, who had no idea of these issues, who got a generic that didn't perform so well, assumed progesterone was a bust and just accepted their continued suffering?

Again, I don't *know* that the Bionpharma drug was the problem. But trying to be a responsible medical citizen, I filed a MedWatch complaint—a complaint to the FDA about problems with a prescription drug—in hopes they'd check it out. (I figured that was more likely if others had complained, too.) I was bowled over by what happened next. I got an email from the FDA:

> This letter is in response to MedWatch Report...that you submitted on 1/19/18.
>
> We have communicated your complaint to the firm (Bionpharma), which is preparing to investigate the problem

> further. However, to continue, the firm has requested an sample of the product. Please provide the information requested and return it in the enclosed prepaid envelope (see attached prepaid mailing label).

In a word, OMG. The watchdog-turned-purse-dog FDA was leaving the investigation of this drug to the company that produced it! I'm sure if the company finds (or already knows about!) any problems with their drug, they'll jump right on ordering themselves to do a multimillion-dollar drug recall!

JUDGING YOUR GENERIC

Should you suspect you're taking a generic that's not doing its job, the Graedons offer helpful advice in their 2011 book, *Top Screwups Doctors Make and How to Avoid Them*. Below are some of their tips I find particularly valuable, with my take added in.

- **"Make no assumptions"**: Don't assume a generic is flawed just because it's a generic, they remind us.
- **"Keep track of the manufacturer"**: They advise asking the pharmacist to always include the manufacturer's name on your prescription bottle. Kaiser, my HMO, does this automatically. (For a long time, I also saved every empty bottle of OMP.)
- **"Keep records"**: They explain that "objective measurements" like blood sugar and blood pressure "will allow you to track progress" of a drug. For OMP or estrogen, take stock of how well it's alleviating your symptoms. (You should also consider whether you might need a higher dose.) If, however, your previous generic had your symptoms pretty much under control and the new generic seems feeble, ask for a different one. Use language like I used to ask the pharmacist to swap out my drug:

  > "I've read that generics aren't always the equivalent of the brand or each other. This generic I just got is not working on my insomnia and other symptoms like the previous generic. Could I bring this drug in, and would you swap it for the brand I had before?"

- **"Challenge and rechallenge":** I'd call this "compare and contrast," since it involves using the brand drug as the standard to determine whether the generic is working. They explain, "If generic drug X causes a headache, going back on the brand name should solve the problem." To confirm that the difficulty lies with the generic, take it again and see whether the symptom reappears.
- **"Seek allies":** Ask your doctor or the pharmacist "to go to bat for you if your insurance company balks at paying for the brand name."

Regarding the last bullet, there *are* a number of doctors and pharmacists out there who do daily battle on behalf of patients with what seem to be deny-all-requested-approvals health insurance companies. They're heroes. But other pharmacists are just too busy or not motivated to fight the fight on the level required.

For decades, I've gotten my prescriptions at the same small Kaiser pharmacy, simply because it was closest to my house. But, over the years, I've gotten to know the pharmacists, and I'm often grateful to them—and let them know. They've consistently been extremely kind to me and gone *waaay* above and beyond to resolve problems.

It occurs to me that it's wise to become a "regular" at a particular pharmacy, kind of like being a regular at a bar, and develop a relationship with your pharmacist, who's basically your prescription-drug bartender. Sure, it's a pharmacist's job to look out for *all* their customers; however, if there's some hideous problem with one of your prescriptions, it probably helps if you're a person the pharmacist knows and likes—as opposed to a stranger attached to a medical record number.

PART 5

MENOPOWER!

— 28 —

THE AMAZING ERASE

Rebelling against the mass cancellation of women in menopause

THERE'S THIS TREND now—in op-eds, blog posts, and celebrity interviews—to complain that "menopause gets a bad rap." It does. And it completely deserves it!

For a lot of us, starting in perimenopause, "My body is my temple" becomes "My body is a tenement some slumlord is letting decay into rubble." And sure, there are those symptom-free "Didn't even notice it" types like my friend Simone. But for a number of us, perimenopause and menopause are a daily hellshow. We're sick; we're sleepless; our emotions are flinging themselves around like drunk grasshoppers; and our vagina's auditioning for a role as the Gobi Desert. Parts of our body that were youthfully plump, like our lips, thin out, while parts that were taut—like the skin on our face—start to sag like an old house. And then there's this awful day, the first day you look in the mirror and notice—horrors!—the beginnings of Droopy Dog jowls.

Because we women are judged to a great extent by our appearance, the "menopause transition" is very often a downward slide in status and importance. *New York Times* film critic Manohla Dargis nailed it in her review of the coming-of-older-age movie, *Hello, My Name Is Doris*: "Wrinkles have a way of making women disappear one crease at a time."

MENOPAUSED

The disappearance of women, one wrinkle at a time, that Dargis describes spills over into many menopausal women's professional lives, draining them of their authority and stalling their career.

There's that 1980s Wall Street commercial, "When E.F. Hutton talks, people listen." Well, when aging women talk, people talk over them. It's easy to suspect this only happens to meek women and shallow empty-heads. In fact, it happens to the meek, the shallow, and the accomplished bigmouths alike. One of those accomplished bigmouths is Ayelet Waldman, a Harvard-trained lawyer turned stay-at-home mom turned novelist and screenwriter. She talked to columnist Deborah Copaken about the professional invisibility she experienced upon turning 50:

> I'm not some gorgeous woman who's used to owning the male gaze, but I have a big personality, and I have a certain level of professional competence, and I'm used to being taken seriously professionally. And, suddenly, it's like I just vanished from the room. And I have to yell so much louder to be seen, and I feel like, Oh my God, this is what they mean when they say about women all the time, "Oh, she's crazy." She's not crazy, she's just yelling so that you can see her! Because you didn't notice that she's sitting at the conference table!

It isn't just aging that drives the invisibilizing. It's views about menopause and the insulting and obviously absurd notion that the end of fertility is the end of women's usefulness: time to shove a woman out on the curb like an old couch.

In reality, industrial-organizational psychologist Alicia Grandey notes that the average age of menopause around the globe (around 51) "coincides with a mid-to-late career stage when organizational leaders typically emerge, with the average age for top leaders in the United States being 54." Male and female "leader emergence occurs at this stage because employees are seeking new identity and meaning in their later careers."

However, highly accomplished women have men like former CNN anchor Don Lemon at the ready to reduce them to the sum of their closed-for-business ovaries. Upon learning that the 51-year-old former South Carolina Governor and US Ambassador to the United Nations Nikki Haley was vying for the

2024 Republican nomination for President, Lemon cut her down to size for the viewers: "Nikki Haley is not in her prime, sorry. A woman is considered to be in her prime in her 20s and 30s and maybe 40s."

Sure, Don—in a world where *The Handmaid's Tale* is a documentary.

Men and women alike will also sneer about a female politician's looks and clothing in ways they just don't about the Grand Old Men of the Senate. These sneers are directed at women of any age, but female politicians who appear to be in menopause or on the approach to it often have their mental health called into question as well.

Yes, some of us do experience mood swings, but these tend to take place for just a few years in perimenopause—and can be treated with drugs and managed to some degree with diet, exercise, and de-stressing techniques. However, because menopause and perimenopause are such unknowns to many women and the general public, as well as being taboo topics, ugly stereotypes about menopausal women being emotionally unstable are broadly applied.

These menopausal stereotypes cast shade on older women at the highest levels. During the 2016 presidential campaign, Hillary Rodham Clinton's ability to lead was called into question: "Do we want a menopausal woman with her finger on the button?" was the headline summing up a letter to the editor in the *Modesto Bee*. Clinton was 67 at the time.

Psychiatrist Ronald Heifetz, at Harvard's Kennedy School of Government, gave Clinton low marks for the ability to be a decisive presidential leader. Clinton has an excess of empathy—along with "thin personal boundaries," wrote Heifetz in the *LA Times*. This "makes it difficult to make decisions, because at the presidential level, almost every decision...causes grief. And Clinton hates causing pain."

Are these shortcomings due to menopause? Well, that's, shall we say, *highly unlikely*—because the Clinton that Heifetz was describing was then-President Bill!

Hillary, on the other hand, is an iron-willed battle-ax: tough, driven, decisive, highly competitive, and unsentimentally tireless in pushing her agenda. Political consultant James Carville described Hillary's bulldozer-ish mettle: She "won't run you down for fun, and she won't run into a ditch to avoid scratching your fender, but if you are blocking something we need to get done you'll get run over in a hurry."

Hillary had that in common with a powerful menopausal battle-ax across the pond, the late British Prime Minister Margaret Thatcher—a tough, tenacious, lower-middle-class young woman who rose through the ranks of soft, posh men. Thatcher unflaggingly shepherded the revitalization of the British economy and stood up in no uncertain terms against Russia's creeping military expansionism, leading a Russian newspaper to denounce her as the "Iron Lady."

This nickname immediately caught on in the British press—coming off as a sort of advertisement for Thatcher's strength, as did world leaders' attempts at poo flinging: "What does she want, this housewife? My balls on a tray?" fumed French President Jacques Chirac. Terror honcho Yasser Arafat lamely referred to her as "the Iron Man." But the best one comes from former Member of Parliament Clement Freud: "Attila the Hen."

What was that again about *menopausal women* being too emotionally afflicted to lead?

WAKE UP, WORLD, AND NOTICE THE BIRTH CONTROL

In addition to the misogynistic notion that our hormones cause us to be unhinged, research by Grandey and other scholars suggests that the stereotype of menopausal women as irrational and unstable also traces to the demeaning notion that our real value is our fertility.

Supposedly, we women entering menopause mourn its loss, staring, grief-stricken, into the sudden empty meaninglessness of our post-fertile lives. Of course, this is obviously ridiculous to anyone who knows women in menopause and has noticed the incredible contributions of older women to human society. Yet, psychologist Joan Borysenko, writing about the midlife metamorphosis of women, noted in 1996, "Reading popular magazines would lead one to believe that menopausal women...go berserk prior to entering deep depressions." Though we no longer see that particular caricature, lingering remnants of the belief that women go nuts in menopause continue to poison the well for women today.

This stereotype paints menopausal women as the crazylady antithesis of the strong, authoritative leader who has "his emotions" under tight control, notes Grandey. (And it's "his" emotions, because people tend to picture leaders as male.)

But the very basis of this belief—the notion that menopausal women fall into deep despair when their bodies will no longer make babies—does not hold up. It may have been the case for some women in the past: generations of women born *prior* to the Baby Boom generation (which extends from just after World War II, in 1946, to 1964, the year I was born), whose identity might've been more wrapped up in being a mother.

But something changed in 1960. The pill was approved by the FDA, and for the first time in history, women had access to highly reliable birth control. Further advances in fertility control followed, including the copper IUD, approved by the FDA in 1984 and available in the US since 1998.

Once women had the means to control their fertility—to decide if and when they would become mothers—they began to put an end to it "long before menopause," explains sociologist Heather Dillaway. This changed the *nature of menopause* for countless women, from the end of fertility to "an end to contraceptive use and menstruation."

Being done with birth control, fear of pregnancy, periods, and the accompanying funfest of symptoms *can* evoke some strong emotions—the sort that lead a woman to yell "Woohoo!"

Setting aside the symptoms, this explains the positive view so many women now have of menopause as a life stage—as was reflected in interview-based research Dillaway conducted in 2005. Dillaway spoke with 45 middle-class, heterosexual women in Michigan, ages 38 to 60; three-quarters of whom were white and one-quarter mostly African American—all in menopause or perimenopause.

Forty of the 45 were mothers, and 44 had shut down their fertility by choice "long before menopause"—with contraception, by having their tubes tied, or by deciding with a male partner that he would have a vasectomy.

Like the women in Dillaway's 2005 sample—the first generation "to have full access to the birth control pill and other contraceptive technologies"—many of us going into menopause today probably take for granted how remarkable this level of control is. We have autonomy over our bodies and lives unlike women have *ever* had throughout human history.

Accordingly, "It was difficult for many interviewees to fathom feeling a loss upon menopause, because they purposefully... ended their reproductive capacity many years" before it, Dillaway explains.

Lenora, an African American woman, said "Final for me was a tubal that I had when my 22-year-old son was born.... I guess I just don't think about (menopause) a whole lot."

Mary, a white woman who had been on the pill since the birth of her youngest child, then 16, said, "I've been looking forward to menopause [since] the day I knew I had my last baby."

Many of Dillaway's interviewees reported enjoying sex more than ever because "the hassles of contraception and menstruation" were no longer weighing on them. Many said they felt "sexier" and more "womanly" and had more sexual energy and a level of sexual confidence they'd never had before.

Women also viewed hitting menopause as what one of Dillaway's interviewees, Valerie, described as getting to "good old"—as opposed to the "bad old" of ill health. "For Valerie," like other women Dillaway interviewed, "menopause enhanced freedom, choice, and ability, while other aging processes signified restriction, lack of choice, and the loss of ability. Conceptualized this way, menopause becomes the opposite of other aging experiences."

Conceptualized this way, men might wish they could go through it!

Well... except for harsh downside.

"The negative side to menopause should not be overlooked," Dillaway concedes. "Menopause did bring forth many problematic symptoms, somewhat uncontrollable bodies, and regular doctor's visits for some interviewees."

Note that last bit: "Regular doctor's visits."

Because you now understand the unscientific state of practice standards for menopause and perimenopause, you know exactly how futile doctor visits can be. Futile... or even harmful, as menopausal and perimenopausal symptoms brought to doctors are undiagnosed and untreated or misdiagnosed and mistreated in women—into the millions.

But, this book, through empowering you with scientific knowledge, allows *you* to be in charge of your health and get your symptoms in hand so you'll have nothing impeding your superpowers. And no, I'm not suggesting you or any of us will moonlight as a Marvel character. I mean something you'll see constantly if you just start looking for it: the everyday superpowers of older women—putting ourselves out into the world as the full-on powerful women we've become.

— 29 —

OLD IS THE NEW BLACK

THERE'S AN OLD saying, "A lady never tells her age."

In fact, a "lady" who is 5 or 8 or 22 will readily tell you her age. Consider the ugly subtext of "never tells": A lady *never lets you know her proximity to menopause* (age 50 and her fifties being a proxy for it).

The problem is, by hiding our age, we become accomplices in our own devaluation, covering up our unsightly mere existence at an age when society deems us to have outlived our usefulness.

As many see it, for a post-fertile woman, aging appropriately—or as it's put, "aging gracefully"—means going quietly: fading into the background and staying there, though they *will* let us back in to deliver the occasional plate of homemade cookies to the break room. Legally, they can't tell us ageism has taken over, but they show us: No promotion for you. Please have a clue and leave so we don't have to shove you out the door.

This "going quietly" business extends to how older women are supposed to look; for example, in blog posts devoted to "Don't dress like this if you're over 50!"—lest you seem the fool. Goodwill the short skirts, cut your hair, tone down the makeup, and buy suitable attire: drapey taupe and beige. (We're effectively expected to wear curtains to cover up our older-lady bodies.) Some might protest that older women *want* to dress this way. Sure, some do. But the cultural poison—"older women icky!"—leeches into the consciousness of others, and they simply comply, in a sort of wardrobe Stockholm syndrome.

Even Halle Berry is considered too unsightly to be seen uncurtained. In 2023, at 56, Berry Instagrammed a shot of herself naked on her balcony drinking wine: "I do what I wanna do," she captioned the shot. "Happy Saturday." Well, it was an outraged Saturday for a locust swarm of menopausal stereotype bearers. "Imagine being in your 50s, still posting nudes for attention in menopause when you should be chilling with the grandkids. Aging with dignity is no longer a thing," one man tweeted.

In light of all of those who are quick to come down on an older woman who doesn't "know her place," the impulse to keep mum about one's age is understandable. Humans evolved to try to avoid social devaluation; to conceal things about ourselves that make us seem unacceptable, unappealing, disgusting, lest we get rejected by others.

Well, I reject this rejection.

Or less politely put: Screw that shit.

We set the tone for how people see and treat us. We can't singlehandedly erase widespread negative beliefs about menopausal women. However, we can challenge people around us to think differently by loudly and actively rebelling against the notion that we're "over" once our ovaries go out of business.

To be fair, not every woman can bear the costs of age transparency. A woman I know who writes for TV would give you the password to her bank account before she'd tell anyone her age. She's terrified that she won't get hired if showrunners know how old she is. It isn't for any of us to demand she go all, "Screw the mortgage payment!" and take one for the team. Additionally, not every woman is comfortable going loud, and that's okay. But I hope those of us who can *will*. I see each of us who *does* moving the needle just a little, inspiring other women to follow suit—and, collectively, moving it a lot.

Personally, starting in my mid-40s, I wore my age like body glitter, defiantly casting off the notion that I was gradually leaking out all my value, birthday after birthday. Searching my Twitter, in 2022 alone, I tweeted my age (then 58) 41 times. I'm now 60, and I constantly blurt that out—shoving it into cocktail party conversations as insistently as people who let you know they attended Harvard before your martini glass makes it to your lip.

As I got older, announcing my age became not just a protest but a brag: a way to announce, "I'm SOMEBODY." Somebody old and fabulous—and, in fact, somebody more fabulous because I'm old.

There's the temptation to argue, "Wait—50 isn't old" or "60 isn't old." Well, no—compared with 90—but consider the source of our knee-jerk defensiveness: the notion that old is *bad*—in fact, ruinous if you're a woman. Sure, that is a belief people have, but do *you* believe that?

Giving that some thought, I realized old is actually *better*. Again, no fan of some of the physical effects, but at 60, I'm a vastly better person than I was at 20, 30, or 40: wiser, kinder, more confident, and more "*bien dans ma peau*"—"comfortable in my skin," as the French saying goes. And not randomly or by accident, but by creation: because I put in decades of emotionally grubby work to become this person.

As a kid, I grew up without friends—not one—till I was 15. I was terribly lonely and so desperate to be liked that I spent much of my first few decades on the planet showing people that there was no amount of backward that was too far for me to bend over in service of that.

Eventually, it occurred to me that I lacked self-respect: a quality I saw allowed other people to be real, to have opinions, to say no—and to have real friends. I had no idea how to develop it, so I did what I figured was the next-best thing: repeatedly acting like somebody who had it. This was terrifying, and there was a good deal of backsliding. But the more I stood up—for myself, for others, and for causes I believe in—the more standing up became the norm for me. I now live in the world like I deserve to be here and have a say in things.

At 59, I'm proudly bossy. Yes, *proudly*—as in, "just say no" to that ill-conceived "ban bossy" campaign that sent women the ludicrous message, *You're powerful! Just not powerful enough to shrug off a word.* (Men don't have campaigns to ban "jerk" or "asshole.")

Just as I bludgeon people with my age, I started referring to myself as "bossy" in my early 50s—in a (bossy!) tone that says I *celebrate* my bossyhood: reclaiming the word from people who use it to warn assertive women, "Sit down and shut up, or else!"

Or else what? You won't like me? Guess what: I'm powerful enough and *somebody* enough to be unlikable—if that's what it takes to say what needs to be said. In fact, I welcome being called "bossy" or a "bitch"—or any of the other words people use to smear women who take charge.

I'm equally proud to announce that I'm frequently insecure, as well as high-strung, congenitally messy, annoying, impatient, prone to arrive at events a day early or a day late, and unable to clap on the beat. And yes, I'm *proud* to reveal all of that because working to become powerful led me to go from being secretive about anything that casts me in the slightest bad light to being comfortably vulnerable: willing to reveal pretty much anything about myself that doesn't compromise somebody else's privacy. This is technically called self-acceptance, but it's actually much more than that: It's self-love—loving all of yourself, including your flaws, because you're a package deal.

Your history—your mistakes and failures—are part of you as much as your strong points and probably made you grow and become much more of a person than you would if more of life had been easy-peasy for you. Leonard Cohen understood this. "There is a crack in everything," he sang. "That's how the light gets in." Japanese artisans centuries ago understood it, too. Kintsugi is the Japanese art of fixing broken crockery with golden paste, accentuating the breaks instead of hiding them. I love the message in this—that the breaks make the thing more beautiful—and if you look at kintsugi pieces, you see they really do.

What's been unexpected for me at 60 is how much I love my life and the person I've become. At 40, 50, or 60 and beyond, you, likewise, are not the person you were born, but the person you've created, and it's hugely important to give yourself the props you deserve for that. Few of us do this. We don't even think to do it, because it's easy to forget who we are and what we've accomplished. But it's important to be in touch with that. Understanding who we *were* versus who we now *are* and how far we've come helps us understand where we can go: who we can be in the next stage of our lives.

MIDLIFE CHRYSALIS

The Young Women giggled; the Middle-Aged Women laughed.
They laughed ... as if they had been set free.
—Ursula Le Guin

My evolution in my early 50s reflects what I've heard from so many women over 50: *Something happens in a woman's 50s*.

Just as we've become somewhat sexually invisible, with the broader sort of invisibility that follows, many of us finally find our voice. We figure out who we really are and put it out there.

This isn't to say we were self-censoring nobodies throughout our 20s, 30s, and 40s. But for many of us, there's a sense we get in our 50s that some of the stuff we were terribly worried and guarded about really doesn't matter at all.

When I'm at a party or gathering with women 50-something and up, I go around asking, "What's great about being over 50?" This response—from Erica, 62, an interior designer—is pretty typical: "I know who I am, and like who I am, and can go to a party and talk to people and not be nervous." She loves when people like her, she explained, "but if they don't, it's not going to break me. I don't really care. And it's not [an angry] 'I don't give a fuck' not caring. I'm just okay with it. And now I do something I didn't do when I was younger: I make room for others to speak."

Many women unhook from the expectations of how they're "supposed" to look. For some, this means putting much less effort into their appearance—or retiring from tending to it at all. For me, it means being joyously inappropriate. I wear floor-length sequin evening dresses as daywear. Every day. Everywhere. To the grocery store, the drugstore, to pick up the mail. Like life is a 24-hour gala I'm attending.

In menopause, some women are done with sex and being sexual beings, but a whole lot aren't. In sociologist Heather Dillaway's interviews, one of the women, Patricia, talked about her continuing and even increased interest in sex in her 50s—despite typical menopausal issues like having a harder time reaching orgasm: "I am much more open than I used to be sexually [because I] don't give a shit anymore. Sorry! (laugh)... I just reached a time where it was just like, this is really silly... to have all these inhibitions."

But there's more to this post-50 shift than relaxing on what we previously were uptight about. We go through a coming of age—a coming of *middle-age*—in which there's suddenly nothing standing between us and exercising our power: an inner strength that was always there for the taking. We just needed to strip away the stuff that wasn't ours, that we didn't choose but lugged the weight of, blocking us from the women we could be. *Can* be. Now *are*.

We do this by taking a critical look at others' expectations of us—both individual and societal—our desire to conform to those expectations, and our fear of what would happen if we didn't. Before menopause, for many or most straight and bisexual women—some of whom may not recognize or admit this—the focus is on men looking at us and our managing our "self-presentation" in light of that.

Aging out of sexual attractiveness to men—to some degree or a great degree—though painful, often ends up being a kind of release. For many of us, there's a change in focus. We go from seeking the male gaze to pointing our attention inward: becoming more introspective and rethinking who we are and how we're living.

In adolescence, there's that question: What (and who) do you want to be? That's a question to ask yourself again in your 50s, because "old" just isn't what it used to be. After 50, we can have exciting full lives for decades—and maybe even close to five decades more, with coming advances in science on dementia and other diseases. We know more than ever about eating and living healthy—like lifting weights to avoid the muscle and bone erosion that leads to frailty.

In defiance of the notion of aging as a tragic decline, "Aging," David Bowie told journalist Aaron Hicklin, "is an extraordinary process where you become the person you always should have been." It truly can be—if you seize the opportunity to do it.

Figure out what you want: Have you always longed to live in Paris? A woman I know moved there in her 60s. That's not in the budget for a lot of us, but other places might be. My friend and book cover designer, Little Shiva, moved to this Croatian island, Vis, where she does freelance graphic design for US clients over Zoom, rents her apartment as an Airbnb in the summer, and feeds street cats year-round.

Do you want to make a difference in the world? How will you do that? My wonderfully cranky neighbor, @MrsAbbotKinney, is a literacy volunteer at the Venice library—teaching adults to read. I can't help but tear up when I see her tweets about taking one of the people she's tutored to apply for their first library card.

Some women in their 50s and 60s start a second (or third or fourth!) career. This takes the courage to be a beginner and embrace the possibility of failure—and then pick yourself up and keep trying. A friend who'd always loved making ceramics started doing it professionally in her 60s. In just a few years, she went from making things for friends and selling at Christmas craft fairs to being coveted by interior designers and sold in chichi stores around Southern California. Another friend—a massage therapist—went back to school in her 50s and became a psychotherapist.

Maybe you, too—at 57 or 67 or even in your 70s or 80s—can take on a new career or project that scares the hell out of you, that you're not sure you can succeed at. And maybe trying but not succeeding is beautiful, too.

Maybe menopause, contrary to all the stereotypes, is not a stopping point but a starting point—the entrance to our age of opportunity: the time we finally grow into ourselves and live with the strength and even a ferocity that we weren't able to in the decades before.

ACKNOWLEDGMENTS

THIS BOOK WOULD never have been possible without the enormous generosity of three people: UCLA emeritus epidemiologist and biostatistician Sander Greenland; University of British Columbia endocrinologist Jerilynn Prior, MD; and my amazing agent, Cameron McClure.

The book simply would not exist without Sander Greenland. Sander not only coached me in how to vet scientific studies and critiqued my work and thinking but also sent me numerous papers and news stories that opened my eyes to how unscientific a horrifying amount of our medical care is—and to the horrifying human harms that leads to. His thinking and values deeply inform mine. When I got that first hot flash, it is because of Sander that I knew to dig into the research to see what the science says rather than simply expecting evidence-based medical care from any doctor.

Reading the scientific literature, I discovered the decades of research by endocrinologist Jerilynn Prior on perimenopause and progesterone. Every time you see perimenopause in the news, I would guess the mention has roots in her work—and her fierce commitment to science that led her to fight for perimenopause to be recognized as a unique stage in women's reproductive lives and her companion fight to amass evidence on progesterone's effects and put it out to the world.

My literary agent, Cameron McClure, was simply heroic in selling and shepherding this book (and me!) and has my back in every way—with wisdom, kindness, and her great literary judgment that I am always grateful for. The best way to sum her up is with a tweet I once posted about her: "If I were held at gunpoint and made to choose between some guy I was into and her, I'd give him a nice goodbye fuck and push him out the door."

And then there's Alexa Stevenson, my original BenBella editor, whom I called "my Maxwell Perkins in blonde Minneapolis mom form." (*The Great Gatsby*, without Perkins's edits, would've been *The Sold Two Copies and One Was to Fitzgerald's Mom Gatsby*.) She edited this book early on and it is vastly better because of her wisdom, meticulous edits, and literary judgment, which she imparted with great kindness. I am forever grateful to her.

I am hugely grateful to Glenn Yeffeth, who started a really cool and successful publishing company—and who believed in me and bought my book and the companion book to this one (coming next!). And I'm so grateful to all the people at BenBella, who are so smart about how to sell books and just so NICE. A big thank you to Claire Schultz, my managing editor at BenBella, who has been just hugely kind and supportive; to terrific Victoria Carmody, who came on at the very, very end—and to executive editor Leah Wilson, Adrienne Lang, Sarah Avinger, Jennifer Canzoneri, Kellie Doherty, Alicia Kania, Madeleine Grigg, and Kim Broderick and Monica Lowry, who've all been just awesome.

Scott Calamar copyedited this book, and to tell you how meticulous and great he was at saving me from my moments of subliteracy and grammatical lunacy while also preserving my voice, many of my replies to his queries were COMPLETELY INAPPROPRIATE! ("ILY!" and the occasional comparison with God.)

My cover, which I just love, is thanks to my brilliant graphic designer friend Little Shiva (littleshiva.com), who previously did the terrif cover for *Meangirlology: How to avoid sneak attacks and social ruin*—a curated collection of my syndicated Creators columns on female competition.

I am beyond grateful for Stef Willen and Moon Unit Zappa, my authorfamily and dear friends—both loving, generous, brilliantly insightful, and so talented. They were there with me for months and years in our Google Hangout room, writing on mute all day (until one of us was in need and we turned on the sound). And thanks to the kind, generous Annabelle Gurwitch, who initially had the brilliant idea to do this authors-writing-together-on-mute thing!

Stef and Stephen Margolis were there for me constantly in exactly the ways I needed, basically scraping me up off the floor (when it came to that—and it often came to that!) with their encouragement. Margolis, like Stef, no matter how (INSANELY!) busy he was, unflaggingly called and texted me day after day to keep me positive and energized. Our regular talks about medicine, science, and the pitfalls that lead to medical error were extremely helpful. (He is also one of my "science peeps"—the rest of whom I name below.)

My dear friend "Sher-Sher" was there for me whenever I needed her—for moral support, friendship, and critical reads, and her diplomatic brilliance.

Generous scientists, doctors, and science peeps I am extremely grateful to include: Robert Lufkin, MD; Catherine Salmon, Jessica Hehman, Kaja Perina, James McQuivey, and Scott Alexander, MD; Val Amrhein, Julian Meyer Berger, Gary Taubes, Nina Teicholz, and William Parker, MD; Kevin Knopf, MD; Mary Dan Eades, MD; Michael Eades, MD; Matthew Pirnazar, MD; Michael Okun, MD; Yue Yang, MD; and Randy Nesse, MD; Monica Koehn, Liliane Soares Pereira Carvalho, Rob Sica, Rolf Poulsen, Tim Skellett, James Heathers, Nick Brown, Marcus Crede, Jaimie Arona Krems, and Dave Sanders.

The godmothers of this book are Virginia Postrel, Katiedid Langrock, Kaja Perina, Alessandra Caruso, Amy Dresner, Susan Self, the late Claudia Laffranchi, Shirley Deutsch, and especially Christina Nihira (a truly good human being whose generosity to me over the years blew me away).

The godfathers of this book are Mark Cridland, Rob McMillan, John Campbell, Tim Skellett, and the unbelievably generous Aubrey Ayash, who rose up out of nowhere—again and again. Oh, and Marc Randazza, the greatest Sicilian mofo First Amendment ninja you could ever have defend your bigmouth ass—and then nerd out for you on fair use!

Thanks hugely to Ken Sherman, Reason's Jon Graff, Debbie Levin, and the kind, caring, absolute pro pharmacists at Kaiser Culver Marina. Huge thanks also to all of my brilliant, kind extreme-nerd meetup peeps—but especially Sam, Emmanuel, Frankie, Vishal, Nico, Nathan, Quantum Jonathan, Effective Villainy Eric, Hot Bald Guy, and Professor Jen, and especially-especially-especially Tal Rosenblum (who, over and over, generously helped me with this book's interior design in brilliant ways—including what I call beautiful math!).

Smart, wonderful friends who read this book in its early stages or who were subtitle whisperers are Virginia Postrel, Steve Postrel, Charlotte Allen, Kate Coe, Susan Upton-Douglas, Elizabeth Serrano, Morgan Rhinegelt, and Katiedid Langrock.

Grateful thanks to all my professional non-fic author peeps in Invisible Institute West for all the help and moral support.

There's one more person without whom this book simply could not exist, and it's my hero, Alexandra Elbakyan, the Kazakhstani computer programmer who created and maintains Sci-Hub. This pirate site makes paywalled science accessible to all (as opposed to $39 or $45 per paper, which would've required me to pay probably about $500,000 or more just to read all the science for this book—probably most of it taxpayer-funded research).

Finally, I want to thank all the women who talked with me about their experiences in menopause and perimenopause. Their openness and trust helped me understand the issues they were experiencing and the shortcomings in the field. Hearing the medical betrayals they experienced filled me with rage—very productive rage that drove me to keep going on days when the terrible difficulty and responsibility in writing this book made me want to crawl under my desk and cry.

SELECTED BIBLIOGRAPHY

(Full bibliography at amyalkon.net)

THE FULL BIBLIOGRAPHY for this book is the length of two other whole books—241 pages, total!—which would make this book cost too much (along with requiring a donkey to haul it from the bookstore to your car).

You will find that entire 84,608-word bibliography on my site, amyalkon.net. Because I completely reorganized the information in this book a number of times, some studies in it may be mixed around (listed in a different chapter than the one that now quotes or references the study, though I worked hard to catch all of these and relocate them properly!).

Within the text of the book, I try to name and credit at least the first author of a study whenever possible, and more if I can—balancing that with the readability of the book. "More" works best when researchers are Chinese (Li, Wu, and Liu) and worst when they are German (von Schnitzelgruberschaftensturm).

To search for studies, Google Scholar (scholar.google.com) is probably the easiest option. PubMed at the National Institutes of Health (pubmed.ncbi.nlm.nih.gov) is more difficult to navigate until you get used to it, but it has advanced search options that allow you to narrow the results it delivers by specific criteria (such as only pulling up systematic reviews).

As I mentioned in my acknowledgments, papers will often be paywalled—meaning they require a $39.99 payment to access and read—even when our tax dollars paid for the research, which is often the case. The requirement for this large payment (required for articles that the researchers themselves are not paid for by journals!) makes science inaccessible to most of us.

A Kazakhstani computer programmer, Alexandra Elbakyan, created a pirate site called Sci-Hub that makes countless paywalled papers accessible for free. The site URL changes from time to time, and the currently viable URLs for it are listed on Sci-Hub's Wikipedia page (https://en.wikipedia.org/wiki/Sci-Hub).

To find a study through Sci-Hub, do the following: Paste the exact title, without any extra words or punctuation, into the search box on the site. If it doesn't come up, go back to the paywalled study itself and find and paste the "DOI," the "Digital Object Identifier," into the Sci-Hub search box. That might sound complicated, but most scientific papers and chapters have a string of letters and numbers starting with DOI, like this example—doi.org/10.4061/2010/845180—from a paper Prior co-authored. (You might have to look for and click the word "cite" on some paywalled studies to get them to spit up the DOI. Most but not all have "cite" somewhere on the page that comes up with the paywall.)

— 1 —
THE AWAKENING
(All night, every night)

Genazzani, Andrea R., Patrizia Monteleone, Andrea Giannini, and Tommaso Simoncini. "Hormone Therapy in the Postmenopausal Years: Considering Benefits and Risks in Clinical Practice." *Human Reproduction Update* 27, no. 6 (2021): 1115–1150.

Monteleone, Patrizia, Giulia Mascagni, Andrea Giannini, Andrea R. Genazzani, and Tommaso Simoncini. "Symptoms of Menopause—Global Prevalence, Physiology and Implications." *Nature Reviews Endocrinology* 14, no. 4 (2018): 199–215.

Prior, Jerilynn C., Christine L. Hitchcock, Poornima Sathi, and Marg Tighe. "Walking the Talk: Doing Science with Perimenopausal Women and Their Health Care Providers." *Journal of Interdisciplinary Feminist Thought* 2, no. 1 (2007): 6.

Prior, Jerilynn C. "Women's Reproductive System as Balanced Estradiol and Progesterone Actions—A Revolutionary, Paradigm-Shifting Concept in Women's Health." *Drug Discovery Today: Disease Models* 32 (2020): 31–40.

— 2 —
WHY YOU WON'T WANT TO BELIEVE ME
AND WHY YOU SHOULD

Allchin, Douglas. "Is Science Self-Correcting?" *American Biology Teacher* 78, no. 8 (2016): 695–698.

Gawande, Atul. "Overkill." *The New Yorker*, May 11, 2015.

Gigerenzer, Gerd. *Risk Savvy: How to Make Good Decisions*. Penguin, 2015.

Teicholz, Nina. "The Scientific Report Guiding the US Dietary Guidelines: Is It Scientific?" *BMJ* 351 (2015): h4962.

Weintraub, Pamela. "The Doctor Who Drank Infectious Broth, Gave Himself an Ulcer, and Solved a Medical Mystery." *Discover* (2010): 1–3.

— 3 —
THE MAJOR ERROR DOCTORS AND RESEARCHERS MAKE BY VIEWING PERIMENOPAUSE AS MENOPAUSE LITE

Prior, Jerilynn C. "Perimenopause: The Ovary's Frustrating Grand Finale." BC Diabetes Foundation. May 19, 2018.

Prior, Jerilynn C., and Christine L. Hitchcock. "The Endocrinology of Perimenopause: Need for a Paradigm Shift." *Frontiers in Bioscience* 3 (2011): 474–486.

Santoro, Nanette. "Perimenopause: From Research to Practice." *Journal of Women's Health* 25, no. 4 (2016): 332–339.

— 4 —
PERIMENOPAUSE AND MENOPAUSE
Two distinct symptomatic stages, not one big meno-blob

Green, Robin, and Nanette Santoro. "Menopausal Symptoms and Ethnicity: The Study of Women's Health Across the Nation." *Women's Health* 5, no. 2 (2009): 127–133.

Harlow, S. D., S-A. M. Burnett-Bowie, G. A. Greendale, et al. "Disparities in Reproductive Aging and Midlife Health Between Black and White Women: The Study of Women's Health Across the Nation (SWAN)." *Womens Midlife Health* 8, no. 3 (2022).

Maki, Pauline M., Ellen W. Freeman, Gail A. Greendale, Victor W. Henderson, Paul A. Newhouse, Peter J. Schmidt, Nelda F. Scott, Carol A. Shively, and Claudio N. Soares. "Summary of the NIA-Sponsored Conference on Depressive Symptoms and Cognitive Complaints in the Menopausal Transition." *Menopause (New York, NY)* 17, no. 4 (2010): 815.

Prior, Jerilynn, C. "Progesterone for Treatment of Symptomatic Menopausal Women." *Climacteric* 21, no. 4 (2018): 358–365.

— 5 —
PERIOD DRAMA
The vital prequel to understanding perimenopause and menopause

Bull, Jonathan R., Simon P. Rowland, Elina Berglund Scherwitzl, Raoul Scherwitzl, Kristina Gemzell Danielsson, and Joyce Harper. "Real-World Menstrual Cycle

Characteristics of More Than 600,000 Menstrual Cycles." *NPJ Digital Medicine* 2, no. 1 (2019): 1–8.

Prior, Jerilynn C. "Documenting Ovulation with Quantitative Basal Temperature (QBT)." CEMCOR.ca.

Prior, Jerilynn C. "The Quantitative Basal Temperature Method for Determining Ovulation and Luteal Phase Length." CEMCOR.ca.

Prior, Jerilynn C., and Christine L. Hitchcock. "The Endocrinology of Perimenopause: Need for a Paradigm Shift." *Frontiers in Bioscience* 3 (2011): 474–486.

— 6 —

JOAN OF ENDOCRINOLOGY

Dr. Jerilynn Prior's crusade to have perimenopause recognized, studied, and treated appropriately

Fugh-Berman, Adriane J. "The Haunting of Medical Journals: How Ghostwriting Sold 'HRT.'" *PLoS Medicine* 7, no. 9 (2010): e1000335.

Houck, Judith A. "'What Do These Women Want?': Feminist Responses to Feminine Forever, 1963–1980." *Bulletin of the History of Medicine* (2003): 103–132.

Ioannidis John P. "Why Science Is Not Necessarily Self-Correcting." *Perspectives on Psychological Science* 7, no. 6 (November 2012): 645–654.

Prior, Jerilynn C., Yvonne M. Vigna, Martin T. Schechter, and Ann E Burgess. "Spinal Bone Loss and Ovulatory Disturbances." *New England Journal of Medicine* 323 (1990): 1221–1227.

— 7 —

IT'S NOT THE MONEY, IT'S THE MONEY

Women are prescribed a cheap progesterone imitator with multiple awful side effects—including increased cancer risk

Bethea, Cynthia L. "MPA: Medroxy-Progesterone Acetate Contributes to Much Poor Advice for Women." *Endocrinology* 152, no. 2 (2011): 343–345.

Carroll, Jason S., Theresa E. Hickey, Gerard A. Tarulli, Michael Williams, and Wayne D. Tilley. "Deciphering the Divergent Roles of Progestogens in Breast Cancer." *Nature Reviews Cancer* 17, no. 1 (2017): 54–64.

de Lignières, Bruno. "Oral Micronized Progesterone." *Clinical Therapeutics* 21, no. 1 (1999): 41–60.

Gompel, A. "Micronized Progesterone and Its Impact on the Endometrium and Breast vs. Progestogens." *Climacteric* 15, no. sup1 (2012): 18–25.

Stanczyk, Frank Z., and Milan R. Henzl. "Use of the Name 'Progestin.'" *Contraception* 64, no. 1 (2001): 1–2.

— 8 —

A BRIEF HISTORY OF A SCIENTIFIC MESS
Why progesterone got misclassified as a progestin and how that still misinforms our medical care today

Allen, Willard M. "Progesterone and 'The Pill.'" *International Journal of Gynecology & Obstetrics* 8, no. 4P2 (1970): 613–616.

Allen, Willard M. "Recollections of My Life with Progesterone." *Gynecologic and Obstetric Investigation* 5, no. 3 (1974): 142–182.

Piette, P. "The History of Natural Progesterone, the Never-Ending Story." *Climacteric* 21, no. 4 (2018): 308–314.

Prior, Jerilynn C. "Progesterone or Progestin as Menopausal Ovarian Hormone Therapy: Recent Physiology-Based Clinical Evidence." *Current Opinion in Endocrinology, Diabetes and Obesity* 22, no. 6 (2015): 495–501.

Stuenkel, C. A. "Compounded Bioidentical Menopausal Hormone Therapy—a Physician Perspective." *Climacteric* 24, no. 1 (2021): 11–18.

— 9 —

NOW I LAY ME DOWN TO THRASH
Insomnia all night, brain fog all day

Krause, Adam J., Eti Ben Simon, Bryce A. Mander, Stephanie M. Greer, Jared M. Saletin, Andrea N. Goldstein-Piekarski, and Matthew P. Walker. "The Sleep-Deprived Human Brain." *Nature Reviews Neuroscience* 18, no. 7 (2017): 404–418.

Maki, Pauline M., and Victor W. Henderson. "Cognition and the Menopause Transition." *Menopause* 23, no. 7 (2016): 803–805.

Polo-Kantola, Päivi, Risto Erkkola, Hans Helenius, Kerttu Irjala, and Olli Polo. "When Does Estrogen Replacement Therapy Improve Sleep Quality?" *American Journal of Obstetrics and Gynecology* 178, no. 5 (1998): 1002–1009.

Schüssler, P., M. Kluge, A. Yassouridis, M. Dresler, K. Held, J. Zihl, and A. Steiger. "Progesterone Reduces Wakefulness in Sleep EEG and Has No Effect on Cognition in Healthy Postmenopausal Women." *Psychoneuroendocrinology* 33, no. 8 (2008): 1124–1131.

— 10 —

HOT FLASHES AND NIGHT SWEATS
There's a dumpster fire burning and it's inside us

Fan, Yubo, Ruiyi Tang, Jerilynn C. Prior, and Rong Chen. "Paradigm Shift in Pathophysiology of Vasomotor Symptoms: Effects of Estradiol Withdrawal and Progesterone Therapy." *Drug Discovery Today: Disease Models* 32 (2020): 59–69.

Freedman, Robert R., and Marappa Subramanian. "Effects of Symptomatic Status and the Menstrual Cycle on Hot Flash-Related Thermoregulatory Parameters." *Menopause* 12 (2005): 156–159.

Freeman, Ellen W., Mary D. Sammel, and Richard J. Sanders. "Risk of Long Term Hot Flashes After Natural Menopause: Evidence from the Penn Ovarian Aging Cohort." *Menopause (New York, NY)* 21, no. 9 (2014): 924.

McEwen, Bruce S. "What Is the Confusion with Cortisol?" *Chronic Stress* 3 (2019): 2470547019833647.

Prior, Jerilynn C., Andrea Cameron, Michelle Fung, Christine L. Hitchcock, Patricia Janssen, Terry Lee, and Joel Singer. "Oral Micronized Progesterone for Perimenopausal Night Sweats and Hot Flushes a Phase III Canada-wide Randomized Placebo-Controlled 4 Month Trial." *Scientific Reports* 13, no. 1 (2023): 9082.

— 11 —

BLOW UP AND THROW UP

Nausea, migraines, bloating, and inflammation run wild

Grunfeld, Elizabeth, and Michael A. Gresty. "Relationship Between Motion Sickness, Migraine and Menstruation in Crew Members of a 'Round the World' Yacht Race." *Brain Research Bulletin* 47, no. 5 (1998): 433–436.

Ornello, Raffaele, Valeria Caponnetto, Ilaria Frattale, and Simona Sacco. "Patterns of Migraine in Postmenopausal Women: A Systematic Review." *Neuropsychiatric Disease and Treatment* 17 (2021): 859.

Prior, Jerilynn C. "Preventive Powers of Ovulation and Progesterone." Center for Menstrual Cycle and Ovulation Research (2018).

Svec, Carol. *Balance: A Dizzying Journey Through the Science of Our Most Delicate Sense*. Chicago Review Press, 2017.

— 12 —

NEEDLESS GUTTING

Countless unnecessary hysterectomies for fibroids and heavy menstrual bleeding

Armeli, Alicia. "Are Fibroids the Cause of Perimenopausal Heavy Flow? Interview with Jerilynn Prior." *Ask4UFE*. Center for Menstrual Cycle and Ovulation Research (CeMCOR.ca).

Chen, Beatrice A., David L. Eisenberg, Courtney A. Schreiber, David K. Turok, Andrea I. Olariu, and Mitchell D. Creinin. "Bleeding Changes After Levonorgestrel 52-mg Intrauterine System Insertion for Contraception in Women with Self-Reported Heavy Menstrual Bleeding." *American Journal of Obstetrics and Gynecology* 222, no. 4 (2020): S888–e1.

Gompel, A. "Micronized Progesterone and Its Impact on the Endometrium and Breast vs. Progestogens." *Climacteric* 15, no. sup1 (2012): 18–25.

Prior, Jerilynn C., Marit Naess, Arnulf Langhammer, and Siri Forsmo. "Ovulation Prevalence in Women with Spontaneous Normal-Length Menstrual Cycles–a Population-Based Cohort from HUNT3, Norway." *PloS One* 10, no. 8 (2015): e0134473.

— 13 —

MENOPAUSE BY SCALPEL

Side-effect-laden gyno cancer protection for high-risk women promiscuously applied to all

Erekson, Elisabeth A., Deanna K. Martin, and Elena S. Ratner. "Oophorectomy: The Debate Between Ovarian Conservation and Elective Oophorectomy." *Menopause* 20, no. 1 (2013): 110–114.

Parker, William H., Vanessa Jacoby, Donna Shoupe, and Walter Rocca. "Effect of Bilateral Oophorectomy on Women's Long-Term Health." *Women's Health* 5, no. 5 (2009): 565–576.

Reade, Clare J., Ruaidhrí M. McVey, Alicia A. Tone, Sarah J. Finlayson, Jessica N. McAlpine, Michael Fung-Kee-Fung, and Sarah E. Ferguson. "The Fallopian Tube as the Origin of High Grade Serous Ovarian Cancer: Review of a Paradigm Shift." *Journal of Obstetrics and Gynaecology Canada* 36, no. 2 (2014): 133–140.

Secoşan, Cristina, Oana Balint, Laurenţiu Pirtea, Dorin Grigoraş, Ligia Bălulescu, and Răzvan Ilina. "Surgically Induced Menopause—a Practical Review of Literature." *Medicina* 55, no. 8 (2019): 482.

Verhoeff, Kevin, Kimia Sorouri, Janice Y. Kung, Sophia Pin, and Matt Strickland. "Opportunistic Salpingectomy at the Time of General Surgery Procedures: A Systematic Review and Narrative Synthesis of Current Knowledge." *Surgeries* 5, no. 2 (2024): 248–263.

— 14 —

SEX, LIBIDO, AND DESERT VAGINA

Basson, Rosemary. "A Model of Women's Sexual Arousal." *Journal of Sex & Marital Therapy* 28, no. 1 (2002): 1–10.

Lorenz, Tierney K. "Interactions Between Inflammation and Female Sexual Desire and Arousal Function." *Current Sexual Health Reports* 11, no. 4 (2019): 287–299.

Prior, Jerilynn C. "Perimenopause and Menopause as Oestrogen Deficiency While Ignoring Progesterone." *Nature Reviews Disease Primers* 1, no. 1 (2015): 15031.

Santen, Richard J. "Vaginal Administration of Estradiol: Effects of Dose, Preparation and Timing on Plasma Estradiol Levels." *Climacteric* 18, no. 2 (2015): 121–134.

— 15 —
CRAZY IS SOMETIMES A STATE OF OVARIES
Mental and cognitive health

Alexander, Scott. "SSRIs: Much More Than You Wanted to Know." 2014. Slate Star Codex.

Maki, Pauline M., Susan G. Kornstein, Hadine Joffe, Joyce T. Bromberger, Ellen W. Freeman, Geena Athappilly, William V. Bobo, et al. "Guidelines for the Evaluation and Treatment of Perimenopausal Depression: Summary and Recommendations." *Menopause* 25, no. 10 (2018): 1069–1085.

Nesse, Randolph M., S. Bhatnagar, and Bruce J. Ellis. "Evolutionary Origins and Functions of the Stress Response System." *Stress: Concepts, Cognition, Emotion, and Behavior* (2016): 95–101.

Prior, Jerilynn C. "Perimenopause: The Time of 'Endogenous Ovarian Hyperstimulation.'" University of British Columbia Centre for Menstrual Cycle and Ovulation Research.

— 16 —
MENOPAUSE BRAIN
Untangling what estrogen does and doesn't do

Dennerstein, Lorraine, and Claudio N. Soares. "The Unique Challenges of Managing Depression in Mid-life Women." *World Psychiatry* 7, no. 3 (2008): 137.

Hara, Yuko, Elizabeth M. Waters, Bruce S. McEwen, and John H. Morrison. "Estrogen Effects on Cognitive and Synaptic Health over the Lifecourse." *Physiological Reviews* 95, no. 3 (2015): 785–807.

Maki, Pauline M., and Rebecca C. Thurston. "Menopause and Brain Health: Hormonal Changes Are Only Part of the Story." *Frontiers in Neurology* 11 (2020): 562275.

Maki, Pauline M., and Victor W. Henderson. "Cognition and the Menopause Transition." *Menopause* 23, no. 7 (2016): 803–805.

Studd, John. "Why Are Estrogens Rarely Used for the Treatment of Depression in Women?" *Gynecological Endocrinology* 23, no. 2 (2007): 63–64.

— 17 —
RETHINKING ESTROGEN

Epel, Elissa, Rachel Lapidus, Bruce McEwen, and Kelly Brownell. "Stress May Add Bite to Appetite in Women: A Laboratory Study of Stress-Induced Cortisol and Eating Behavior." *Psychoneuroendocrinology* 26, no. 1 (2001): 37–49.

Genazzani, Andrea R., Patrizia Monteleone, Andrea Giannini, and Tommaso Simoncini. "Hormone Therapy in the Postmenopausal Years: Considering Benefits and Risks in Clinical Practice." *Human Reproduction Update* 27, no. 6 (2021): 1115–1150.

Kaunitz, Andrew M. "More Evidence Backs the Hormone Therapy Timing Hypothesis." *Journal Watch*. December 10, 2018.

Naftolin, Frederick, Hugh S. Taylor, Richard Karas, Eliot Brinton, Isadore Newman, Thomas B. Clarkson, Michael Mendelsohn, et al. "The Women's Health Initiative Could Not Have Detected Cardioprotective Effects of Starting Hormone Therapy During the Menopausal Transition." *Fertility and Sterility* 81, no. 6 (2004): 1498–1501.

— 18, 19, 20 —
LONG-TERM HEALTH PROTECTION
Estrogen, Progesterone, and Hearts, Breasts, and Bones

Bethea, Cynthia L. "MPA: Medroxy-Progesterone Acetate Contributes to Much Poor Advice for Women." *Endocrinology* 152, no. 2 (2011): 343–345.

Clarkson, Thomas B., Giselle C. Meléndez, and Susan E. Appt. "Timing Hypothesis for Postmenopausal Hormone Therapy: Its Origin, Current Status, and Future." *Menopause* 20, no. 3 (2013): 342–353.

Hodis, Howard N., and Wendy J. Mack. "Menopausal Hormone Replacement Therapy and Reduction of All-Cause Mortality and Cardiovascular Disease: It Is About Time and Timing." *Cancer Journal* 28, no. 3 (2022): 208–223.

"Inflammation, Nutritional Ketosis, and Keto-Immune Modulation: New Insights into How Virta Can Reverse Type 2 Diabetes." Virta Health. June 8, 2023.

Mueck, A. O. "Postmenopausal Hormone Replacement Therapy and Cardiovascular Disease: The Value of Transdermal Estradiol and Micronized Progesterone." *Climacteric* 15, no. sup1 (2012): 11–17.

Prior, Jerilynn C. "Progesterone Within Ovulatory Menstrual Cycles Needed for Cardiovascular Protection: An Evidence-Based Hypothesis." *Journal of Restorative Medicine* 3, no. 1 (2014): 85–103.

— 21 —
THE TROPIC OF BREAST CANCER

Abenhaim, Haim A., Samy Suissa, Laurent Azoulay, Andrea R. Spence, Nicholas Czuzoj-Shulman, and Togas Tulandi. "Menopausal Hormone Therapy Formulation and Breast Cancer Risk." *Obstetrics & Gynecology* 139, no. 6 (2022): 1103–1110.

Bluming, Avrum Z., Howard N. Hodis, and Robert D. Langer. "'Tis but a Scratch: A Critical Review of the Women's Health Initiative Evidence Associating Menopausal Hormone Therapy with the Risk of Breast Cancer." *Menopause* (2023): 10–1097.

Goldštajn, Marina Šprem, Mislav Mikuš, Filippo Alberto Ferrari, Mariachiara Bosco, Stefano Uccella, Marco Noventa, Peter Török, Sanja Terzic, Antonio Simone Laganà, and Simone Garzon. "Effects of Transdermal versus Oral Hormone Replacement

Therapy in Postmenopause: A Systematic Review." *Archives of Gynecology and Obstetrics* 307, no. 6 (2023): 1727–1745.

Gompel, A., and G. Plu-Bureau. "Progesterone, Progestins and the Breast in Menopause Treatment." *Climacteric* 21, no. 4 (2018): 326–332.

Stringer-Reasor, Erica M., Ahmed Elkhanany, Katia Khoury, Melissa A. Simon, and Lisa A. Newman. "Disparities in Breast Cancer Associated with African American Identity." *American Society of Clinical Oncology Educational Book* 41 (2021): e29–e46.

— 22 —
DEM BONES
How to avoid smoking a hip joint

Erviti, Juan. "Bisphosphonates: Do They Prevent or Cause Bone Fractures." *Drug and Therapeutics Bulletin of Navarre* 17 (2009): 65–75.

Feskanich, Diane, Haakon E. Meyer, Teresa T. Fung, Heike A. Bischoff-Ferrari, and Walter C. Willett. "Milk and Other Dairy Foods and Risk of Hip Fracture in Men and Women." *Osteoporosis International* 29, no. 2 (2018): 385–396.

Prior, Jerilynn C. "Progesterone for the Prevention and Treatment of Osteoporosis in Women." *Climacteric* 21, no. 4 (2018): 366–374. *Climacteric* 21, no. 4 (2018): 366–374.

Seifert-Klauss, Vanadin. "Influence of Progestagens on Bone Health. Bone Changes Related to Ovulatory Disturbances and Low Progesterone Levels." *Drug Discovery Today: Disease Models* (2020).

— 23, 24, 25, 26 —
HOW TO HELP YOUR DOCTOR GIVE YOU EVIDENCE-BASED CARE

Christianson, Mindy S., Jennifer A. Ducie, Kristiina Altman, Ayatallah M. Khafagy, and Wen Shen. "Menopause Education: Needs Assessment of American Obstetrics and Gynecology Residents." *Menopause* 20, no. 11 (2013): 1120–1125.

Dillaway, Heather E. "Menopause is the 'Good Old': Women's Thoughts About Reproductive Aging." *Gender & Society* 19, no. 3 (2005): 398–417.

Fisher, Max. "Irony Lady: How a Moscow Propagandist Gave Margaret Thatcher Her Famous Nickname," *Washington Post,* April 8, 2013.

"Menopause Practitioner Directory." The Menopause Society. Menopause.org.

Prior, Jerilynn C. "Cyclic Progesterone Therapy." Center for Menstrual Cycle and Ovulation Research. CEMCOR.ca.

Prior, Jerilynn C. "Ovarian Hormone Therapy in the Twenty-First Century." CEMCOR.ca (Centre for Menstrual Cycle and Ovulation Research).

Stute, Petra, J. Neulen, and L. Wildt. "The Impact of Micronized Progesterone on the Endometrium: A Systematic Review." *Climacteric* 19, no. 4 (2016): 316–328.

— 27 —
GENERIC DRUGS ARE THE SAME AS BRAND DRUGS (EXCEPT WHEN THEY'RE NOT)
How to know when you've gotten a bum generic and get it replaced

Bate, Roger, Aparna Mathur, Harry M. Lever, Dinesh Thakur, Joe Graedon, Tod Cooperman, Preston Mason, and Erin R. Fox. "Generics Substitution, Bioequivalence Standards, and International Oversight: Complex Issues Facing the FDA." *Trends in Pharmacological Sciences* 37, no. 3 (2016): 184–191.

Eban, Katherine. "Are Generics Really the Same as Branded Drugs?" *Fortune*, January 10, 2013.

Eban, Katherine. *Bottle of Lies: The Inside Story of the Generic Drug Boom*. New York: HarperCollins Publishers; 2019.

McDonald, Kathryn M., Cindy L. Bryce, and Mark L. Graber. "The Patient Is In: Patient Involvement Strategies for Diagnostic Error Mitigation." *BMJ Quality & Safety* 22, no. Suppl 2 (2013): ii33–ii39.

Graedon, Joe, and Teresa Graedon. *Top Screwups Doctors Make and How to Avoid Them*. Harmony, 2011.

— 28, 29 —
MENOPOWER!

Christianson, Mindy S., Jennifer A. Ducie, Kristiina Altman, Ayatallah M. Khafagy, and Wen Shen. "Menopause Education: Needs Assessment of American Obstetrics and Gynecology Residents." *Menopause* 20, no. 11 (2013): 1120–1125.

Dillaway, Heather E. "Menopause is the 'Good Old': Women's Thoughts About Reproductive Aging." *Gender & Society* 19, no. 3 (2005): 398–417.

Fisher, Max. "Irony Lady: How a Moscow Propagandist Gave Margaret Thatcher Her Famous Nickname," *Washington Post,* April 8, 2013.

INDEX

A
Abenhaim, Haim, 304–305
ACOG. *See* American College of Obstetricians and Gynecologists
advocating for self with doctors. *See* doctor-patient relationship.
aging, female, rethinking and embracing
   announcing our age instead of hiding it, 385
   middle-aged self-reinvention, 390
   older is better: aging into our best selves, 387
   finding our voice and power in our 50s and beyond, 388–391
age- and menopause-related stigma
   age-related sexism closing doors to women, 380–381
   Berry, Halle, criticized for nude photo at 56, 385
   CNN's Don Lemon calls Nikki Haley "not in her prime," 380–381
   "invisibilizing" of menopausal women, 379–380, 388
   myth of menopausal women as emotionally unfit to lead, 381–382
      Hillary Clinton, Margaret Thatcher, powerhouses among soft men, 381–382
Alba, Bianca, 192
Allchin, Douglas, 19–20
Allen, Willard, 85–89

Alzheimer's disease. *See also* dementia
   cortisol, chronically elevated, as contributor, 207–208
   dementia, 217–218
   estrogen timing: early initiation for "healthy cell bias," 244–245
   estrogen, neuroprotective effects, 225–226, 247
      "biological plausibility" of estrogen's protectiveness and benefits for cognition, 229–230
      longer lifetime exposure to estrogen, cognitive and protective benefits, 230
   medroxyprogesterone acetate (MPA), neurotoxic effects, 211–212
   mitochondrial dysfunction, 228
   neurotoxin accumulation from poor sleep, 111
   surgical menopause as contributor to, 174
   Women's Health Initiative study, distortion of risk, 219–222, 244–246
American College of Cardiology (ACC)'s mea culpa on saturated fat, 22
American College of Obstetricians and Gynecologists (ACOG), 96–98, 100–101,
   confused progestins and progesterone, 96

ACOG (*continued*)
  leading source of gynecological practice standards, 18, 96
  made "viewing symptoms as disorders" error, dangerous to patients, 98
  recommendation for safer morcellation in gynecological surgeries, 163
  recommendation for opportunistic salpingectomies (prophylactic fallopian tube removal), 179
Anderson, Britta L., 15
androgens ("male" hormones, such as testosterone), androgenic treatments and conditions, 165, 197
  DHEA (dehydroepiandrosterone), dryness-alleviating vaginal suppository, 197
  Mirena levonorgestrel IUD, androgenic (male hormonal) side-effects, 170
  polycystic ovary syndrome (PCOS), excessive androgen levels, 240
  testosterone, symptoms from lack or excess, 240
  testosterone tests, 241
  testosterone therapy, menopausal, 240–241
anovulatory (no ovulation) menstrual cycles, 53, 145, 254, 263, 304, 327. *See also* ovulation, Quantitative Basal Temperature
  health risks from, 57, 63, 95, 148, 263, 304, 325, 327
  myth that ovulation occurs on day 14 of menstrual cycle, 54
  myth that intense exercise causes anovulation, 62
  oral micronized progesterone (OMP) as treatment, 95
antidepressants
  "discontinuation syndrome" (*also* tapering, withdrawal), 137, 215, 369–370
  hot flash and night sweat treatment, non-hormonal, 98, 137, 369–370
    certain antidepressants diminish hot flashes by 50% or more, 137
    side-effects may outweigh, as with other non-hormonal drugs for hot flashes, 137, 369, 212–213
  may mask underlying disorders, 98
  menopausal women's poorer response to some antidepressants, 213
  mental health treatment, 212–215, 369–370
    buproprion (Wellbutrin) for perimenopausal women, 212
    desvenlafaxine effective in perimenopause and menopause, 213
    desvenlafaxine, unpublished and hidden findings, 213
    major depressive disorder, perimenopause and menopause, 213
    side-effects, 137, 369, 212–213
    premenstrual dysphoric disorder (PMDD) and, 215
    selective serotonin reuptake inhibitors (SSRIs), 213, 215, 369
    serotonin-norepinephrine reuptake inhibitors (SNRIs), 213, 369
    primary care doctors and gynecologists prescribing outside their expertise, 213
Archer, David, 136
Art and Science of Low Carbohydrate Living, The, Volek, Jeff, and Phinney, Stephen, 287
Asada, Noboru, 324
assertiveness, 350–352. *See* doctor-patient relationship
Astur, Robert, 225
asymptomatic women, hormone therapy to protect hearts, bones, brains, and other organs and tissues, 9. *See also* specific subject areas
atherosclerosis (blocked arteries). *See* detailed entry, cardiovascular health and disease
atrophic vaginitis (vaginal atrophy), 187–188. *See* genitourinary syndrome of menopause
Ayerst (Wyeth-Ayerst), 65–69

INDEX

B

Baik, Seo H., 247–248
Baker, Fiona, 110
Barrett, Lisa Feldman, 84
Barron, Mary Lee, 55
basal body temperature (BBT) readings, 55–56
    inaccuracy for predicting ovulation, 55
    medical provider websites recommend use, despite flaws exposed
        Cigna, 55
        Kaiser Permanente, 55
        Quantitative Basal Temperature (©CEMCOR), 56, 290, 304, 348–350, 357
Basson, Rosemary, 188–189
Baye, Drew, 287–289
Beaudin, Jeannie Collins, 272
Berry, Halle, 185, 385–386
Besins-Iscovesco, 88
biases,
    availability bias (in diagnosis), 17
    confirmation bias, 92, 353
    controlling for, 13
    medical outsiders, objectivity of, 21–22, 24–25
    risk of (in research), 228
Biglia, Nicoletta, 125
Bikman, Benjamin, 285–286, 301
"bioidentical" hormones, 78–79
    compounded "bioidenticals" may be ineffective, unsafe, adulterated, 78
    definition of, 78
    estrogen (as estradiol), 366
    estradiol patch (transdermal estradiol), 248, 269, 304, 366,
    marketing term, not scientific term, 79
    oral micronized progesterone (OMP), 81
    progesterone, 80, 88–89, 305
    researchers beginning to use term, 79
bisphosphonates (bone drugs), 320–322, 325–326. *See also* bone
Blaine, Judith, 167
Blank, Joani, 192
bloating
    ovarian cancer symptom, 179
    perimenopausal symptom, 5, 71, 148, 202,
    progesterone, possible temporary effect of, 359
blocked arteries (atherosclerosis). *See* cardiovascular health and disease, atherosclerosis
blood clots, 270–271. *See* cardiovascular health and disease
blood sugar, 249, 253, 260, 279. *See* cardiometabolic health and disease
blood pressure. 270, 281–283, 290–291, 295, 300, 374. *See also* cardiovascular health and disease
high blood pressure,
    accomplice in cardiovascular ruin, 249, 259–263
    combined oral contraceptives associated with, 171
    damage to arteries when chronically high, 259–264
    smoking, including e-cigarettes, 151
    hysterectomy increases risk, 159
    elevates heart disease and diabetes risk, 249
    in supposedly healthy but elderly and infirm Women's Health Initiative participants prior to study, 244
    in menopause more than in perimenopause, 47
    metabolic syndrome, 281, 291
    prevention of, 252–253
    racial differences, 260
    hypothalamus of brain as blood pressure manager, 128
    medroxyprogesterone acetate (MPA) and, 264
Bluming, Avrum, 221, 222, 301–303, 313
Bolland, Mark, 330
bone, 315–332. *See also* osteoporosis, osteopenia
    arbitrary standard for healthy bone, 318
    bone density. *Also* bone mineral density (BMD), 63, 76, 316–320
    bone health relationship to total health, 330

bone (continued)
  calcium and, 329–330. See also
      calcium myth, the
  collagen, 319
  corticosteroids destructive to, 324
  drugs prescribed for osteoporosis,
      315–318,
    bisphosphonates, 320–322
      as cause of microcracks, 320
      "drug holidays" (time off) from,
          322
      increased risk of osteonecrosis
          (death of jawbone) from
          injectable bisphosphonates,
          321.
      increased risk of spontaneous
          hip fracture from, 321
  estrogen and bone health, 325–326
  exercise for, 287–289, 328–329
  falls, greatest risk factor for fracture,
      322–323
  hip fracture in elderly women,
      potentially deadly, 317
  hysterectomies destructive to, 324
  Merck pharmaceuticals creates a
      disease to expand narrow market
      for Fosamax, 316–317, 319–321
  National Osteoporosis Foundation
      distorting fracture risk, 318
  osteopenia, not a disease or predictor
      of fracture, 326
  osteoporosis as mere fracture risk
      factor vs. a disease, 316–319
  progesterone and bone health,
      325–328
  protein, dietary, 282, 330
    myth that protein harms healthy
        kidneys, 330
  race, impact of, 331–332
  scans for bone density or bone mineral
      density (BMD) via dual X-ray
      absorptiometry (DEXA), 319
    myth that scanners predict fracture
        risk, 319–320
    scanners' inability to assess bone
        quality, 320
  smoking destructive to, 330
  supplements supporting bone health,
      330

Borg, Walter P., 137
Borysenko, Joan, 382
Bowie, David, 390
brain. See also cognitive health, mental
    health
  ADHD-like symptoms in menopause in
      women not previously diagnosed,
      227
  estrogen
    "biological plausibility" of
        enhancing brain function, 229
    boosts blood flow and glucose
        transport, supporting healthy
        function of memory, 224, 227–
        228
    boosts brain connectivity, 227
    greater lifetime estrogen exposure,
        less shrinkage of gray matter,
        225–226
  medroxyprogesterone acetate (MPA),
      paired with
    neurotoxic effects, 211–212
    progesterone, compared with,
        significantly less damage
        in brain-injured rats,
        210–211
      improvements in brain-injured
          humans, 211
  timing of estrogen initiation in
      menopause, early critical
      window
  "healthy cell bias" (of estrogen
      action in brain), 245–246,
      265–266
  vital to brain, McEwan, Naftolin, 222
  Women's Health Initiative trial, errors
      and distortions in memory and
      cognition arm, 218–222
brain fog, 44, 47, 109–110, 127, 229,
    357
brand drugs vs. generics, 371–375
breast cancer, 299–314
  anovulatory cycles, effect of, 304
  BRCA and other mutations, 299
  dense breasts, 308
  estrogen therapy
    conflicting findings on risk due to
        variations in methodology,
        309

estrogen therapy alone not
associated with increased
breast cancer risk, 305
fear disproportionate to risk, 300
in healthy women, 303
timing hypothesis for early-
menopause estrogen initiation,
303
greater risk of death from heart
disease, greater fear of breast
cancer, 300–301
hysterectomy (surgical uterus removal)
to decrease breast cancer risk, 176
medroxyprogesterone acetate (MPA)
associated with increased breast
cancer risk, 305
oophorectomy, bilateral, both ovaries
removed to decrease breast cancer
risk, 176
progesterone
conflicting findings
does not cause breast cancer
but may feed and spread
existing cancer (Horwitz,
Sartorius, 2020), 313
inhibited tumor formation in
estrogen-driven (ER+)
breast cancers in mice
(Mohammed, 2015), 313
high levels of progesterone
associated with decreased
risk of breast cancer, 30
preventive cell differentiation
and specialization
instigated by, 52, 311–314
safety of oral micronized
progesterone (OMP) over
medroxyprogesterone
acetate (MPA), 304
racial, ethnic differences in risk, 307,
311
risk calculator, 306
risks, 299–304, 306–311
Women's Health Initiative study claim
of increased risk of breast cancer
based on methodological error,
302
Brinton, Roberta Diaz, 210–211, 228,
244–245

Brown, Roxanne, 301
Buehler, Gary, 371
Bull, Jonathan, 54, 55
Bulun, Serdar, 156
Burger, Henry G., 30
Butenandt, Adolf, 86
Byambaa, Enkhmaa, 296

C

Cagnacci, Angelo, 126, 182
calcium myth, the, 329–330.
calcium need far lower than advised,
330
excessive calcium intake increases
fracture risk, 329–330
heart attack risk even from low doses,
329
cancer. *See also* breast cancer, gynecologic
cancers: cervical, ovarian, uterine
(endometrial), vaginal, vulvar
colon, 174
lung, 174
risks increased by surgical menopause,
174
cardiometabolic health and disease
(cardiovascular and metabolic),
277–297
blood sugar, 249, 253, 260, 279.
cardiometabolic cluster of conditions,
280–281
inflammation overload, 277–280
insulin resistance, 281–282
lab tests measuring cardiometabolic
health and disease, 289–297
fostering willpower, 283–284
Trifecta, Estrogen, Diet, and Exercise,
285–289
Baye, Drew, 287–289
high-intensity training (HIT), slow-
speed weightlifting, 285–289.
See also exercise as medicine,
285–289
inflammatory overload, preventing,
286
immune response-boosting effects,
285–286
insulin resistance, reduction of, 286
ketogenic diet, 282–283
visceral fat, 234–236

cardiovascular health and disease, 8, 151, 258, 290–291.
   atherosclerosis (blocked arteries), 257–259
   endothelium (arterial lining), key to cardiovascular and total health, 151, 257–262, 265, 267, 269, 277, 290, 294, 367
   cardiovascular risks,
      blood clots, 16, 167, 169, 197–198, 247–248, 262, 264, 268, 273. 277, 296
      by race, 261
      high blood pressure, 259–261. *See also* detailed section, blood pressure
      insomnia, 271
      plaque, 7, 252, 257, 259, 261, 263, 265–269, 177, 290, 294, 296–297
      stroke, 7–8, 47, 126, 151, 160, 207, 235, 238, 244–245, 250, 252, 257, 260, 264, 267–268, 271, 273, 277, 281, 305, 329.
   estrogen, 252, 261–275
      cardioprotective when initiated early in menopause, 261–262
      critical window for initiating, 264–269, 246
      delivery form, 269–272
      dosage, 272–275
      preserve receptors, 264–265
      protects endothelium, 262, 264–269
   lab tests measuring cardiovascular health and disease, 289–297
   medroxyprogesterone acetate (MPA), 264
   progesterone, oral micronized progesterone (OMP)
      anovulatory menstrual cycles, lacking progesterone, associated with heart attacks, 261–263
      cardioprotective, perimenopause, menopause, 262–264
Carroll, Jason, 76, 303–304
Carville, James, 381
Caufriez, Anne, 113

CBT (cognitive behavioral therapy), 138, 215
CBT-i (cognitive behavioral therapy for insomnia), 119–120
CEE, 65, 220, 246–247, 269–270, 274, 302–305, 309–310, 366–367. *See also* conjugated equine estrogen, Provera
Centre for Menstrual Cycle and Ovulation Research (CeMCOR), 60
cervical cancer. *See* cervix, gynecological cancers
cervix,
   as source of lubrication for sexual intercourse, 175
   cancer, 179–180
      prevalence in Hispanic women, 180
      preserving through prophylactic salpingectomy (fallopian tube removal), 178
   surgical removal of, 175
Chen, Rong, 132, 133, 209
cholesterol, 270, 292–294. *Also* lipids
   estrogen and progesterone, steroid hormones, made from cholesterol, 74
   healthy ratios, 293
   healthy vs. unhealthy levels, 281, 291
   lipid measures that matter, 291–293
   myths, 293
   treating lab numbers instead of patient health, 294
   oxidized (degraded), unhealthy LDL cholesterol, 150
   lab tests, 294–297
Chua, Alexander, 295
Ciarambino, Tiziana, 280
Cidlowski, John A., 312–313
Clarkson, Thomas, 267
Clinton, Hillary Rodham, 381–382
Cochrane, Archibald, 95–96
Cochrane Collaboration (for assessing research), 171, 214, 235, 270–271
cognitive behavioral therapy (CBT), 138, 215
cognitive behavioral therapy for insomnia (CBT-i), 119–120

INDEX

cognitive health. *See also* Alzheimer's disease, brain, dementia, mental health
attention deficit hyperactivity disorder (ADHD) becoming worse at menopause, 227
ADHD-like symptoms in menopausal women without ADHD, 227
ADHD drug Vyvance, 227
brain fog, 44, 47, 109–110, 127, 229, 357
chronically elevated stress hormones erode cognition, 207
estrogen and estrogen therapy, 226–230
associated with improved verbal memory
associated with less brain shrinkage, 226
benefits for cognition, 228–229
"healthy cell bias of estrogen action" in brain, estrogen timing, 265
improves "executive function," higher reasoning, 226
increases blood flow and fuel to brain, 228
reversed cognitive decline upon replacement after estrogen blockers, 229
Women's Health Initiative Study, methodological cheating to falsely deem estrogen harmful, 220–222
hundreds of studies find estrogen beneficial, 220–221
medroxyprogesterone acetate (MPA)
diminishes protective effects of estrogen, 211
exacerbates neurotoxic effects, 211
fails or compares poorly with oral micronized progesterone (OMP), 210
may degrade cognitive function, contribute to Alzheimer's disease, 211
may suppress brain plasticity, 212
memory
deficits associated with declines in estrogen, 224
erosion at menopause, 223–224
estrogen receptors, higher density associated with worse performance, 224
protected by estrogen, 223
types of, 223–225
oral micronized progesterone (OMP)
"brain-stabilizing, calming hormone" (Dr. Prior), 209
protective in brain-injured, 211
Cohen, Leonard, 388
Collip, James Bertram, 64–65
colon cancer (*also* colorectal cancer) 174, 247, 281
communicating with your doctor, 353–360. *See also* doctor-patient relationship
compounded drugs
issues with safety, purity, effectiveness, and untested drug combinations, 78
Pharmacy Compounding Accreditation Board, 78
progesterone capsules made without peanut oil for the allergic, 358–359
confirmation bias, 92–93. *See also* biases
conjugated equine estrogen, 65, 220, 246–247, 269–270, 274, 302–305, 309–310, 366–367. *See also* CEE, Provera
Consumerlab.com, independent supplement testing company, 120, 167
Copaken, Deborah, 380
Corner, George, 85–86
Cornutiu, Gavril, 222
cortisol,
benefits and necessity of, 125–126, 236
brain's hypothalamus as cortisol monitor and control center, 128, 132
chronically-elevated cortisol vandalizes health, 126–127, 207–208
cumulative health detriments, 126
increased risk of serious health conditions, 207
role in "inflammaging," 278

cortisol (*continued*)
   cortisol-reducing interventions, 208, 138–139
   estrogen
      estrogen spiking and diving (withdrawal), cortisol spiking, 236
      menopausal estrogen decline and loss of control over cortisol release, 235
      McEwen, Bruce, 125–126, 220, 222, 225–227, 230, 236
Coulam, Carolyn, 303–304
Cowan, Linda, 303–304
critical window (for initiating estrogen), 243–244, 266–269. *See also* timing hypothesis
Cummings, Steve, 326, 332

D

Dargis, Manohla, *New York Times, The*, 379
de Lignières, Bruno, 95, 357, 362
dementia. 207, 217–222. *See also* Alzheimer's disease
   blanket (umbrella) term including Alzheimer's, 217
   estrogen, neuroprotective effects of, 226, 245, 247
   progesterone, neuroprotective effects, 247
   risk increased by surgical menopause, 174
   risk increased by chronically elevated cortisol (stress hormone), 207
   risk mischaracterized by Women's Health Initiative study, 218–222, 244
   statistics, 217–218
   Willen, Stef, "Column 17: Wonderfully Ordinary," *McSweeney's*, 217
de Milliano, Inge, 166
Dennerstein, Lorraine, 209
Depo-Provera (high-dose MPA in injectable birth control), 70–71, 75, 77, 166,
   associated with acne and weight gain, 71
   side-effects falsely attributed to progesterone, 70
   shrinks and prevent fibroids, 164
   often increases bone density to higher levels when stopped, 327
   temporarily decreases bone density in high amounts, 326–327
depression, depressive symptoms, 204–205. *See* mental health
DesignWrite drug marketing agency behind ghostwritten studies, 69
desvenlafaxine antidepressant, 137, 213–214, 369. *See also* antidepressants
Desyrel (generic as trazodone, off-label for sleep), 121
Devries, Michaela, 330
DEXA (dual X-ray absorptiometry) bone scans, 319. *See* bone
DHEA, dehydroepiandrostenone, vaginal suppository to treat painful intercourse due to vaginal atrophy, 197–198
diabetes, 8, 21, 23, 249, 260, 280–281
diagnosis
   artificial intelligence improving accuracy, 17
   based on outdated treatment guidelines, 17–19
   critical thinking needed for, 16–17
   diagnostic reasoning not formally taught in medical school, 16–17
   differential (à la Dr. House), 17
diet, 281–284. *See also* cardiometabolic health and disease, Trifecta, Estrogen, Diet, and Exercise,
   heart disease, 251, 253–255
   inflammation, 146–151, 187–188, 206, 235, 249, 252–253, 260–262, 265, 277, 279, 281–282, 285–287, 289–291, 296, 325
   insulin resistance, 277–295, 301, 324
Dillaway, Heather, 383–384, 389
Djerassi, Carl, 88
doctor-patient relationship,
   doctor-patient power imbalance, tools for shifting, 343–352
   assertiveness, 350–352
   data you collect about yourself, 347–350
   knowledge about menopause, perimenopause, and medicine empowering you, 344–346
   your attitude shapes your doctor's, 353–355

fighting Kaiser to get evidence-based treatment, 31–33, 89–101
finding a knowledgeable doctor
  Menopause Society certified practitioners list, 341–342
  nurse recommendation, 342
go in informed about drug amounts, timing, frequency, 361
  antidepressants in place of hormones, 369–370
  estrogen, 365–368
  progesterone, 361–364
    oral micronized progesterone (OMP) for sleep, 357
    cautions about OMP, 358
    women with liver issues, 358
    peanut allergies, 358
    rare vaginal bleeding, menopause, 359
    initial but passing side-effects, 359–360
informed consent, 346
partnering with your doctor, 353–357
shared decision-making, 248
six questions to ask your doctor before agreeing to treatment, 345–346
what your doctor doesn't know *can* hurt you, 361
why doctors rely on prepared fact sheets and practice standards, 32–33
Dolitsky, Shelley, 133
Dresner, Amy, 337–340
Dubeau, Louis, 178
Duggal, Niharika, 285, 286

E

Eades, Mary Dan, 33, 281–282, 292, 293, 296
Eades, Michael, 32–33, 139, 150, 281–282, 294
Eban, Katherine, 79, 371–372
Ekin, Murat, 195
Ellis, Albert, 119–120, 152, 355
endometrium (uterine lining), 50
Epel, Elissa, 236
Epperson, C. Neill, 227
Erekson, Elisabeth, 176
Erkkola, Risto, 117
estradiol, 51, 117, 144, 195, 269–272, 366–367. *See also* estrogen

estrogen, 51. *See also* estradiol
critical window (for initiating estrogen), 8, 243–244, 266–269. *See also* timing hypothesis
"deficiency disease," 66, 233–240
estrogen and estradiol, terminology, 51. *See also* estradiol
estrogen types, dosage, alternatives, 365–368
  antidepressants for hot flashes as substitute for hormones, 369
  estrogen, estradiol doses, 272–275
  exceptions to Prior's advice against estrogen in perimenopause, 114, 215
  oral estrogen, estradiol, 247, 269–272
  transdermal estradiol, 117, 136, 144, 247–248, 269–275, 366–367
  systemic estrogen (throughout the body), 119, 186, 195–197, 366–368
  vaginal estrogen, estradiol (locally acting), 186, 195–197, 270, 365–366, 368
    systemic vaginal, Femring, 270, 366
    FDA fact sheet wrong, 197
fear of taking, 8–9
menstrual cycle, 50–51
rethinking estrogen after Women's Health Initiative errors and distortions exposed, 233–248
sleazy marketing of, 65–69
  Wilson, Robert, 66–68
  ghostwritten journal articles, 68–69
symptoms estrogen can be prescribed for, 365
evidence-based medicine,
"authority-based medicine" vs., 95
calling out unwarranted practice standards, 24–25
Cochrane, Archibald, 95
deceptive marketing of estrogen vs., 64–69
doctors' mistaken beliefs, 5–8
"evidence"-based care, 13–17
Gelman, Andrew, 14
Gigerenzer, Gerd, 14–16, 23–24
Graber, Mark L., 16–17

evidence-based medicine (*continued*)
    Marshall, Barry; Warren, Robin; and H. pylori, 20
    medical outsiders, objectivity of, 21–22, 24–25
    medical schools failing to train doctors
        diagnostic reasoning, 16–17
        how to read and assess scientific studies, 13–14
        even older doctors lack the ability, 14–15
        risk assessment, 14–16
        minimum statistical literacy, 14–16
    modern history of evidence-based medicine, 95–96
    outsiders' objectivity, 21, 24–25
    persistence of scientific errors, 19–20, 81–84
    panels to assess evidence for medical institutions, 23
    practice standards often lack scientific foundation, 17–19, 22–25, 100–101
    Semmelweis, Ignaz, pre-surgery handwashing, 95
    Women's Health Initiative study (WHI), failings of. *See entry*
exercise, 285–289. *See also* Trifecta, Estrogen, Diet, and Exercise, exercise, 285–289
    as medicine, 285–289
        immune response-boosting effects, 285–286
        insulin resistance, reduction of, 286
        inflammatory overload, preventing, 286
        high-intensity training (HIT), slow-speed weightlifting, 285–289.
        Prior's study on women runners, debunking myth that exercise kills menstrual periods, 62

F

fallopian tube removal (proactive salpingectomy) to prevent ovarian cancer, 177–179
falls (top source of fracture), 322–323
Fehring, Richard, 55
Feldman, Dave, 289–290
Feminine Forever, Wilson, Robert, 67
Ferriss, Tim, 122
fibroids, 155–166
    age of first appearance, typical, 156
    black women: more and larger fibroids, more symptoms, suffering, 156, 158–159
    drugs commonly prescribed shrink but do not eliminate, 164–166
    estrogen's role, 155–157
    four types of, 157
    heavy menstrual bleeding (menorrhagia) wrongly associated with, 158.
    endometrial ablation, surgical procedure, 161
    hysterectomies wrongly given to treat heavy menstrual flow, 161
    leiomyosarcoma, rare cancer among fibroids, 162
    surgical procedures for fibroids, often unnecessary, 158–163
    which fibroids *can* require surgery, 158–160
Fisher, James, 286–287
follicles, ovarian, 50
follicle-stimulating hormone (FSH), the "get the egg out of bed" hormone, 39–40, 52, 56
follicular phase (of menstrual cycle), 51–52, 85. *See also* menstrual cycle
Ford, Betty, 312
Fosamax (bisphosphonate brand drug for osteoporosis), 317, 320
Fournier, Agnès, 303
Franceschi, Claudio, 147, 277–279
Freedman, Robert R., 129–130
Freeman, Ellen W., 115, 247
Fried, Itzhak, 110
Friedenreich, Christine, 139
FSH. *See* follicle-stimulating hormone
Fugh-Berman, Adriane, 69, 317
funding
    denied for research questions contrary to status quo beliefs, 62–63, 114, 133, 136, 187–188, 214, 311, 327
    pharma-funded
        conferences, 318
        disease creation, 317
        supporting technology, 319

foundations, 318
research, 213–214, 320–321
    disappeared and hidden results, 213–214
    pooled results changing the finding, 214, 221–222

G

gamma-aminobutyric acid (GABA), 112, 209
Gawande, Atul, 12
Gelman, Andrew, 14
Genazzani, Andrea, 245, 248
generic drugs, 79, 371–375
  Bottle of Lies, Eban, Katherine: tainted generics from corrupt Indian drug companies, 339
  generics not necessarily equivalent of brand drugs, 371–375
  judging your generic, 374–375
  "People's Pharmacy, The," Joe and Teresa Graedon radio show, column, 372, 374
  Budeprion XL 300, withdrawn extended-release antidepressant (generic for Wellbutrin XL 300), 372
genitourinary syndrome of menopause (GSM), 181–199
  diagnosis of, 182
    AGATA genital atrophy study, getting women to open up about symptoms, 182
  estrogen therapy
    bladder issues may not be addressed, 186
    systemic, 186. *See* estrogen, detailed entry
    vaginal, 186, 195, 196, 365–366, 368
    vaginal estrogen falsely accused by FDA of systemic estrogen's effects, 197
  non-hormonal therapies for vaginal dryness alone
    vaginal lubricants, 193–194
    vaginal moisturizers, 193–195
  potential causes of, 186
  symptoms of, 181–193
    clitoral changes, 184–185, shrinkage, loss of sensitivity, 190
    narrowing of vagina, 185
    nocturia, 186
    overactive bladder (OAB), 186
    urinary, leakage/incontinence, 184, 186–188
    vaginal dryness, 181–187, 193–195
    vaginal tissue thinning, 184–185
  sexual issues. *See also* libido
    female cycle of sexual desire different, not broken (Basson), 188–189
    hypoactive sexual desire disorder (HSDD), low or absent sexual desire: "a made-up condition" used to market drugs (Nappi), 189–190
    HSDD drugs, dangerous side-effects, barely work, 189-190
  treatments for painful intercourse and other symptoms of vaginal atrophy, 188–199
    estrogen, 195–197
    non-hormonal therapies
    DHEA, 197–198
    ospemifine (generic for oral drug Osphena), selective estrogen receptor modulator (SERM), 198
    myth, sexual activity with a penis as cure, 192–193
    vaginal lubricants, 193–194
    vaginal moisturizers, 193–195
    vaginal "rejuvenation" laser procedure, 198–199
    vibrators, 190–192
Gerris, Jan, 95–96
Gianni, Lorenzo, 145
Gigerenzer, Gerd, 14–16, 23–24
glands, 51 FIX
glucose tests, 291–292 FIX
glutamate, 210–211 FIX
Golding, John, 145
Good Vibrations (store), 191–192
Graber, Mark L., 16, 17
Grady, Denise, 162
Graedon, Joe, 372, 374–375
Graedon, Teresa, 372, 374–375
Grandey, Alicia, 380, 381

INDEX

Greenland, Sander, 11–12, 23–24, 221, 230, 310
Grob, Gerald, 329
GSM. *See* genitourinary syndrome of menopause
Gunter, Jen, 192–196, 198, 199
Gusberg, Saul, 67
gynecologic cancers and their symptoms, 173–180
   cervical, 179–180
   ovarian, 175–180
      many ovarian cancers originate in fallopian tubes, 178
      prophylactic bilateral salpingectomy (fallopian tubes surgically removed) to prevent, 177–179
   uterine (usually endometrial, cancer in uterine lining)
      oral micronized progesterone, 179–180
         counterbalances estrogen, decreasing uterine (endometrial) cancer risk, 52, 57, 313–314
         erroneous claim progesterone causes uterine (endometrial) cancer, 82
         lack of adequate progesterone in perimenopause may increase risk, 98
         progesterone creams do not offer adequate endometrial protection, 116
      estrogen prescribed in perimenopause possibly increases risk, 58
      morcellation for fibroid removal can be deadly to woman with undiagnosed uterine cancer, 161–163
   racial differences in cancer prevalence, 180, 339
   vaginal, 179–180
   vulvar, 179–180

H

Hain, Timothy, 145
Haley, Nikki, 380–381
Hanley, Gillian E., 178–179
Harper, Joyce, 28
Healthwise medical "fact" sheets, 31, 32
Heaney, Robert P., 330
heart disease. *See* cardiovascular health and disease, cardiometabolic health and disease
Heifetz, Ronald, 381
Hello, My Name Is Doris, Showalter, Michael, dir., 379
Herbert, Carol, 135
Hicklin, Aaron, 390
high-intensity training (HIT), slow-speed weightlifting, 285–289.
Hippocrates, 101
histamine, 146. *See also* inflammation
HIT, (high-intensity training), slow-speed weightlifting, 285–289
Hitchcock, Christine, 40, 117, 364
Hodgson, Ruth, 164
Hodis, Howard, 264–268, 274, 302, 367
Hogervorst, Eef, 205
Holzer, Gregor, 187
hormones. *See also* individual hormones (estradiol, progesterone, cortisol, testosterone)
   chemical imitators of steroid hormones like medroxyprogesterone acetate (MPA) in action, 74–75
   defined, 51
   hormones in action, 74
   steroid hormones, 74, 88, 125, 210,
Horwitz, Kathryn, 312, 313
hot flashes and night sweats, 4, 123–139
   antidepressants. *See* non-hormonal treatments, below
   black women's intense hot flashes, 45
   non-hormonal treatments
      antidepressants, 137, 369, 212. *See also* antidepressants, individual entry
      other non-hormonal drugs, 137
      unproven natural remedies, 136–137
      stress-reduction, drug-free
         cognitive behavioral therapy, 138
         deep breathing, 138–139
         exercise, 139
   duration of, 46, 123–125
   embarrassment, 124
   estrogen's effect on, 129–132

estrogen withdrawal mimics drug withdrawal, 131–132
health detriments of, 125–127
    frequent hot flashes and harm to cardiometabolic and overall health, 126
    increased risk of cardiovascular disease, heart attacks associated with severe, 126
hormone treatments
    estrogen most powerful hot flash relief, 7
    estrogen-progestin more powerful than estrogen alone, 133
    dose necessary to control hot flashes and night sweats, 115, 363
    medroxyprogesterone acetate (MPA) therapy, 133–134
    oral micronized progesterone (OMP) therapy, 132–136
        as stand-alone treatment, 114, 117–118, 132–133, 364
        dose necessary to control hot flashes and night sweats, 115, 363
hypothalamus of brain in charge of temperature control, 128–129
intensities of, 123–124
KNDY signaling molecules inciting hot flashes, 137–138
menopausal, 117, 123–125
perimenopausal, 27, 46, 123, 132–136
statistics, prevalence of hot flashes, night sweats, 123
stress hormones' role, 125–126, 130–132, 208–209
stress-reduction, drug-free
    cognitive behavioral therapy, 138
    deep breathing, 138–139
    exercise, 139
thermoneutral zone shrunken in women with hot flashes, 129
How to Stubbornly Refuse to Make Yourself Miserable About Anything—Yes Anything! Ellis, Albert, 152
Hull, Sarah, 335–336
hunger, raging perimenopausal, 5, 234
Hunt, Van, 185
hysterectomies (surgical removal of uterus), 155, 159, 174–177, 325

I

IAPMD (International Association for Premenstrual Disorders), 214, 215. *See also* premenstrual dysphoric disorder, PMDD.
"inflammaging," low-grade chronic inflammation, significantly raising risk of disease, premature death, 147, 149, 277–278, 285–286
inflammation, 146–152
    chronic systemic inflammation, 147, 277
        associated with atrophic vaginitis (vaginal atrophy) and other urogenital issues, 188
        contributing to "inflammaging," 278. *See also* inflammaging
    versus acute inflammation (targeted healing),147, 277
    decreasing inflammation, 150–153, 277–279. *See also* Trifecta, Estrogen, Diet, and Exercise
    factors in, 150–153, 277–279
    histamine, 146
    lab tests, C-reactive protein (CRP) and high-sensitivity CRP (hs-CRP), to measure inflammation, 291
    muscle and bone as immune- and inflammation-regulatory organs, 285–287
        factor in preventing insulin resistance, 285–286
    runaway inflammation and cardiovascular disease, 249
    vicious circle of perimenopausal and menopausal symptoms and chronically elevated inflammation, 127
inhibin B, a "brake" in hormone form, 56. *See also* perimenopause
insomnia, 5, 109–122. *See also detailed entry* sleep
insulin, 279–280
insulin resistance, 280, 287. *See also* Trifecta, Estrogen, Diet, Exercise
insulin response, 249, 279–281
International Association for Premenstrual Disorders (IAPMD), 214, 215

Ioannidis, John, 14–15
Izano, Monika, 322

J
John, Esther M., 307
Jones, Arthur, 288
Jones, Kirtly Parker, 195

K
Kaiser Permanente, 18, 23, 31, 32, 55, 89–95, 99–100, 328
Kaunitz, Andrew M., 197, 305, 369
Kazdin, Alan E., 343
Kelleher, Susan, 318
ketogenic diet, 282–284. See cardiometabolic health and disease, Trifecta, Estrogen, Diet, Exercise
Khedezla, antidepressant for hot flash relief (generic as desvenlafaxine), 137, 213. See also Pristiq (generic as desvenlafaxine).
Kim, J. Julie, 83
Kirschbaum, Clemens, 208
knee surgery, pointless, 18–19, 148–149
Kofoed, Klaus Fuglsang, 265
Kuhl, Herbert, 269, 274

L
Labrie, Fernand, 197
lab and other tests for cardiovascular, cardiometabolic health, 289–297
    Apolipoprotein A (ApoA1), 296
    Apolipoprotein B (ApoB), 296
    coronary artery calcium test (CAC), 295
    C-reactive protein, 291
    glucose, 291–292
    high-sensitivity C-reactive protein, 291
    insulin, fasting, 292
    lipid panels, 292–297
        black women's lower triglyceride levels, higher HDL, 295
    lipoprotein(a) [Lp(a)], 296
        black people's higher Lp(a), 297
        reducing Lp(a), 297
        PLAC Test for Lp-PLA2, more predict-worthy test for black women, 295
    monitoring cardiovascular health with, 290–291
    nonprofit service for, 289–290
    particle size tests, LDL and HDL, 293–294
Langrock, Katiedid, 11
laser vaginal "rejuvenation," 198–199. See also genitourinary syndrome of menopause, vaginal "rejuvenation" laser procedure
Laws of Medicine, The, Mukherjee, Siddartha, 314
Lean, Michael, 239
LeDoux, Joseph, 203
Le Guin, Ursula, 388
leiomyosarcoma, rare cancer among fibroids, 162. See also fibroids
Lemon, Don, 380–381
Leng, Gareth, 207
Libby, Peter, 277
libido. See genitourinary syndrome of menopause, sexual desire
Lo, Joan C., 331
Lonnée-Hoffmann, Risa, 174
Love, Susan, 60, 66
Lufkin, Robert, 22
lung cancer, 151, 174, 176, 247
luteal phase (of menstrual cycle), 52, 53, 56, 62, 327, 348–349, 366. See also menstrual cycle.
luteinizing hormone, triggers ovulation, 40.
Lyubomirsky, Sonja, 151–152

M
Mack, Wendy, 264–268, 367
Maddalozzo, Gianni, 328–329
magnesium for constipation, 167
Maki, Pauline, 120, 205, 212–213, 223–224, 227–229, 246, 266
Mani, Shailaja, 83
Markman, Art, 284
Marsh, Erica, 156
Marshall, Barry, 20
Matyi, Joshua, 230, 245
McEvoy, Maggie, ACOG, 96–97
McEwen, Bruce, 125–126, 220, 222, 225–227, 230, 236
medical practice standards (diagnostic criteria and treatment standards). See practice standards, medical
medroxyprogesterone acetate (MPA), 7, 74

INDEX 423

bone health, 326–328
breast cancer, 303–305
cost of, 77
FDA fact sheet wrong, 76–77
heavy periods, 171
hot flashes and night sweats, 132–134
mental health, 210–212
misclassification harming female patients and tainting research, 81–84
oral micronized progesterone (OMP) vs., 74–84
progestins confused with progesterone, wrongly used interchangeably, 73–77
side effects of, 76–77
memory, 113, 218–225. *See also* brain, cognitive health
menopause, 6–8, 33–35, 46–48
American College of Obstetricians and Gynecologists (ACOG) guidelines, 18
cessation of periods for 12 months straight, 31, 34, 43, 246, 264, 289,
clitoral changes, 184–185,
shrinkage, loss of sensitivity, 190
dismissing of women in, 379–384
distinction between perimenopause and, 27–28, 31–35, 47–48
estrogen levels, 28
night sweat-driven insomnia, 117–119
natural (vs. surgical), 173–176
no simple test to predict or confirm, 40
oral micronized progesterone (OMP) and sleep, 114
surgical, 159–160, 173–176
symptoms of, 7, 46–48. *See also* specific symptom chapters
insomnia, 109
hot flashes and night sweats, 123
nausea, migraines, bloating, and inflammation, 141
fibroids and heavy bleeding, 155
genitourinary symptoms, 181
mental and cognitive health, 201
additional brain effects 217
Menopause Manifesto, The, Gunter, Jen, 193, 198, 199
The Menopause Society, previously the North American Menopause Society (NAMS), 341
menstrual cycle, 49–56
age at menopause, average, 34
anovulatory (no ovulation) cycles, 53, 263, 304, 327
basal body temperature (BBT) inaccurate for fertility prediction, 54–56,
cessation of periods prior to menopause, 33–34
12-months-straight standard, 34
follicular phase (of menstrual cycle), 51–52, 85.
heavy, prolonged menstrual periods (menorrhagia), 29, 158, 166–172
hormones affecting, 50–52
length of, 54–55
luteal phase (of menstrual cycle), 52, 53, 56, 62, 327, 348–349, 366
myth of 28-day menstrual cycle, 54
ovulation, 52, 56–57
oral micronized progesterone (OMP) for heavy bleeding, Prior's clinical experience, 172
Prior's research on, 59–64
Stages of Reproductive Aging Workshop (STRAW), flawed standard of irregular menstrual cycles as start of perimenopause, 36–38
treating heavy menstrual bleeding (menorrhagia), 166–172
combined oral contraceptives, 171
extra fluid and salt, 168
ibuprofen, 167–168
iron, 168–169
magnesium for any ibuprofen-driven constipation, 167
Mirena IUD, 170
oral micronized progesterone (OMP), 172
oral progestins, 171
tranexamic acid, 169-170
vitamin D, 169
Quantitative Basal Temperature readings (QBT, ©CEMCOR), 56, 290, 304, 348–350, 357

mental health, 201–215
   antidepressants, 212–215, 369–370. *See also* detailed entry, antidepressants
   depression vs. depressive symptoms, 204–205
   estrogen treatment, 223, 228–230
   GABA, gamma-aminobutyric acid, promoting calm, 112, 209
   medroxyprogesterone acetate (MPA), adverse effects on mental health, brain health, 210–212
   mood swings, 201–208
   progesterone and oral micronized progesterone (OMP) treatment, 208–212, 359
   premenstrual dysphoric disorder (PMDD), 214–215
   resilience, psychological, 151–153
   stress in men and animals, 208
   "smoke detector principle" of emotional reactivity (Nesse), 204
   symptoms
      anger, 3–5, 44, 70, 98, 132, 201–202, 205. Also rage
      anxiety, 203–204
      chronic stress, 205–208
      depression, 204–205
      mood swings, 38, 41, 44, 53, 117, 202, 205, 208–210, 224, 229, 336, 381
      rage, 201–202, 20
migraines, 143–145, 363–364
Million Women Study, 310
Mintzes, Barbara, 319
Mirena progestin-only IUD, 170–171
Moen, Mette Hass, 29
Mohammed, Hisham, 313
Mona Lisa Touch (vaginal laser), 198
Mosconi, Lisa, 224, 226, 230
motion sickness, 141–145
   betahistine (generic for Serc), 100
MPA. *See* medroxyprogesterone acetate
Mukherjee, Siddartha, 313
muscle, 236–238, 285–286

N

Naftolin, Frederick, 222, 289
Napoli, Maryann, 317–318, 320–321
Nappi, Rossella E., 189, 190

naturalistic fallacy (if it's natural, it's good), 78
naturopaths recommending scientifically unverified treatments, 136–137
nausea, 141–143
Nedergaard, Maiken, 111
Nesse, Randolph, 97–98, 203–204
night sweats. *See* hot flashes and night sweats
nocturia, 118. *See* genitourinary syndrome of menopause
Nolan, Brendan J., 115
Noorchashm, Hooman, 162
norethisterone,
   first progestin synthesized for birth control, 88,
   prescribed for heavy menstrual bleeding, 171
   with oral estradiol in 10-year Danish randomized controlled trial, 288
North American Menopause Society (NAMS), now The Menopause Society, 40, 78, 80, 89, 134, 246–248, 272, 341

O

O'Brien, Katie M., 309
Ohayon, Maurice, 123–124
Oliver-Williams, Clare, 271
OMP. *See* oral micronized progesterone and progesterone
oophorectomy (surgical removal of ovaries), 173, 176–177, 325
   associated health risks, 159–160
   bilateral (both ovaries), prophylactic, 173
   bone fragility, 325
   increased overall deaths, 177
   partnered with hysterectomy, 177
   surgical menopause 159–160
   symptoms caused by, 176–177
   salpingo-oophorectomy, fallopian tubes surgically removed with ovaries, 178
   unilateral (one ovary), 173
oral micronized progesterone (OMP), 73
   confused with progestins, wrongly used interchangeably, 31–32, 73–77, 79–84, 85–101

cost of, 77
development of, 88–89
dosage, 115, 361–363
effectiveness, 114–115
MPA vs., 74–84
progesterone creams vs., 116
sleep aids if more than OMP is needed
in menopause, 120–122
precautions, 358–360
prescribing of, 77–78, 89–95, 172,
361–364,
safety of, 122–114
Ornato, Joseph, 250
Ortiz, Arisa E., 199
osteomalacia, confused with osteoporosis,
329
osteopenia, not a disease or predictor of
fracture, 326
osteoporosis, 316–318, 324–328, 329, 331.
See also detailed entry, bone
Ott, Susan, 325–326
Ouanes, Sami, 207
ovarian cancer, 176–179. *See* gynecologic
cancers
ovarian hormones. *See* estrogen and
progesterone.
ovaries, 50–57, 173, 176
ovulation, 50–56. *See also* anovulatory (no
ovulation) menstrual cycles
ownyourlabs.com (discount lab tests), 169,
289–291, 295

P

Packer, Milton, 13–14
pamidronate (generic for Aredia),
injectable osteoporosis drug,
320–321
risk of osteonecrosis (rotting and
death) of jaw, 321. *See also* bone
Panay, Nick, 311
Parker, William, 176–178
Parsanezhad, Mohammad Ebrahim, 165
PCOS (polycystic ovary syndrome), 239,
240
perimenopause, 6, 27–45
confusion of progesterone and
progestins by researchers and
doctors, 58, 73–84
diagnosing yourself, nine changes,
39–42

distinction between menopause and,
27–28, 31–35, 47–48
DIY diagnosis of anovulatory
menstrual cycles, 55–56
duration of, estimated by Prior and
colleagues, 42–43
estrogen in, 6–7, 28–31, 56–57, 75
hunger, raging, 5, 234
insomnia in, 110–116. *See also* sleep
markers of start of, 36–37
medroxyprogesterone acetate (MPA)
and other progestins, 75–84
no simple test to predict or confirm,
40
oral micronized progesterone (OMP),
75–84
practice standards lack scientific
foundation, 24–25
progesterone, 7, 29, 55–57
soaring estrogen levels in many
women, 28
Stages of Reproductive Aging
Workshop (STRAW),
flawed irregular menstrual
cycles standard for start of
perimenopause, 36–38
symptoms of, 3–6, 36–38, 40–46,
47–48, 70–71, 355–356. *See also*
specific symptom chapters
insomnia, 109
hot flashes and night sweats, 123
nausea, migraines, bloating, and
inflammation, 141
fibroids and heavy bleeding, 155
genitourinary symptoms, 181
mental and cognitive health, 201
temporary nature of perimenopausal
suffering, 44–45
periods, menstrual, *See* menstrual cycle
Pfizer, 65
Phinney, Stephen, 282–283, 287
placebo, definition, 18
used in research, 19, 118, 136,
"placebo effect," 18, 148–149, 367,
PMDD (premenstrual dysphoric disorder),
210, 214–215
Politi, Mary C., 46
polycystic ovary syndrome (PCOS), 239,
240
Popp, Julius, 207

426 INDEX

"postmenopause" absurd term in need of retirement, 36
practice standards, medical (diagnostic criteria and treatment standards). *See also* treatment guidelines
    can be based on outdated science, 18–20, 23
    pointless medical care, 12, 18–20
    developed by medical practice organizations
        American College of Obstetricians and Gynecologists, 18, 96–97
        American College of Cardiology, 22
    errors can persist for decades, 5–9, 19–24
    institutional requirement to adhere to, 100–101
    wrongly treat perimenopause as "menopause lite," 28, 57–58
Premarin, 65–66, 68, 368
Premature menopause, menopause before age 40, 34
Prempro, 65, 68
premenstrual dysphoric disorder (PMDD), 210, 214–215
Prior, Jerilynn C., 59–64, 69–71
    calling out scientists ignoring high perimenopausal estrogen in their own data, 30
    CeMCOR, nonprofit Center for Menstrual Cycle and Ovulation Research, 60
    correcting error by STRAW (Stages of Reproductive Aging Workshop), 37
    physiologically accurate perimenopause and menopause staging, 42–43
    correcting myth of perimenopausal estrogen deficiency, 29
    fight to have perimenopause recognized, studied, and treated appropriately, 59–64
    harsh early years shaped her as a scientist, 59–64
    progesterone as first line of therapy for perimenopausal women, 57
    Quantitative Basal Temperature (©CEMCOR), 56, 290, 304, 348–350, 357
    taking on the unscientific lumping-together of perimenopause and menopause, 28
    massive dose of estrogen led her to question the scientific status quo, 70
Pristiq antidepressant for hot flash relief (generic as desvenlafaxine) 137, 213. See also Khesdezla (generic as desvenlafaxine).
progesterone. *See also* oral micronized progesterone therapy
    bioidentical, 73, 88–89.
    cream does not protect endometrium, 116, 187, 338–340
    daily vs. cyclical, 363–364
    dose, timing, and frequency, 361–364
    safety of huge doses, 209–210
    false claims about, 70
    menstrual cycle, 50–52
    mental health affected by, 208–210
    misclassified as a progestin, 31–32, 73–77, 79–84, 85–101
        misclassification harming female patients and tainting research, 82–84
    oral lacked bioavailability for many years, 87
    micronization, 88–89
    safety, 99, 112–13, 304–305, 358–360, 363–364
    taken without estrogen, 364
progestins, 79–81. *See also* medroxyprogesterone acetate (MPA), norethisterone
    development of, 85–88
    progesterone misclassified as a progestin, 31–32, 73–77, 79–84, 85–101
    progestins and progesterone wrongly used interchangeably, 73–77
    misclassification harming female patients and tainting research, 82–84
    Makena progestin, 17a-hydroxyprogesterone caproate (17-OHPC), assumed to be progesterone to tragic effect, 81–82

progestogens, 80–81
skin, 187
Prometrium (generic as oral micronized progesterone), 90, 358

Q

Quantitative Basal Temperature (©CEMCOR), 56, 290, 304, 348–350, 357. *See also* basal body temperature (BBT), 56, 290, 304, 348–350, 357

R

race and ethnicity
  most research conducted on middle-class white women, 35, 310
  racial physiological differences ignored, unstudied, lead to undertreatment, overtreatment, 35, 45–46
    bone density, 316
    bone health, 331–332
    breast cancer risk-increasing BRCA mutations in groups beyond Ashkenazi Jews, 307
    cardiovascular disease, 260
    fibroids, 156, 158–159
    gynecologic cancers, 180, 310
    heart disease, 249
    lipids (cholesterol, triglycerides), 294–295
    lipoprotein(a) [L(p)a], 296–297
    menopausal symptoms, 226
    metabolic syndrome, 281
    waist circumference, 281
  SWAN, Study of Women's Health Across the Nation, diverse research participants, 45
Rahn, David, 196
Rational Emotive Behavior Therapy (REBT), 119–120, 152
Reaven, Gerald, 280
Reed, Amy, 162
Reid, Ian, 330
resilience, psychological, 151–153. *See also* mental health
Resnick, Susan M., 227–228
Rethinking Diabetes, Taubes, Gary, 23
Rhee, Mary, 292
Richards, Ann, former Texas governor, 240

risk
  absolute, 16, 218–219. *See also* risk, relative, this section
  doctors unable to correctly calculate, 14
  Gigerenzer, Gerd, 14
  medical schools failing to produce risk-literate graduates, 14–16
  myth of careful risk-benefit analysis driving treatment advice, 13
  relative, 16, 218–219. *See also* risk, absolute, this section
Roche, Kara Long, 178
Romero, Roberto, 81, 82
Roof, Robin, 210–211
Ross, Robert, 238–240
Roter, Debra, 345
Rubinow, David R., 228
Ruddock, Nicole K., 81
Russo, Eleonora, 186
Rutherford, Sharlene, 62
Rylance, PB, 263–264

S

Sackett, David, 13
Salami, Minna, 35
Salmon, Catherine, 331
Salpeter, Shelley, 268
salpingectomies (proactive fallopian tube surgical removal), 177–179. *See also* ovarian cancer.
Santoro, Nanette, 28, 37, 40, 94, 123, 125, 185–186
Sarrel, Philip M., 302
Sartorius, Carol, 313
Schierbeck, Louise Lind, 268
Schmidt, Peter J., 214, 215
Schoenfeld, Brad, 289
Schumacher, Michael, 89
Schüssler, Petra, 117
Scialli, Anthony, 89
Scott, Timothy, 68
Seaman, Barbara, 65
Secosan, Cristina, 174
selective serotonin reuptake inhibitors (SSRIs), 213, 215, 369. *See also* antidepressants
self-respect, 387
Selye, Hans, 207. *See also* stress
Semmelweis, Ignaz, 95

Seritan, Andreea, 203
serotonin-norepinephrine reuptake inhibitors (SNRIs), 213, 369. *See also* antidepressants
Shanmugan, Sheila, 227
Shapiro, Samuel, 310
Simpkins, James, 211–212, 220–221, 230, 243
Six Questions, The, six questions to ask your doctor before agreeing to treatment, 345–346
Sitruk-Ware, Regine, 89
skin, estrogen and progesterone for, 187, 242
sleep. *See also* insomnia
  apnea, 116–117
  apps, 347–348
  bladder issues
    nocturia, interruption of sleep with urge to urinate, 119
  cognitive behavioral therapy for insomnia (CBT-i), 119
    apps and workbooks, CBT-i, 120
    national and international directories of therapists, 120
    if oral micronized progesterone (OMP) no longer sufficient, 120–122
    sleeping pills, 120-122
  "disturbed sleep" in perimenopause and menopause, 110
  estrogen, indirect benefits for sleep through diminishing night sweats, 117, 271
    improvement of some bladder issues that stop sleep, 118–119
  glymphatic system, the brain's janitor
    brain fog from disturbed sleep, 110–112
    neural trash accumulation from disturbed sleep, 111
  medroxyprogesterone acetate (MPA) lacks progesterone's modulation of sleep-promoting neurotransmitter GABA, 112
  menopause, new sleep disturbances, 46, 120
    estrogen plus oral micronized progesterone (OMP), 117–118

  oral micronized progesterone (OMP) alone, 117–118
  oral micronized progesterone (OMP) for sleep
    alleviates perimenopausal insomnia, 75, 112
    dose, timing, 113, 115
    effectiveness, 114
    falsely accused of causing sleeplessness, 84
    FDA approved capsules, not sketchy creams, 116
    lacks harmful side-effects, 357
    positive modulator of GABA, gamma-aminobutryic acid, sleep-promoting inhibitory neurotransmitter, 112
    promotes healthy sleep rather than sedation (of sleeping pills), 113
    safety, 112–113
    sans estrogen in menopause for sleep, 117–118
  perimenopause,
    oral micronized progesterone (OMP) a sleep savior, 112, 110–116
  sleep induction vs. sleep maintenance, 120
  sleeping pills, 120–122
Slotta, Karl, 86
smoking, 150–151, 260
Snow, Christine M., 328–329
SNRIs (serotonin-norepinephrine reuptake inhibitors). 213, 369. *See also* antidepressants
Society of Gynecological Oncology, 179
Spaczyński, Robert, 262–263
SSRIs (selective serotonin reuptake inhibitors). *See also* antidepressants
Stages of Reproductive Aging Workshop (STRAW), 37, 41–42. *See also* menstrual cycle, perimenopause
Stanczyk, Frank, 81, 82, 89, 210–211
statistical literacy, 14–16
Steele, James, 286–287
Steward, Elizabeth, 159
Stoffregen, Thomas, 142
STRAW (Stages of Reproductive Aging Workshop), 37, 41–42

Streeter, Leslie Gray 153
stress, 205–208
    chronic, 5, 205–206
        associated with serious health problems, 207
    cortisol (stress hormone), 125–127
    drug-free stress reduction, 138–139
    estrogen withdrawal and stress hormone release, 130–132
    hot flashes, night sweats, as bursts of stress chemicals, 125–127, 138
    in men given estrogen and then solving math problems aloud, 208
    norepinephrine, stress neurotransmitter, 125, 129, 132, 208–209
    oral micronized progesterone (OMP) suppresses stress hormones, 132, 208–210
    perimenopausal estrogen spikes, 208
    provoking anxiety, 132
    resilience, psychological, 151–153. *See also* mental health
    Selye, Hans, 207
stroke risk, 7–8, 47, 126, 151, 160, 207, 235, 238, 244–245, 250, 252, 257, 260, 264, 267–268, 271, 273, 277, 281, 305, 329. *See also* cardiovascular health and disease
Study of Women's Health Across the Nation (SWAN), 45–46, 124, 204
Stuenkel, Cynthia, 79
Stute, Petra, 362
Sundström-Poromaa, Inger, 209–210
surgical menopause (removal of both ovaries, bilateral oophorectomy), 159–160, 173–177. *See also* menopause, oophorectomy
    cardiovascular and cardiometabolic damage, 260
    depressive symptoms, 229
    estrogen prescription upon surgical menopause mitigates some health effects, symptoms, 229
    greater symptomatic suffering, 173–176
    increased risk of migraines, 143
    serious long-term health risks, 159–160, 173–176

T

Taubes, Gary, 21, 23, 24, 61, 279, 282, 283, 293, 305
Tavris, Carol, 221
Teicholz, Nina, 21
testosterone, 240–241. *See* androgens
Thatcher, Margaret, 382
Thomas-White, Krystal, 118–119
Thornton, M. Julie, 242
thyroid, 240
    endocrine gland, 51
    hyperthyroidism (excess of thyroid hormone), 240
        black women prone to, 331
    hypothyroidism (low thyroid hormone levels), 240
        possible cause of fatigue in perimenopause, 116
        associated with increases inflammation-promoting Lp(a), 296
    thyroid disorders spike follicle stimulating hormone (FSH), 41
timing hypothesis, critical window for estrogen to help, not harm, 243–246, 267, 303. *See also* estrogen, critical window. *See also* cardiovascular health and disease, estrogen: cardioprotective and critical window
Top Screwups Doctors Make and How to Avoid Them, Joe Graedon and Teresa Graedon, 374–375
trazodone (generic for Desyrel), prescribed off-label for sleep, 121–122
treatment guidelines. *See also* practice standards
Trifecta: Estrogen, Diet, and Exercise, 277–297
    diet, 281–284
    exercise, 285–289
    current and long-term health-protective, 106–107, 253–255
triglycerides, 126, 260, 270, 279, 281, 291–295. *See also* cardiovascular disease
Turner, Erick, 213–214

U

United States Pharmacopeia (USP), 340
USP (United States Pharmacopeia), 340

uterine cancer, 82, 162, 179, 180
Utian, Wulf, 243

V

vaginal issues. *See* genitourinary syndrome of menopause (GSM)
van de Mortel, Laurens, 225–226
Vandenboom, Rene, 237–238
Van Dongen, Hans, 111
van Wingen, Guido, 226
vaping, 150–151. *See also* smoking.
Verhoeff, Kevin, 179
Vesco, Kimberly K., 181
vibrators, 190–192
"viewing symptoms as diseases" error, 98
visceral fat, 234–236
vitamin D, 169
Volek, Jeff, 282–283, 287
Vollman, Rudolf, 348

W

waist size, factor in metabolic health, 238–240
Waldman, Ayelet, 380
Walker, Matthew, 113, 122
Warren, Michelle P., 237
Warren, Robin, 20
Webb, Paul, 235–236
WebMD, false claims about progesterone side-effects, 70
weight gain, 5, 21, 29, 41, 44, 47, 53, 61–62, 70–71, 77, 147, 126–127, 137, 165–166, 169, 202, 213, 234–240, 260

Weintraub, Pamela, 20
Wellbutrin, 212–213, 372
WHI. *See* Women's Health Initiative study
Why We Get Sick, Bikman, Benjamin, 285–286, 301
Wickelgren, Ingrid, 220–221
Wilkin, Terence J., 319, 329
Willen, Stef, 217
Willett, Walter, 330
Wilson, Robert A., 66–66, 68
Wilson, Thelma (wife of Robert), 68
Winner, Brooke, 163
Winters-Stone, Kerri, 328–329
Wolfman, Wendy, 187–188
Women's Health Initiative study (WHI), 7–8, 218–222, 243–247, 301–303, 309–310
Wray, Nelda P., 18
Wright, David, 211
Wyeth-Ayerst, 65–69

Y

Yang, Xin, 308
Yen, Samuel, 131

Z

zoledronic acid (generic for Reclast), injectable osteoporosis drug, 320–321
  risk of osteonecrosis (rotting and death) of jaw, 321
Zuckerman, Diana, 160–161

ABOUT AMY ALKON

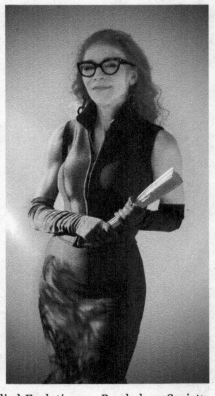

AMY ALKON IS an independent investigative science writer specializing in "applied science": using scientific evidence to solve real-world problems. Alkon critically evaluates and synthesizes research across disciplines and then translates it into everyday language, empowering regular people to make scientifically informed decisions for the best of their health and well-being.

For 25 years, Alkon wrote an award-winning, science-based, nationally syndicated advice column, distributed by Creators. With *Going Menopostal*, Alkon has authored five books—most recently, her "science-help" book *Unf*ckology: A Field Guide to Living with Guts and Confidence* (St. Martin's Press, 2018).

She is the past president of the Applied Evolutionary Psychology Society, which brings evolutionary science to public policy, education, and medicine. Alkon has given invited talks to academics on applied science at scientific conferences and to large groups at universities. She has given two TED talks, and the Los Angeles City Attorney's Office hires Alkon, a State of

California–certified mediator, to do behavioral science–based dispute resolution talks and training videos.

Alkon has been profiled in *The New York Times*, *TIME*, *The Washington Post*, *The Independent/UK*, and *Maclean's*. Alkon has appeared on numerous national TV and radio shows, including *Good Morning America*, *Today*, *NPR*, *CNN*, *Nightline*, *Anderson Live* with Anderson Cooper, *Coast to Coast*, and Canada's *The Agenda* with Steve Paikin, along with podcasts by Adam Carolla, Joe Rogan, Michael Shermer, Robert Wright, and Scott Barry Kaufman.

Alkon lives in Venice, California. Follow Amy on X: @AmyAlkon. Her website: AmyAlkon.net